Science and Football VIII

T0373626

Science and Football VIII showcases the very latest scientific research into the variety of sports known as 'football'. These include soccer, the national codes (American football, Australian rules football and Gaelic football), and the rugby codes (union and league). Bridging the gap between theory and practice, this book is by far the most comprehensive collection of current research into football, presenting important new work in key areas such as:

- the physiology of training
- performance analysis
- fitness assessment
- nutrition
- biomechanics
- injury and rehabilitation
- youth football
- environmental physiology
- psychology in football
- sociological perspectives in football.

Science and Football VIII is an essential resource for all sport scientists, trainers, coaches, physical therapists, physicians, psychologists, educational officers and professionals working across the football codes.

Jens Bangsbo is Professor in Human Physiology and Exercise Physiology in the Department of Nutrition, Exercise and Sports at the University of Copenhagen, Denmark.

Peter Krustrup is Professor in Human Physiology in the Department of Nutrition, Exercise and Sports at the University of Copenhagen, Denmark.

Peter Riis Hansen is Consultant Invasive Cardiologist at Gentofte University Hospital, Denmark, and Associate Professor of research at the University of Copenhagen, Denmark.

Laila Ottesen is Associate Professor in the Department of Nutrition, Exercise and Sports at the University of Copenhagen, Denmark.

Gertrud Pfister is Professor Emeritus in the Department of Nutrition, Exercise and Sports at the University of Copenhagen, Denmark.

Anne-Marie Elbe is Associate Professor for Sport Psychology in the Department of Nutrition, Exercise and Sports at the University of Copenhagen, Denmark.

Science and Football VIII

The Proceedings of the Eighth World Congress on Science and Football

Edited by Jens Bangsbo, Peter Krustrup,
Peter Riis Hansen, Laila Ottesen,
Gertrud Pfister and Anne-Marie Elbe

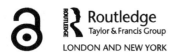
Routledge
Taylor & Francis Group
LONDON AND NEW YORK

First published 2017
by Routledge
2 Park Square, Milton Park, Abingdon, Oxon OX14 4RN

and by Routledge
605 Third Avenue, New York, NY 10017

First issued in paperback 2021

Routledge is an imprint of the Taylor & Francis Group, an informa business

British Library Cataloguing in Publication Data
A catalogue record for this book is available from the British Library

Library of Congress Cataloging-in-Publication Data
Names: World Congress of Science and Football (8th : 2015 :
    Copenhagen, Denmark) | Bangsbo, J. (Jens), editor.
Title: Science and football VIII : [proceedings] / edited by Jens Bangsbo,
    Peter Krustrup, Peter Riis Hansen, Laila Ottesen, Gertrud Pfister,
    Anne-Marie Elb.
Other titles: Science and football 8 | Science and football eight
Description: Abingdon, Oxon ; New York, NY : Routledge, 2016. |
    Papers originally presented at the 8th World Congress on Science and
    Football held May 20–23, 2015, in Copenhagen, Denmark. | Includes
    bibliographical references.
Identifiers: LCCN 2016015217 | ISBN 9781138947061 (hardback) |
    ISBN 9781315670300 (e-book)
Subjects: LCSH: Football—Congresses. | Soccer—Congresses. | Rugby
    football—Congresses. | Football—Physiological aspects—Congresses. |
    Soccer—Physiological aspects—Congresses. | Rugby football—
    Physiological aspects—Congresses.
Classification: LCC GV940 .W674 2015 | DDC 796.334—dc23
LC record available at https://lccn.loc.gov/2016015217

ISBN 13: 978-0-367-78726-4 (pbk)
ISBN 13: 978-1-138-94706-1 (hbk)

Typeset in Times New Roman
by Apex CoVantage, LLC

Contents

PART I
Physiology and sports medicine
Training and testing

Physiology   59

Injuries   105

PART II
Humanities and social sciences
Social sciences   127

Figures

Tables

Contributors

Per Aagaard is Appointed Professor in Biomechanics at the Institute of Sports Science and Clinical Biomechanics at University of Southern Denmark, Odense. He has previously worked for the Danish Elite Sports Organization (Team Danmark), providing physiological research, testing and supervision of Danish elite athletes within the fields of strength/power training and neuromuscular training adaptation. He has published more than 200 peer-reviewed research articles and book chapters.

Nicholas G. Allen is a Research Student with the Sport & Exercise Discipline Group at the University of Technology Sydney, Australia, investigating interval training and chronic systemic inflammation.

Jesper Løvind Andersen (PhD) is a Researcher at the Institute of Sports Medicine, University of Copenhagen, Bispebjerg Hospital, Copenhagen, Denmark, where he specializes in muscle physiology and power training. He has worked as power training coach for more than ten years for FC Copenhagen, and is now working for Brøndby IF. He is an instructor for the Danish FA, UEFA and AFC at Pro license level.

Kevin Ball is affiliated to the Institute of Sport, Exercise and Active Living (ISEAL), Victoria University, Melbourne, Australia. Kevin is currently the Australian junior AFL kicking coach, the South Sydney Rabbitohs kicking coach and consults to a number of AFL clubs. He is also on the editorial board of *Sports Biomechanics*, a director of the International Society of Biomechanics in Sport, an associate member of the AFL Sport Science Advisory Group and is a member of the AFL kicking skill acquisition group.

Jens Bangsbo is Professor in Human Physiology and Exercise Physiology at the Department of Nutrition, Exercise and Sports at the University of Copenhagen, Denmark. He is the Head of the Copenhagen Centre of Team Sports and Health. UEFA pro-license coach and FIFA, UEFA, and AFC instructor. Author of over 300 scientific articles and more than 20 books, he is recognized as a world expert in training physiology and testing on account of his ability to translate scientific knowledge into practice.

Søren Bennike is a PhD student at the Department of Nutrition, Exercise and Sports at the University of Copenhagen, Denmark. He is working within the section of Sport, Individual & Society and is affiliated with the Copenhagen

Centre for Team Sport and Health. His research focus is in the implementation of research and organisational studies in a sporting context.

Mario Bizzini (PhD, MSc, PT) is a Research Associate at the Schulthess Clinic, a private orthopedic and sports medicine center in Zurich (Switzerland), and for the FIFA Medical Research and Assessment Centre. His research interests focus on hip and knee rehabilitation/training, football injuries and sports injury prevention, and he has published extensively in these areas.

Carlo Castagna (PhD) is a Sports Scientist in the Italian Football Referees Association, head of the Fitness Training and Biomechanics Laboratory of the Technical Department of the Italian Football Federation, and a researcher at the School of Sport and Exercise Sciences, University of Rome Tor Vergata.

John Connolly is a Senior Lecturer at Dublin City University, Ireland. His research interests include figurational–sociological approaches to sport, organizations and advertising.

Brian Dawson is a Professor in Sport and Exercise Physiology at the School of Sport Science, Exercise and Health, University of Western Australia, and West Coast Eagles Football Club, Australia. Brian has published over 220 refereed papers and supervised over 100 honours, masters and doctoral students since 1982. He is also a Level 3 accredited Australian football coach.

Paddy Dolan is a Sociologist at the Faculty of Business, Dublin Institute of Technology, Ireland. His research interests include figurational sociology, sport, emotions, consumerism and childhood.

Rob Duffield is an Associate Professor at the Sport and Exercise Discipline Group, University of Technology Sydney, Australia. His research areas relate to sports performance and the role of exercise in chronic systemic inflammation.

Anne-Marie Elbe (PhD) is an Associate Professor of Sport Psychology at the University of Copenhagen, Denmark. She is also section editor on the *International Journal of Sport and Exercise Psychology* and is vice-president of FEPSAC, the European Federation of Sport Psychology.

Matteo Fiorenza is a PhD student at the Department of Nutrition, Exercise and Sports at the University of Copenhagen, Denmark, and at the Department of Neurological, Biomedical and Movement Sciences at the University of Verona, Italy. His research areas include the physiological and performance adaptations to intense intermittent exercise training. He has also worked as a fitness coach of a professional Italian football club.

Colin Fuller is a Consultant in Sports Risk Management with Colin Fuller Consultancy Ltd, Sutton Bonington, UK. Colin provides expert research and management support to several international and national sports governing bodies.

Gerald R. Gems is affiliated to North Central College, Naperville, Illinois, USA. Gerald is the past president of the North American Society for Sport History and the current vice-president of the International Society for the History of Physical Education and Sport. He is the author of a dozen books and was designated a Fulbright scholar by the US government.

Peter Riis Hansen (MD, PhD, DMSc, FESC) is Consultant Invasive Cardiologist at Gentofte University Hospital, Denmark, Associate Professor of research at the University of Copenhagen, Denmark, and cardiology specialist adviser to the Danish Health and Medicines Authority. His primary research interests are inflammatory mechanisms in cardiovascular disease, clinical investigations of cardiovascular effects of exercise in children and adults, and pharmaco-epidemiological studies.

Richard Hawkins holds a PhD in Sports Science and is Head of Athletic Training Services at Manchester United Football Club, UK. He has been involved in professional football for the past 19 years working as a fitness coach and sport scientist.

F. Marcello Iaia holds a PhD in Sport and Exercise Science and he is Assistant Professor/Researcher at the School of Exercise Sciences, Department of Biomedical Sciences for Health, University of Milan, Italy. He is the author of scientific articles focusing on training physiology and performance and has worked in elite football as fitness coach and sport scientist.

Takahito Iga is a Research Associate of Biomechanics in the Faculty of Sports and Health Science, Fukuoka University, Japan. He won the New Investigator Award at the 31st International Congress of Biomechanics in Sports; he is also the secretary of Japanese Society of Science and Football.

Koichiro Inoue is a Lecturer in Sport Biomechanics at the Faculty of Education, Art and Science, Yamagata University, Japan. After studying at Chukyo University (2004–7) and Nagoya University (2008–12), he worked as a research assistant at Kokugakuin University (2013–14). He won the New Investigator Award at the congress of Japanese Society of Biomechanics (2012).

Maria Kavussanu (PhD) is a Senior Lecturer in Sport and Exercise Psychology at the School of Sport, Exercise & Rehabilitation Science, University of Birmingham, UK. Her main area of research is morality in sport, which she has been studying for over 15 years. She has published over 80 journal articles and book chapters, is associate editor of the *Journal of Applied Sport Psychology* and editor-elect of *Sport, Exercise and Performance Psychology*.

Peter Krustrup is affiliated to the Department of Nutrition, Exercise and Sports, Copenhagen Centre for Team Sport and Health, University of Copenhagen, Denmark. Peter has authored 200 original research articles, including 80 on physical–tactical–technical match analyses, fatigue, training and testing in elite football and another 80 on his pioneering research about fitness and health effects of recreational football. He has played football since the age of 5 and is hoping that he is just about halfway through his career. He has played 200 matches in the Danish 2nd and 3rd League and has been a football coach for a total of 15 years. He was assistant coach for the Danish Women's National Team winning a bronze medal in the Euro 2013 and is currently participating in the UEFA Pro-license course.

Paul Larkin holds a research position in the Faculty of Education and Social Work at the University of Sydney, Australia. He received his PhD in 2013 from the University of Ballarat, and conducts applied research in many football codes, with specific interest in talent identification, player development, and perceptual–cognitive performance.

Amy E. Mendham is a Research Fellow in the Division of Exercise Science and Sports Medicine, Department of Human Biology, University of Cape Town, South Africa. Amy investigates mechanisms underlying insulin resistance in Indigenous populations.

Magni Mohr is Associate Professor at the Faculty of Natural and Health Sciences, University of the Faroe Islands and at the Department of Food and Nutrition, and Sport Sciences, University of Gothenburg, Sweden. He is a leading expert in soccer science and has authored four books and 85 original research articles, of which 65 deal with physical match analyses, training and testing in soccer, as well as muscle metabolism and fatigue development during intense exercise and its link to muscular adaptations to training. He is a former elite soccer player and coach, and has worked as match analyst for AC Juventus (1999–2003) and scientific consultant for Chelsea FC (2008–11). He is a FIFA instructor and teaches on Pro Diploma coaching courses all over the world.

Siegfried Nagel is full Professor at the University of Bern, Switzerland, and vice-director of the Institute of Sport Science. His main fields of interest are sport development and sport organization research, particularly sport club development, as well as sport participation and life course research.

George Nassis has a PhD in Exercise Physiology with special experience within elite-level football. He is currently in charge of the National Sports Medicine Programme Excellence in Football Project at Aspetar Orthopaedic and Sports Medicine Hospital, Doha, Qatar. Prior to that, he served as head of the soccer performance laboratory at Panathinaikos FC.

Hiroyuki Nunome is currently Professor of Biomechanics in the Faculty of Sports and Health Science, Fukuoka University, Japan. Hiro is president of the Japanese Society of Science and Football and a member of the International Steering Group of Science and Football. He is well known as a world expert on soccer kicking biomechanics, having published a number of articles on the subject.

Lars Nybo is a Professor in Human Physiology in the Department of Nutrition, Exercise and Sport Sciences, University of Copenhagen, Denmark. His main research area relates to fatigue mechanisms and performance optimization with special reference to exercise in the heat. Studies include highly specialized and invasive lab experiments as well as applied field studies. Furthermore, he is involved in guidance of national and international athletes preparing for competitions in adverse environmental settings.

Donna O'Connor is an Associate Professor and the course coordinator of the postgraduate program in Sports Coaching at the Faculty of Education and Social Work, University of Sydney, Australia. A former strength and conditioning coach, Donna publishes and presents on her research interests which focus on sports expertise, and athlete and coach development. Her current project focuses on the development of decision-making skills in players. Donna has worked with a number of teams and coaches in the various football codes in translating theory into practice.

Laila Susanne Ottesen is an Associate Professor in the Department of Nutrition, Exercise and Sports at the University of Copenhagen, Denmark. Her research is affiliated with the Copenhagen Centre for Team Sport and Health. Her main area of research is sociology of sport, policy and health ranging from individual life style change to more organizational changes.

Gertrud Pfister is Professor Emeritus in the Department of Nutrition, Exercise and Sports at the University of Copenhagen, Denmark, and was involved in the FREE project (Football Research in an Enlarged Europe), funded by the EU.

Sébastien Racinais has a PhD in Exercise Physiology and is Head of Research Operations within the "Athlete Health & Performance" research pillar at Aspetar Orthopaedic and Sports Medicine Hospital, Doha, Qatar. He has developed a research program on the adaptations of the human body to hot ambient conditions and their repercussions on sport performance. He initiated and runs a Special Interest Group of physiologists with a strong interest in environmental physiology. Sébastien has also been collaborating with various national and international sports federations on consensuses on exercising in hot ambient conditions.

Lars Tore Ronglan is Associate Professor in Sport Sociology at the Department of Coaching and Psychology, Norwegian School of Sport Sciences, Norway. Lars' research interests are leadership, learning and coaching in sport. His PhD thesis was a sociological analysis of a performance group in elite team sport. Among his recent publications are co-edition of *The Sociology of Sports Coaching* (Routledge, 2011) and *Managing Elite Sport Systems: Research and Practice* (Routledge, 2015).

Torsten Schlesinger is Senior Lecturer at the Institute of Sport Science of the University of Bern, Switzerland. His research interests relate to sport club development, analyzing decision-making processes in sport organizations, and human resource management in voluntary sport clubs.

Hironari Shinkai is Associate Professor of Sports Biomechanics at the Faculty of Education, Arts and Sports Sciences Division, Tokyo Gakugei University, Japan. He is and executive board member of the Japanese Society of Science and Football, and is vice editor-in-chief of the international online journal *Football Science*. He had received many domestic and international young investigator awards for his work.

Albrecht Sonntag is Director of the EU–Asia Institute at ESSCA School of Management, Angers, France. Over the last 15 years he has published extensively on the sociocultural and political dimensions of international football. He was the initiator and scientific coordinator of the FREE Project, a large transnational and interdisciplinary research project supported by the 7th European Framework Programme. He is now the series editor of the Football in an Enlarged Europe book series (Palgrave Macmillan).

Lone Friis Thing is an Associate Professor at the Department of Nutrition, Exercise and Sports at the University of Copenhagen, Denmark. She is a researcher in health promotion in relation to sport and physical activity through the work with lifestyle and innovative culture strategies for organizational changes in Danish secondary schools.

Preface

The 8th World Congress on Science and Football was held in Copenhagen on May 18–23, 2015 with more than 450 participants from 46 countries.

We would like to thank all the delegates for their contributions to the success of the congress. We are very happy that so many scientists within the field of football gathered to present their newest findings. The results from numerous disciplines clearly showed that science in football is developing exponentially, and it was a great pleasure for us to experience that our strategic focus on the human and social sciences was very well received. We enjoyed the great interactions that took place between researchers from the various scientific disciplines, and the large participation in the social program of the Congress. We believe that this builds a strong foundation for the future, where the need for a multidisciplinary approach becomes stronger and stronger in order to examine and, we hope, solve some of the complex questions that arise from football. An obvious example is the studies focusing on the beneficial effects of recreational soccer showing that soccer not only is an effective means of broad spectrum prevention and treatment of a number of non-communicable diseases, but also provides the participants with psychological well-being and social networks.

In this volume we have collected 23 contributions from selected invited speakers at the Congress in order to provide the reader with high-level scientific information to be used on a daily basis on the football field or as a foundation for further research, perhaps to be presented at the next World Congress on Science and Football in Melbourne in 2019.

Enjoy reading!

Jens Bangsbo, Peter Krustrup, Peter Riis Hansen,
Laila Ottesen, Gertrud Pfister, Anne-Marie Elbe
Copenhagen Centre for Team Sport and Health,
University of Copenhagen, Denmark

Acknowledgement

We would like to thank the reviewers of the book's manuscript for their great contribution: Thomas Bull Andersen, Mario Bizzini, Joao Brito, Carlo Castagna, Brian Dawson, Rob Duffield, Barry Drust, Svend Sparre Geertsen, Per Hølmich, Jesper Lundbye-Jensen Klaus Madsen, Magni Mohr, Bente Rona, Dawn Scott and Mathew Weston.

Introduction

Modern technology has made a marked difference in the analysis of matches and training, and has led to more efficient training and tactical strategies during matches as described in a number of physiologically oriented chapters in Part I of the proceedings from the 8th World Congress on Science and Football, Copenhagen 2015. However, the practical use of such information and, ultimately, the cost-effectiveness of implementation strategies should be carefully evaluated and future studies should focus on those variables that are most important for selected purposes, and on how to condense the increasing information in an appropriate way as addressed in the book. The current book also provides valuable information about how various types of tests can supply useful information about the players' physical capacity, and how various types of training can improve players' performance. In addition, specific issues related to women's soccer and football refereeing are addressed in the book, together with other physiological and health-related issues relevant to the various codes of football including Australian rules football, rugby, Gaelic football, American football and soccer. For example, injuries in football remain a serious challenge for any team, and it has been shown, perhaps not surprisingly, that elite teams with few injuries are the most successful ones. Fortunately, the book provides a number of chapters focusing on how to avoid and treat sport injuries.

Another main topic of this book is football for health. The activity profile and physiological demands of recreational football participation for untrained 6–80-year-olds is described along with interesting new scientific evidence that small-sided football training with 4–14 players is an effective prevention of lifestyle diseases, as it combines elements of high-intensity interval training, endurance training and strength training. Specifically, this book provides information on the cardiovascular, metabolic and musculoskeletal effects of small-sided recreational soccer and rugby for sedentary healthy individuals and also the potential of football in the treatment of hypertension, type 2 diabetes and prostate cancer. These findings are of great public interest, considering the popularity of football as well as the sociological and psychological findings about how the positive motivational and social factors in team sports that may facilitate compliance and persistence with the sport and contribute to the achievement and maintenance of a physically active lifestyle of the world population.

Part II of the book focuses on the human and social sciences. In total, there are ten chapters from the disciplines of sociology, history and psychology. The first seven chapters address historical developments and current scientific focus areas of football and soccer. Part II includes chapters looking at both females and males and addressing different football codes, i.e. European soccer, but also Gaelic and American football. In addition, research about a new fitness concept in Denmark 'Soccer Fitness' and its benefits are described. Volunteering in soccer clubs and the group dynamics in soccer teams are further topics. Moreover, soccer viewed not only as an activity, but also as a social display is a theme that is discussed and highlights the role and interaction between soccer consumers and fans.

The psychological contributions focus on three different aspects. Chapter 21 illustrates how soccer physical activity interventions can elicit flow experiences and that these flow experiences seem to be important for long-term adherence to regular physical activity. Chapter 22 investigates the coaching behaviors and practice activities of coaches from various football codes at different playing levels and provides recommendations for coaching practice. Chapter 23 investigates soccer players in three European countries and highlights the importance of moral factors for preventing doping of soccer players.

Part II of the book presents a large spectrum of research from sociological, historical and psychological perspectives with regard to football, thus complementing Part I and demonstrating the full range of current research relevant to the various codes of football.

Part I

Physiology and sports medicine

Training and testing

1 Muscle power training in soccer

Jesper Løvind Andersen and Per Aagaard

Soccer has become more and more intense and the physical demands are increasing. Therefore, the physiological strain imposed on players is also progressively increasing (Barnes et al., 2014). Thus, in addition to a high aerobic capacity, soccer players need to develop their 'explosive' movement abilities to improve performance in actions such as accelerations, decelerations, side-cutting and other rapid changes of direction movements and sprinting. On top of that, players have to develop high muscle force in single actions such as tackling, kicking, heading and jumping. Thus, optimization of muscle strength and power may have a strong focus in training for soccer players.

Maximal muscle strength and power, including explosive strength (rate of force development: RFD) can be maximized by means of resistance training, however different types of training may lead to differential gains in one or the other parameter (Aagaard, 2003). Heavy-resistance strength training (HRST) has been demonstrated to lead to increased levels of contractile muscle strength in both youth and adult elite soccer players during isometric, concentric and eccentric muscle actions of maximal voluntary effort (Aagaard et al., 1996; Helgerud et al., 2011; Rønnestad et al., 2011; Sander et al., 2013; Silva et al., 2015). Corresponding effects of HRST on maximal muscle power production in elite soccer players have also been reported (Aagaard et al., 1994a, 1994b), while more specialized types of resistance training (i.e. plyometric exercises) may also help to additionally facilitate gains in maximal muscle power production.

The low incidence of maximal-velocity sprints combined with a high number of short-lasting player actions of maximal acceleration over 10–20 meters (Aughey and Varley, 2013; Bangsbo et al., 2006; Barnes et al., 2014; Dalen et al., 2016; Mohr et al., 2005) suggest that muscle power training in elite/sub-elite soccer should have a strong focus on improving muscular RFD since a high RFD is particularly important in the short-duration fast sprints with maximal acceleration rather than in the longer sprints approaching maximal running speed.

What is the evidence for increased performance with muscle power training in soccer?

Robust evidence exists to show increased muscle power performance (including enhanced concentric–eccentric muscle strength and RFD) in response to prolonged regimes of HRST (Aagaard, 2003) also when performed in soccer players (Hoff and Helgerud 2004; Silva et al., 2015). Nevertheless, most studies examining muscle power training have been conducted on untrained or moderately trained subjects, and typically in subjects who did not perform concurrent types of training (i.e. resistance training in parallel with aerobic training). The adaptation to muscle power training in the elite or semi-elite soccer setting has been scarcely examined, but in more recent times a number of scientific studies of this nature have appeared.

By the early 1990s we and others demonstrated that by adding an HRST regimen to the regular training of elite players it was possible to change muscle fiber characteristics, isometric and dynamic (concentric–eccentric) muscle strength and power in a favorable direction (Aagaard et al., 1994a, 1994b, 1996; Andersen et al., 1994). Wisløff et al. (2004) demonstrated a strong positive correlation between maximal lower limb muscle strength vs. short sprint velocity and jumping ability in adult elite soccer players. Over the last ten years, several studies in both youth and adult players have confirmed that muscle power training either in the form of pure HRST or plyometrics or by using a combination of them integrated in normal soccer training is capable of increasing the performance of players in various muscle power-related tests relevant in soccer (Brito et al., 2014; Christou et al., 2006; Rønnestad et al., 2008, 2011; Thomas et al. 2009; Wong et al., 2010).

Definition of muscle power training in soccer

When working with soccer players, HRST is a key element for improving maximal muscle strength, RFD and power output, respectively, but we suggest broadening this training focus using the generalized term 'Muscle power training' (Bangsbo and Andersen, 2013). Within this definition, muscle power training includes three levels: (1) *basic muscle power training* which refers to training that aims at increasing muscle mass, strength and power; (2) *transference power training* which aims at improving the ability to perform maximal or near-maximal soccer-related movements; (3) *soccer power training* which aims to improve muscle power output during intense, soccer-specific actions (Bangsbo and Andersen, 2013).

Basic muscle power training

The aim of *basic muscle power training* is to increase neuromuscular drive, muscle mass, muscle strength and RFD. Basic muscle power training should lead to improvements in soccer performance elements such as: acceleration capacity, running speed, ability to repeatedly sustain high running speed and maximal vertical jumping ability. It also serves to reduce the risk of injuries where the latter aspect is addressed separately in Chapter 13. Basic muscle power training may involve the use of free weights, machines or other devices that in a safe manner can provide a high external load on the muscle. Typical exercises are: squat, leg press, leg curl, knee extensions, lunges, dead-lift (Bangsbo and Andersen, 2013).

Transference power training

The aim of *transference power training* is to optimize the use of basic muscle power training in specific playing actions during the game. It focuses on transferring the basic muscle strength achieved during basic muscle power training to explosive movements that have functional relevance for the game of soccer. Thus, transference power training should lead to increased acceleration, higher running speed, better jumping abilities, reduced ground contact time in sprint running and jumping and increased performance in side-cutting manoeuvers and other movements involving rapid changes in running direction. Transference power training involves specific muscle contractions performed at maximal or near-maximal velocity with low or no external loads. Plyometric training may be considered an important element of transference power training. Typical exercises are: jumping hurdles, drop jumps, various cone jumps, jumping with low load barbells or similar, loaded accelerations and steep uphill running (Bangsbo and Andersen, 2013).

Soccer power training

The aim of *soccer power training* is to increase players' power capacity in specific game situations. With soccer power training, gains in muscle strength obtained through basic muscle power training and transference power training are utilized in soccer-specific activities such as: acceleration, deceleration, change of direction sprints, ball kicking and vertical jumping. All exercises are performed without external loads, using own body weight only. Typical exercises are: acceleration in-between cones, sprints with change of direction, sprints with repeated accelerations and decelerations, dribbling with high speed alternating with rapid stop-and-acceleration actions and maximal heading exercises (Bangsbo and Andersen, 2013).

Power training types are linked

The three types of muscle power training described above are obviously closely linked and provide a complementary supplement to one another. Basic muscle power training provides the basis for muscle strength in soccer and should in adult players be conducted prior to involving the other types of power training (transference power training, soccer power training) in order to maximize the adaptive effect. Nevertheless, both transference power training and soccer power training can stand alone, and are especially useful in children and young players (Bangsbo and Andersen, 2013).

The focus and amount of muscle power training should be modulated during the playing season as well as in the preceding preparatory periods. Typically, the preparation period should contain a relatively high amount of basic muscle power training, which should be continued throughout the preparation period and gradually be reduced during the playing season, where it should be supplemented by increasing amounts of transference power training and soccer specific power training. However, it is important to sustain a certain amount of basic muscle power training (for instance involving 1–2 weekly training sessions) throughout the playing season in order not to lose significant amount of the muscle strength gained at the preparation period (Rønnestad et al., 2011).

Planning of muscle power training in soccer

It is important to realize that muscle power training is only one of several types of physical, technical and tactical training aspects that a soccer player has to address in order to achieve improvements in physical capacity and soccer skills, or to ensure that these skills are maintained at the highest level. When planning muscle power training for soccer players one is faced with the traditional dilemma of wanting to increase both muscle strength, power and RFD and to some extent perhaps also increase skeletal muscle mass, along with keeping up a relatively high level of aerobic fitness. Thus, strict and precise planning of muscle power training has to occur, to avoid potentially negative interference effects between these two opposing modes of exercise (Wilson et al., 2012). Given that the time available to the coach and the player is typically limited, muscle power training in its most ideal form may not be possible to reach (see Table 1.1).

Most often the pre-season preparation training period is when most time is available for conducting muscle power training (with a strong focus on basic muscle power training). The pre-season preparations are often shorter than what is needed for generating large improvements in muscle strength and muscle mass and therefore the training conducted has to be carefully and efficiently incorporated into the general regime of soccer exercise if improvements serving as basis for the playing season are to be reached (see Table 1.1).

The more difficult part of the planning of muscle power training is to transfer the improvements achieved in the pre-season into the playing season. The question often asked is: how much muscle power training is enough to keep up the acquired muscle strength throughout the entire playing season? In a soccer setting, this question has only been addressed on the basis of a scientific setting in very few studies. One study that does provide some information seems to indicate that one basic muscle power session a week during the season is sufficient to retain maximal muscle strength for several months into the playing season, whereas a single session performed every second week led to decreases in maximal muscle strength and power (Rønnestad et al., 2011). On the other hand, other studies indicate that concurrent endurance and strength training (as is the case with muscle power training performed in a soccer setting) may dampen the improvements in muscle strength, muscle power and muscle mass. In addition, this dampening effect is increased as the volume of endurance-type training goes up (for review, see Wilson et al., 2012). Bearing this in mind, the number of basic muscle power sessions need to be at least once a week, and possibly more to countermeasure the potential negative interference from the high amounts of aerobic training being performed by high-level soccer players.

Table 1.1 Distribution and priority of muscle power training during a full season in professional adult/post-adolescent players

	Types of muscle power training (priority)	Frequency (times per week)	Intensity (sets x repetitions)	Timing
Early preparation period	BMPT; high	BMPT; 2–3	BMPT; 4 x 8–12	BMPT; last activity of the day
	TPT; low/medium	TPT; 1		TPT; mid-session
	SPT; low	SPT; 0–1		SPT; after warm-up
Late preparation period	BMPT; medium	BMPT; 2	BMPT; 3–4 x 6–10	BMPT; last activity of the day
	TPT; medium/high	TPT; 1–2		TPT; mid-session
	SPT; low/medium	SPT; 1		SPT; mid-session
Match season	BMPT; low/medium	BMPT; 1–2	BMPT; 3 x 4–6	BMPT; when convenient
	TPT; medium	TPT; 1		TPT; mid-session
	SPT; medium/high	SPT; 1–2		SPT; mid-session/after warm-up
Intermediate period (summer)	BMPT; high/medium	BMPT; 2–3	BMPT; 4 x 8–12	BMPT; last activity of the day
	TPT; low/medium	TPT; 0–1		TPT; mid-session
	SPT; low	SPT; 0–1		SPT; after warm-up
Match season	BMPT; low/medium	BMPT; 1–2	BMPT; 3 x 4–6	BMPT; when convenient
	TPT; medium	TPT; 1		TPT; mid-session
	SPT; medium/high	SPT; 1–2		SPT; mid-session/after warm-up
Individualized training periods (no team training)	BMPT; high	BMPT; 2–3	BMPT; 4 x 8–12	BMPT; last activity of the day
	TPT; low	TPT; 0–1		TPT; when convenient
	SPT; very low	SPT; 0		SPT; not relevant

Notes
BMPT: basic muscle power training
Frequency: times per week that the specific activity should be conducted (duration 10–60 min depending on activity)
Intensity: for basic muscle power training
sets x repetitions: timing; recommendations for activity in individual training sessions; recommendations are very broad, periodization and necessary individualized variations in training volume/intensity are not included
SPT: soccer power training (for more details, see chapter text)
TPT: transference power training

Muscle power training on post-match days

On post-match days soccer players often conduct very limited amounts of physical activity only aimed at restitution, typically consisting of low-intensity aerobic work, various types of gymnastic exercises (or similar) and physiotherapeutic treatment or massage.

Studies have shown that glycogen deposits in the leg muscles of soccer players are reduced to 50–60 per cent of pre-match levels on post-match day, and may remain reduced to 60–70 per cent up to two days after the game (Bangsbo et al., 2006). This could be an argument for not conducting training sessions that will further tax the glycogen deposits on post-game days, especially if playing a mid-week match subsequent to a weekend match. Nevertheless, in the frequently tight match programs it may be difficult to find the correct point in time to conduct the necessary basic muscle power training. Thus, conducting resistance training with a limited number of sets and repetitions should theoretically be less harmful to the already low glycogen deposits than engaging in different types of aerobic training. In this context, performing basic muscle power training on post-game days may serve several purposes, including not only maintenance of muscle strength and muscle mass but also allowing muscle glycogen levels to restore.

In practical terms, part of or all of the ordinary post-game restitution training may be successfully substituted with basic muscle power training exercises. In our hands, post-match power training session(s) would include only two to four different basic muscle power training exercises, typically some of the traditional resistance exercises aiming at multiple muscle groups in the legs at once (e.g. squats, leg presses). Players would perform three to four sets of four to eight reps not to fail using 4–8RM loads that are reduced 10–15 per cent in comparison to the loads lifted during their basic muscle power training sessions on 'ordinary' training days. Thus, these sessions can be considered more as a 'maintenance' than an 'improvement' stimulus on muscle strength, power and muscle mass, which nevertheless plays an important role in preventing a drop in muscle strength/power/RFD during the playing season.

Conclusions

In conclusion, muscle power training is an effective and necessary tool in the training of elite and sub-elite soccer players, both in an attempt to improve on-pitch playing performance, but also to enable players to tolerate high amounts/intensity of physical training and match play, respectively, without sustaining overload injuries in the musculo-skeletal system (Lauersen et al., 2014; see also Chapter 13 in this book). Importantly, with proper planning it is possible to incorporate power training that effectively facilitates increases in muscle mass, muscle strength and RFD. In turn, these qualities are transferred to gains in sprinting ability, acceleration/deceleration capacity and vertical jumping performance, which altogether provide a high agility level for the soccer player.

It is likely that training-induced improvement in maximal oxygen uptake may provide some advantages in the performance level of elite soccer players. However, a strong focus on improving anaerobic capacity, muscle power and RFD by means of designated muscle power training may more effectively add to the performance level of top-class soccer players. In the years to come the game of modern soccer most likely will develop even further in a direction towards faster and more intense player actions, in turn imposing progressively increasing demands on maximal muscle strength and power. Consequently, an increasing need exists for developing and implementing effective and individualized regimes of muscle power training in elite soccer.

References

Aagaard, P. (2003). Training-induced changes in neural function. *Exercise and Sport Sciences Reviews, 31*, 61–67.

Aagaard, P. and Andersen, J.L. (2017). Eccentric training as treatment of muscle-tendon injury. In J. Bangsbo et al. (ed.): *Science and Football VIII* (pp. 119–125). London: Routledge.

Aagaard, P., Simonsen, E.B., Trolle, M., Bangsbo, J. and Klausen, K. (1994a). Effects of different strength training regimes on moment and power generation during dynamic knee extensions. *European Journal of Applied Physiology and Occupational Physiology, 69*, 382–386.

Aagaard, P., Simonsen, E.B., Trolle, M., Bangsbo, J. and Klausen, K. (1994b). Moment and power generation during maximal knee extensions performed at low and high speeds. *European Journal of Applied Physiology and Occupational Physiology, 69*, 376–381.

Aagaard, P., Simonsen, E.B., Trolle, M., Bangsbo, J. and Klausen, K. (1996). Specificity of training velocity and training load on gains in isokinetic knee joint strength. *Acta Physiologica Scandinavica, 156*, 123–129.

Andersen, J.L., Klitgaard, H., Bangsbo, J. and Saltin, B. (1994). Myosin heavy chain isoforms in single fibres from m. vastus lateralis of soccer players: effects of strength-training. *Acta Physiologica Scandinavica, 150*, 21–26.

Aughey, R.J. and Varley, M.C. (2013). Acceleration profiles in elite Australian soccer. *International Journal of Sports Medicine, 34*, 34–39.

Bangsbo, J. and Andersen, J.L. (2013). *Power Training in Football – A scientific and practical approach.* Denmark: Bangsbosport.

Bangsbo, J., Mohr, M. and Krustrup, P. (2006). Physical and metabolic demands of training and match-play in the elite football player. *Journal of Sports Sciences, 24*, 665–674.

Barnes, C., Archer, D.T., Hogg, B., Bush, M. and Bradley, P.S. (2014). The evolution of physical and technical performance parameters in the English Premier League. *International Journal of Sports Medicine, 35*, 1095–1100.

Brito, J., Vasconcellos, F., Oliveira, J., Krustrup, P. and Rebelo, A. (2014). Short-term performance effects of three different low-volume strength-training programmes in college male soccer players. *Journal of Human Kinetics, 40*, 121–128.

Christou, M., Smilios, I., Sotiropoulos, K., Volaklis, K., Pilianidis, T. and Tokmakidis, S.P. (2006). Effects of resistance training on the physical capacities of adolescent soccer players. *Journal of Strength and Conditioning Research, 20*, 783–791.

Dalen, T., Ingebrigtsen, J., Ettema, G., Hjelde, G.H. and Wisløff, U. (2016). Player load, acceleration, and deceleration during 45 competitive matches of elite soccer. *Journal of Strength and Conditioning Research, 30*(2), 351–359.

Hoff, J. and Helgerud, J. (2004). Endurance and strength training for soccer players – Physiological considerations. *Sports Medicine, 34*, 165–180.

Helgerud, J., Rodas, G., Kemi, O.J. and Hoff, J. (2011). Strength and endurance in elite football players. *International Journal of Sports Medicine, 32*, 677–682.

Lauersen, J.B., Bertelsen, D.M. and Andersen, L.B. (2014). The effectiveness of exercise interventions to prevent sports injuries: a systematic review and meta-analysis of randomised controlled trials. *British Journal of Sports Medicine, 48*, 871–877.

Mohr, M., Krustrup, P. and Bangsbo, J. (2005). Fatigue in soccer: a brief review. *Journal of Sports Sciences*, *23*, 593–599.

Rønnestad, B. R., Kvamme, N. H., Sunde, A. and Raastad, T. (2008). Short-term effects of strength and plyometric training on sprint and jump performance in professional soccer players. *Journal of Strength and Conditioning Research*, *22*, 773–780.

Rønnestad, B. R., Nymark, B. S. and Raastad, T. (2011). Effects of in-season strength maintenance training frequency in professional soccer players. *Journal of Strength and Conditioning Research*, *25*, 2653–2660.

Sander, A., Keiner, M., Wirth, K. and Schmidtbleicher, D. (2013). Influence of a 2-year strength training programme on power performance in elite youth soccer players. *European Journal of Sport Science*, *13*, 445–451.

Silva, J. R., Nassis, G. P. and Rebelo, A. (2015). Strength training in soccer with a specific focus on highly trained players. *Sports Medicine – open*, *1*, 1–27.

Thomas, K., French, D. and Hayes, P. R. (2009). The effect of two plyometric training techniques on muscular power and agility in youth soccer players. *Journal of Strength and Conditioning Research*, *23*, 332–335.

Wilson, J. M., Marin, P. J., Rhea, M. R., Wilson, S. M., Loenneke J. P. and Anderson, J. C. (2012). Concurrent training: a meta-analysis examining interference of aerobic and resistance exercises. *Journal of Strength and Conditioning Research*, *26*, 2293–2307.

Wisløff, U., Castagna, C., Helgerud, J., Jones, R. and Hoff, J. (2004). Strong correlation of maximal squat strength with sprint performance and vertical jump height in elite soccer players. *British Journal of Sports Medicine*, *38*, 285–288.

Wong, P. L., Chaouachi, A., Chamari, K., Dellal, A. and Wisloff, U. (2010). Effect of preseason concurrent muscular strength and high-intensity interval training in professional soccer players. *Journal of Strength and Conditioning Research*, *24*, 653–660.

2 The application of the Yo-Yo intermittent recovery tests to the soccer population

Jens Bangsbo and Matteo Fiorenza

Introduction

The physical demands in top-class soccer are progressively increasing, requiring greater and greater physical capacity of the players. Thus, the ability to repeatedly perform high-intensity work during a game is of particular importance, as it will allow the players to frequently take part in intense actions, which can be essential for the outcome of the game. Therefore, it is important to evaluate a player's capacity to perform and recover from intense actions. In soccer, traditional laboratory tests, such as treadmill running for determination of the maximum oxygen uptake, have been used or tests with continuously running, e.g. the 12-minute Cooper running test or the shuttle run test, have been applied. However, the type of exercise is different from that experienced in soccer, and this led to the development of the Yo-Yo intermittent tests. The present review will deal with the application of the Yo-Yo intermittent recovery (YY-IR) tests in soccer. The YY-IR test evaluates the players' ability to do repeated intense exercise and has two levels; the level 1 test (YY-IR1) is usually indicated for players with low or moderate fitness capacity, and level 2 (YY-IR2) for players with a high capacity.

Physiological response to Yo-Yo intermittent recovery tests

The physiological responses to the YY-IR tests have been investigated in depth through non-invasive, e.g. heart rate monitoring, and invasive measurements such as muscle biopsies and blood samples, demonstrating that both tests stimulate the aerobic system maximally while the rate of the anaerobic energy contribution is different between the two tests (Krustrup et al., 2003, 2006).

Heart rate increases progressively during the YY-IR1 and IR2 test, reaching values equal to 100 percent and 99 percent, respectively, of the peak heart rate observed during an incremental test to exhaustion (Krustrup et al., 2003, 2006). Accordingly, YY-IR tests can be used to determine the maximal heart rate (HR_{max}), which represents a useful tool for monitoring the internal training load (Bangsbo, 2007; Bangsbo and Mohr, 2014; Halson, 2014). Also, according to the different starting speed of the two tests, heart rate increases faster in the YY-IR2 than in IR1 test. Furthermore, it has been observed that the heart rate response, expressed as percent HR_{max}, during a submaximal version of the YY-IR1, e.g. 6-min. duration, is inversely related to YY-IR1 performance (Krustrup et al., 2003). Thus, a non-exhaustive version of the IR1 test, which can be carried out frequently without being demanding for the players and which can be suitable for injured players during rehabilitation, can provide useful information about the fitness level. Similarly, the heart rate response after two minutes of the YY-IR2 has been reported to be inversely related to YY-IR2 performance in sub-elite players (Ingebrigtsen et al., 2012), suggesting that also a submaximal version of the IR2 test can be used.

In terms of utilization of the anaerobic system, the YY-IR2 test requires a higher rate of anaerobic energy contribution than the IR1 test. The lowering in creatine phosphate (CP) level was greater at the end of the YY-IR2 compared to the IR1 test, with the rate of CP utilization in both the first and the last phase of the YY-IR2 being higher than during the IR1 test (Krustrup et al., 2006). Similarly, the muscle lactate concentration at the end of the test was higher in YY-IR2 than in the YY-IR1 test, with the mean rate of muscle lactate accumulation during the YY-IR1 test being about one-fifth of that observed in the IR2 test (Krustrup et al., 2006). Accordingly, peak blood lactate and the rate of lactate accumulation in the blood were higher in the YY-IR2 compared to YY-IR1 test.

Moreover, a marked reduction of glycogen levels in a significant number of muscle fibers was noted after both the YY-IR1 and YY-IR2 test (Bangsbo et al., 2008), with the rate of glycogenolysis being more pronounced during the YY-IR2 than IR1 test, as reflected by the higher rate of muscle glycogen utilization during the YY-IR2 test (Krustrup et al., 2006). On the other hand, the decrease in muscle glycogen content at exhaustion was less marked after the YY-IR2 compared to the IR1 test (9 percent vs. 23 percent), due to the shorter duration of the YY-IR2 test (Bangsbo et al., 2008). To date, no data have been provided regarding the time needed to replenish the muscle glycogen stores following the YY-IR tests, but considering the minor lowering of muscle glycogen during the tests, it should be expected that muscle glycogen is fully restored ~24 h following the completion of the YY-IR tests.

In summary, both YY-IR tests induce a maximal activation of the aerobic system, with the YY-IR2 test taxing the anaerobic energy system with a higher rate than during the YY-IR1 test.

Yo-Yo intermittent recovery test performance in relation to match performance

The performance of the YY-IR1 test has been shown to be correlated to the distance covered with high speed running during a soccer match for both professional (Bangsbo et al., 2008) and young (Castagna et al., 2009, 2010; Rebelo et al., 2014) players, suggesting that the test result can provide information about a player's potential in a match. Despite the relationship, significant variations occur, which probably reflect that factors other than the physical capacity is affecting performance during a game. These include tactical limitation, e.g. a central defender may not cover as much distance as he could due to his primary role of taking care of the opponent's forward, psychological factors, e.g. a player may be lazy and not be motivated to put the opponent under pressure, and another player may 'save' energy during the game in order to be able to perform at the end of the game. Nevertheless, one would never expect to have a one-to-one correlation as the game is much more complex than the test. The important finding is that the test result appears to reflect the running performance in the game.

Similarly, the YY-IR2 test result was correlated to the peak high speed running distance covered in a five-minute period (Bangsbo et al., 2008). The YY-IR2 test has a significant anaerobic component and apparently reflects the player's ability to perform intense running in a game and to recover rapidly from the intense exercise, i.e. the faster the player recovers from an intense action, the more high-intensity work the player can do during the match. Also for the YY-IR2 test variations in the relation to match performance were observed probably for the same reasons mentioned for the YY-IR1 test.

Yo-Yo intermittent recovery test performance in relation to competitive level

A top-class player covers around 2,400 m in the YY-IR1 and 1,400 m in the YY-IR2 test (Figure 2.1), with the best performance recorded being 3,640 m and

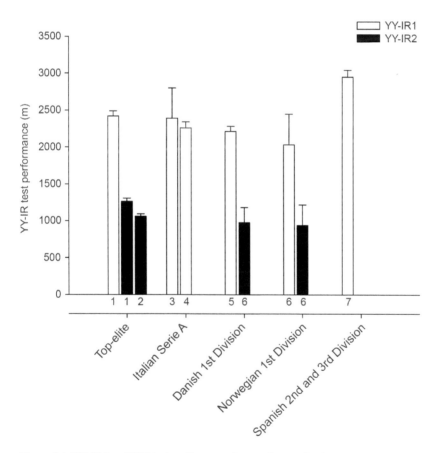

Figure 2.1 YY-IR1 and IR2 test performance in top-class male players

Sources: data from Bangsbo et al., 2008 (study 1); Krustrup et al., 2006 (study 2); Castagna et al., 2013 (study 3); Mohr et al., 2003 (study 4); Krustrup et al., 2003 (study 5); Ingebrigtsen et al., 2012 (study 6); Mohr et al., 2010 (study 7).

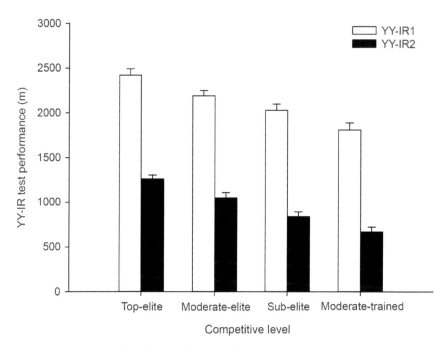

Figure 2.2 YY-IR1 and IR2 test performance for male soccer players in relation to their competitive level

Source: Bangsbo et al. (2008).

about 1,800 m in YY-IR1 and YY-IR2 test, respectively. There are major differences among players in the same squad, but an adult playing at an elite level should be expected to do more than 2,100 and 1,100 m in the YY-IR1 and IR2 test respectively, with the exception of the goalkeeper. There is a clear difference in YY-IR2 test performance between top-elite, moderate-elite and sub-elite soccer players, with greater differences than the ones detected by the YY-IR1 (Figure 2.2) (Bangsbo et al., 2008), suggesting that the higher anaerobic contribution characterizing the YY-IR2 test performance can act as a powerful discriminant among different soccer populations. Furthermore, significantly higher YY-IR2 test scores were observed in the top three teams compared to the bottom three teams of the same Scandinavian National league, while no significant differences were reported in YY-IR1 test performance (Ingebrigtsen et al., 2012). Thus, the YY-IR2 test appears to be sensitive enough to detect differences in high-intensity intermittent exercise performance also between successful and unsuccessful elite teams playing in the same league.

Yo-Yo intermittent recovery test performance in relation to playing position

The playing position does influence YY-IR performance. Among adult male professional players, central defenders usually have a poorer performance in

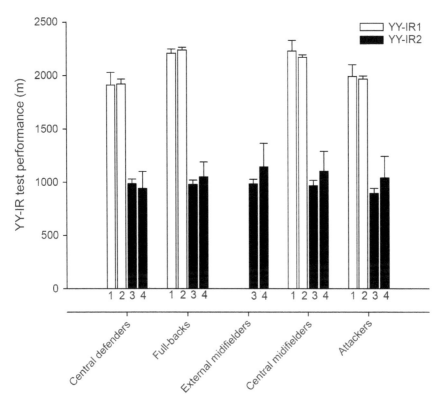

Figure 2.3 YY-IR1 and IR2 test performance in relation to different playing positions. Data from top-elite ((Mohr et al., 2003); study 1), moderate-elite ((Krustrup et al., 2003); study 2), moderate-elite and sub-elite ((Krustrup et al., 2006); study 3), and sub-elite ((Mohr and Krustrup, 2014); study 4) players

YY-IR1 compared to midfielders and full backs, with the full backs also doing significantly better than the attackers (Krustrup et al., 2003). Similar YY-IR1 performance differences in relation to playing roles are reported also in male elite players (Figure 2.3) (Mohr et al., 2003). The lower ability to perform high-intensity intermittent exercise by the central defenders is confirmed by the observation that their YY-IR2 performance was not as good as other outfield positions when studied throughout an entire season (Mohr and Krustrup, 2014).

These findings are in line with the observed lower amount of high speed running done by the central defenders during match play compared to other groups of outfield players (Bradley et al., 2009; Mohr et al., 2003; Rampinini et al., 2007). Furthermore, central defenders have the longest recovery time between intense actions during a game (Carling et al., 2012), suggesting that their lower amount of intense match activities is related to the lower ability to perform intense intermittent exercise as determined by the YY-IR tests.

Yo-Yo intermittent recovery test performance and maximum oxygen uptake

A number of studies have found a relationship between YY-IR1 test performance and maximal oxygen consumption (Table 2.1; VO_{2max}). Thus, a very large correlation between the YY-IR1 and VO_{2max} for male adult players of different competitive levels has been observed (Ingebrigtsen et al., 2012; Rampinini et al., 2010) whereas the relationship appeared to be weaker in elite female players (Krustrup et al., 2005; Martínez-Lagunas and Hartmann, 2014) and young elite male players (Karakoç et al., 2012). Only one study did not find a significant relationship between YY-IR1 performance and VO_{2max} (Castagna et al., 2006).

A weak, but significant, relation between YY-IR2 performance and VO_{2max} has been observed in a heterogeneous sample consisting of both professional and amateur players (Ermanno Rampinini et al., 2010). In addition, Ingebrigtsen et al. (2012) observed that the YY-IR2 test performance was moderately related to VO_{2max} in sub-elite players, with no significant relationship for elite players. The weaker relationships for the YY-IR2 test compared to the YY-IR1 test may be explained by shorter duration and the higher anaerobic contribution characterizing the YY-IR2 test.

Nevertheless, despite the positive correlation between YY-IR1 and VO_{2max}, it has been shown that players with similar VO_{2max} values may have substantial different YY-IR1 test scores (Bangsbo et al., 2008), suggesting that besides maximum aerobic power other physiological factors are important for YY-IR test performance. This also demonstrates that the YY-IR tests provide a different measure than VO_{2max}, and a more valid measure of performance during match play (Krustrup et al., 2003, 2006). For soccer players, training-induced changes are often much greater in YY-IR test performance compared to VO_{2max} (Table 2.2).

The Yo-Yo intermittent recovery tests in relation to repeated sprint ability

There is no real value in comparing one test with another test. Each test has its characteristics and provides information about specific performance abilities and in some cases also about aspects in a soccer game. The finding of a correlation between one and another test should not lead to the conclusion that both tests are equally valid and useful. Nevertheless, such comparisons have been made. Very large correlations have been reported between both YY-IR tests performance and repeated sprint ability (RSA) in elite players, with lower associations observed in sub-elite players (Ingebrigtsen et al., 2012). It is worth noting that, in the study, elite and sub-elite players had similar RSA scores, while YY-IR test performances were significantly lower in the sub-elite players. Hence, the RSA test, in contrast to the YY-IR tests, did not provide a measure sensitive enough to distinguish between players of different competitive levels. Thus, despite a significant correlation between the two tests, the YY-IR tests were able to yield a more accurate determination of the intense intermittent exercise capacity of a player.

Table 2.1 Relationship between YY-IR test performance and VO_{2max}

| Study | Subjects | | | | Relationship with VO_2 max | | | |
| | n | Gender | Age (yrs) | Level | VO_2 max (ml/kg/min) | YY-IR1 (m) | | YY-IR2 (m) | |
						r	Magnitude of the correlation	r	Magnitude of the correlation
Castagna et al. (2006)	24	Male	Adult (26)	Amateur	56.3	0.46	Moderate	—	—
Rampinini et al. (2010)	13 + 12	Male	Adult (25)	Professional + Amateur	58.5 + 56.3	0.74*	Very large	0.47*	Moderate
Ingebrigtsen et al. (2012)	12	Male	Adult (26)	Elite	59.2	0.76*	Very large	0.59	Large
	39	Male	Adult (20)	Sub-elite	61.5	0.73*	Very large	0.48*	Moderate
Karakoc et al. (2012)	12	Male	Young (15)	n.r.	60.0	0.56*	Large	0.53*	Large
Krustrup et al. (2005)	14	Female	Adult (24)	Elite	49.4	0.55*	Large	—	—
Martinez-Lagunas et al. (2014)	18	Female	Adult (22)	Elite	55.0	0.67*	Large	—	—

Note: *indicates significant (P<0.05) relationship with VO_{2max}

Table 2.2 Changes in YY-IR1 and IR2 performance and VO_{2max} following different training interventions for soccer players

Study	Relative change		Effect size	Magnitude	Forest plot
	Variable	Δ change (%)	Hedges' g ± 95% CI	Magnitude of the effect	Forest plot
Castagna et al. (2013)	YY-IR1 (m)	19.5	1.06 ± 0.95	Large	
	VO_{2max} (ml/kg/min)	5.5	0.72 ± 0.91	Moderate	
Ferrari Bravo et al. (2007) [RSG]	YY-IR1 (m)	12.4	0.67 ± 1.04	Moderate	
	VO_{2max} (ml/kg/min)	6.6	1.03 ± 1.09	Large	
Ferrari Bravo et al. (2007) [ITG]	YY-IR1 (m)	27.6	1.06 ± 1.09	Large	
	VO_{2max} (ml/kg/min)	5.0	0.78 ± 1.06	Moderate	
Hill-Haas et al. (2009) [ITG]	YY-IR1 (m)	21.9	1.33 ± 1.31	Large	
	VO_{2max} (ml/kg/min)	2.0	0.26 ± 1.17	Small	
Hill-Haas et al. (2009) [SSG]	YY-IR1 (m)	17.1	0.65 ± 1.16	Moderate	
	VO_{2max} (ml/kg/min)	−0.7	−0.07 ± 1.12	Trivial	
Impellizzeri et al. (2008) [ITG]	YY-IR1 (m)	13.2	1.25 ± 1.20	Large	
	VO_{2max} (ml/kg/min)	4.8	0.87 ± 1.14	Large	
Impellizzeri et al. (2008) [CG]	YY-IR1 (m)	−4.5	−0.48 ± 1.14	Small	
	VO_{2max} (ml/kg/min)	−1.0	−0.36 ± 1.13	Small	
Gunnarsson et al. (2012)	YY-IR2 (m)	10.8	0.34 ± 1.02	Small	
	VO_{2max} (ml/kg/min)	1.0	0.08 ± 1.01	Small	
Wells et al. (2014)	YY-IR2 (m)	10.2	1.95 ± 1.54	Large	
	VO_{2max} (ml/kg/min)	2.3	0.30 ± 1.21	Trivial	

Note: *indicates significant ($P<0.05$) relationship with VO_{2max}.

It is also noteworthy that the relationship between YY-IR performance and RSA is influenced by the number and length of the sprints included in the RSA test protocol. McGawley and Bishop (2014) found that VO_2 increases during 5 x 6-s sprints, with aerobic metabolism contributing from around 10 percent in the first sprint to 40 percent in the last sprint. The aerobic contribution is also higher the longer the sprinting distance (Ingebrigtsen et al., 2014). Therefore, RSA protocols including a high number of and longer sprints might provide a better correlation to YY-IR tests performance because of a larger contribution of the aerobic energy delivery system. This is probably the reason why no significant association was found between YY-IR2 performance and RSA performance using a protocol involving only 5 x 30-m sprints (Krustrup et al., 2006).

The effect of training on the Yo-Yo intermittent recovery test performance

Fitness training in soccer should, during the various phases of the season, focus on, among other things, maintaining or improving the ability of the players to perform high-intensity intermittent exercise (Bangsbo and Mohr, 2013). Whether the fitness training is successful may be measured by the YY-IR tests. Thus, the YY-IR performance has been extensively reported to be sensitive to seasonal changes (Bangsbo, 2007; Krustrup et al., 2003, 2006; Mohr and Krustrup, 2014). Several studies have investigated the effects of training on YY-IR1 (Table 2.3) and IR2 (Table 2.4) performance, however, most of these studies were conducted comparing before-and-after pre-season. Given that prior to the pre-season the players usually come from a detraining period, it is most likely to observe significant improvements during the pre-season due to a low baseline fitness level. Thus, two weeks of detraining in male soccer players are reported to induce a 23 percent impairment in YY-IR2 performance (from 845 to 654 m) (Christensen et al., 2011; Thomassen et al., 2010). Similarly, three to four weeks of inactivity after the competitive season deteriorated YY-IR2 performance by 12 percent and 11 percent in semi-professional (Nakamura et al., 2012) and sub-elite (Krustrup et al., 2006) male players, respectively. It is therefore no surprise that the players improve during the pre-season. The raise in training load, that usually characterizes the pre-season, is expected to induce physiological adaptations that beneficially affect the ability to perform high-intensity intermittent exercise. A 20 percent improvement in YY-IR1 performance (from 2,000 to 2,390 m) for players in an Italian Serie A club has been observed following eight weeks of soccer specific training during the pre-season (Castagna et al., 2013). A similar improvement (20 percent, from 1,510 to 1,808 m) has been shown in sub-elite players after eight weeks of concurrent strength and high-intensity short-intervals training during pre-season (Wong et al., 2010). Comparisons have also been made between the effects of different types of training on YY-IR1 test performance. No significant differences in the improvements were observed when comparing seven weeks of generic training (22 percent, from 1,764 to 2,151 m) and training with small-sided games (17 percent, from 1,488 to 1,742 m) of young elite players (Hill-Haas et al., 2009).

Table 2.3 Effect of training on YY-IR1 test performance

Study	Subjects					Training		
	n	*Gender*	*Age (yrs)*	*Level*	VO_{2max} *(ml/kg/min)*	*Type*	*Protocol*	*Frequency (no. sessions per week)*
Krustrup et al. (2003)	10	Male	Adult (26)	Elite	51.3	Soccer training	Pre-season preparation	5–7
Boullosa et al. (2013)	8	Male	Adult (24)	Elite	n.r.	Soccer training	Technical–tactical training (SSG) + strength and endurance training	5–11
Castagna et al. (2013)	18	Male	Adult (29)	Professional	58.2	Soccer training	13% generic aerobic training 14% anaerobic training	7
Hill-Haas et al. (2009)	9	Male	Young (15)	Elite	60.2	Mixed training	HSIT: 30–60-s at >90% HR_{max} RST: 7 x 35 m sprint with 35s rec) SET: 15–90-s at max intensity Sprint, CoD and agility training	2
	10	Male	Young (15)	Elite	59.3	SSG	3x7 min 2vs2 or 3–6x6–11 min 3vs3 or 3x10–11 min 6vs6 – 1/3-min rec	2
Manzi et al. (2013)	18	Male	Adult (28)	Professional		Soccer training	13% generic aerobic training 14% anaerobic training	7
Wong et al. (2010)	20	Male	Adult (25)	Professional	n.r.	STR + HSIT	STR = gym-based exercisesHSIT = 16 x 15"–15" at 120% MAS	2
Ferrari Bravo et al. (2007)	13	Male	Young (17) + Adult (24)	Professional + Amateur	52.8	HLIT	4 x 4 min at 90–95% HR_{max} – 3 min rec at 60–70% HR_{max}	2
	13	Male	Young (17) + Adult (24)	Professional + Amateur	55.7	RST	3 x (6 x 40-m maximal sprints with CoD – 20 s rec) - 4-min rec	2
Haugen et al. (2014)	6 + 7	Male + Female	Young (17)	Sub-elite	58.2	RST	20–25 x 20-m sprints at 90% maximal intensity – 55-s rec	1
Impellizzeri et al. (2008)	11	Male	Young (18)	n.r.	56.2	HLIT	4 x 4 min at 90–95% HR_{max} – 3-min rec at 60–70% HR_{max}	2–3
	10	Male	Young (18)	n.r.	57.7	Soccer training	Low-intensity Technical–tactical training	2–3

Notes: HR_{max} = maximal heart rate; MAS = maximal aerobic speed; VO_{2max} = maximal oxygen uptake; HSIT = high-intensity short-interval training; HLIT = high-intensity long-interval training; RST = repeated sprint training; SET = speed-endurance training; SSG = small sided games; STR = strength training; CoD = changes of direction; *indicates significant change ($P<0.05$).

Duration (no. of weeks)	Period of the season	Training load (TL) changes/training conducted in addition to the specific training investigated	YY-IR1 test performance				Forest plot
			Distance (m)		Δ change (%)	Effect size (Hedge's g ± 95% CI)	
			Pre	Post			
6	Pre-season	n.r.	1,760	2,211	25.6*	1.99 ± 1.41	
8	Pre-season	Strength, endurance and proprioceptive training included	2,475	2,600	5.1	0.17 ± 1.21	
8	Pre-season	15% Technical training, 21% Technical–tactical training. 8% matches 29% warm-up	2,000	2,390	19.5*	1.06 ± 0.95	
7	Pre-season	2 soccer specific training sessions/wk (4 training sessions/wk in total)	1,764	2,151	21.9*	1.33 ± 1.31	
7	Pre-season	2 soccer specific training sessions/wk (4 training sessions/wk in total)	1,488	1,742	17.1*	0.65 ± 1.16	
9	Pre-season	15% Technical training 21% Technical–tactical training, 8% Matches 29% Warm-up	1,998	2,366	18.4*	1.00 ± 0.94	
8	Pre-season	6–8 training sessions/wk	1,510	1,808	19.7*	0.73 ± 0.87	
7	In-season	n.r. No additional strength/power training	1,850	2,080	12.5*	0.67 ± 1.04	
7	In-season	n.r. No additional strength/power training	1,920	2,450	28.1*	1.06 ± 1.09	
9	In-season	Technical–tactical training SSG	1,583	1,858	17.4*	0.35 ± 1.02	
4	End-season	n.r. No additional strength/power training	1,900	2,150	12.0*	1.25 ± 1.20	
4	End-season	n.r. No additional strength/power training	2,000	1,910	−4.5	−0.48 ± 1.14	

-4 -3 -2 -1 0 1 2 3 4

Effect size

Table 2.4 Effect of training on YY-IR2 test performance

Study	Subjects					Training	
	n	Gender	Age (yrs)	Level	VO_{2max} (ml/kg/min)	Type	Protocol
Ingebrigtsen et al. (2013)	8	Male	Young (17)	Elite	n.r.	SET	1–2 x (5–8 x 30–40 s at 80–100% maximal running speed (with 180° CoD) – 3/4-min rec) – 5-min rec
McGawley et al. (2013)	9	Male	Adult (23)	Semi-professional + Professional	n.r.	Mixed training (HSIT + STR)	RST + SET (1st day), Speed, agility and CoD (2nd day), IT or SSG (3rd day) STR: gym-based exercises (1st and 2nd day) Jumps. core training (3rd day)
	9	Male	Adult (23)	Semi-professional + Professional	n.r.	Mixed training (STR + HSIT)	RST + SET (1st day), Speed, agility and CoD (2nd day), HLIT or SSG (3rd day) STR: gym-based exercises (1st and 2nd day) Jumps, core training (3rd day)
Wahl et al. (2014)	12	Male	Adult (26)	Semi-professional	n.r.	HLIT or SSG	4 x 4-min performed as HLIT or dribbling track orSSG – 3-min rec
Gunnarsson et al. (2012)	18	Male	Adult (23)	Elite	60.6	SET	SET: 6–9 x 30-s all-out – 3-min rec
Nakamura et al. (2012)	13	Male	Adult (23)	Semi-professional	n.r.	Aerobic moderate intensity	30 min at 70–80% HR_{max}
	11	Male	Adult (23)	Semi-professional	n.r.	Plyometric	Plyometric training
	5	Male	Adult (23)	Semi-professional	n.r.	Inactivity	—
Thomassen et al. (2010)	7	Male	Adult (23)	Elite	55.0	SSG + SET	SSG: 8 x 2 min SET: 10–12 x 25–30-s all-out
	11	Male	Adult (23)	Elite	55.0	Inactivity	—
Wells et al. (2014)	8	Male	Adult (21)	Professional	n.r.	HSIT	4 x 60-s or 6 x 35-s or 10 x 10-s at >18 km/h with CoD - 2-min rec

Notes: HR_{max} = maximal heart rate; MAS = maximal aerobic speed; VO_{2max} = maximal oxygen uptake; HSIT = high-intensity short-interval training; HLIT = high-intensity long-interval training; RST = repeated sprint training; SET = speed-endurance training; SSG = small sided games; STR = strength training; CoD = changes of direction; *indicates significant change ($P<0.05$).

Frequency (no. sessions per week)	Duration (no. of weeks)	Period of the season	Training load (TL) changes/ training conducted in addition to the specific training investigated	YY-IR2 test performance Distance (m) Pre	Post	Δ change (%)	Effect size (Hedge's g ± 95% CI)	Forest plot
2	6	Pre-season	4 training sessions/wk including Technical–tactical. SSG. core and balance training (6 training sessions in total)	559	622	11.3*	0.36 ± 1.22	
3	5	Pre-season	2 Technical–tactical training sessions 1 Pilates session (6 training sessions/wk in total)	769	875	13.8*	0.72 ± 1.21	
3	5	Pre-season	2 Technical–tactical training sessions 1 Pilates session (6 training sessions/wk in total)	729	867	18.9*	0.63 ± 1.20	
6	2	Pre-season	4 training sessions/wk including Technical–tactical training	408	505	23.8*	1.83 ± 1.28	
1	5	In-season	+30% TL during the intervention period	778	862	10.8*	0.34 ± 1.02	
2	3	End-season	−67% TL during the intervention period (no additional training was performed except for the IT training)	855	723	−15.4*	−0.67 ± 1.04	
2	3	End-season	−67% TL during the intervention period (no additional training was performed except for the IT training)	860	727	−15.5*	−1.00 ± 1.16	
—	3	End-season	−100% TL	720	632	−12.2*	−0.36 ± 1.29	
5	2	End-season	−30% TL during the intervention period	937	994	6.1	0.28 ± 1.26	
0	2	End-season	−100% TL	845	654	−22.6*	−1.38 ± 1.22	
3	6	n.r.	Soccer specific training (Technical–tactical, SSG, fitness)	896	987	10.2*	1.95 ± 1.54	

-4 -3 -2 -1 0 1 2 3 4
Effect size

YY-IR2 performance has also been shown to be sensitive to pre-season training. Improvements in the range of 15–20 percent have been noted as a result of five weeks of concurrent strength and high-intensity interval training in semi-professional and professional adult players (McGawley and Andersson, 2013). Furthermore, two speed-endurance training (SET) sessions per week during a six-week pre-season training period induced a beneficial change in YY-IR2 performance (11 percent, from 559 to 622 m) in young well-trained players (Ingebrigtsen et al., 2013).

Performances in both the YY-IR1 and YY-IR2 tests do often decline in the final phase of the competitive season compared to starting and mid-season periods (Bangsbo et al., 2008; Mohr and Krustrup, 2014), which may be related to an insufficient level of aerobic and anaerobic training toward the end of the season. This may be a specific problem for players who are taking part in international tournaments, i.e. World Cup or Continental Cups, which usually are played after the end of the competitive season. Carrying out training with high intensity plays a key role, as two to four weeks of high-intensity training seems to be sufficient to improve YY-IR performance following the competitive season. Specifically, two weeks of intensified training conducted as small-sided games and speed endurance production training, with a concurrent reduction in training volume by ~30 percent, has been shown to induce an 11 percent improvement in YY-IR2 test performance (from 937 to 994 m) in sub-elite players (Christensen et al., 2011; Thomassen et al., 2010). Likewise, four weeks of high-intensity long interval training (4 x 4 min at 90–95 percent HR_{max}) with no reduction in training volume, induced a 12 percent increment in YY-IR1 performance in young players (Impellizzeri et al., 2008). Conversely, three weeks of biweekly moderate intensity aerobic training sessions (30-min. continuous running at 70–80 percent HR_{max}) with a concurrent reduction in training volume by 67 percent, are reported to negatively affect YY-IR2 performance in semi-professional players (−15 percent; from 855 to 723 m), with no significant differences compared with three weeks of inactivity (Nakamura et al., 2012). Thus, to improve or restore performance during the season, it appears appropriate to concurrently lower the training volume and to increase training intensity (Mujika, 2010).

It is not always possible to plan a marked reduction in training volume during the competitive season, since most soccer competitions involve one or more matches per week. Nevertheless, it has been shown that, despite a lack in training volume reduction, intense training per se can improve the players' capacity to perform intense intermittent exercise also during the in-season period. In these terms, Gunnarsson et al. (2012) observed that one additional speed endurance production training session a week for a five-week period during the competitive season improved YY-IR2 test performance in elite players (11 percent; 778 vs. 862 m). In addition, Ferrari Bravo et al. (2008) investigated the effect of a seven-week in-season intervention including either biweekly repeated sprint training (RST) or biweekly high-intensity long intervals training (HLIT) in young professional and adult amateur players, showing a greater improvement in YY-IR1 performance following RST (28 percent; from 1,920 to 2,450 m) compared to HLIT (13 percent; from 1,850 to 2,080 m). The reasons for the difference may be that the players during RST not only completed a high number of runs with maximal speed, but often also changed direction, whereas the players performing HLIT had no maximal runs and no changes in directions. Thus, part of the larger improvement in RST may have been due to specific neuromuscular adaptations (Hader et al., 2014). Taken together, both the YY-IR1 and IR2 test are sensitive and can detect high-intensity intermittent performance changes over a training period. However, the YY-IR1 test seems to be more responsive to training than the YY-IR2 test (Fanchini et al., 2014).

Summary

YY-IR tests are incremental tests to exhaustion that stimulate the aerobic system maximally, and also the anaerobic system toward the end of the test. The test results are related to the performance in a game and can detect changes related to training interventions and different level of soccer.

References

Bangsbo, J. (2007). *Aerobic and Anaerobic Training in Soccer – With Special Emphasis on Training of Youth Players. Fitness Training in Soccer I.* 1–231. www.bangsbosport.com (last accessed August 15, 2015).

Bangsbo, J., Iaia, F.M. and Krustrup, P. (2008). The Yo-Yo intermittent recovery test : a useful tool for evaluation of physical performance in intermittent sports. *Sports Medicine (Auckland, NZ)*, *38*(1), 37–51.

Bangsbo, J. and Mohr, M. (2011). *Fitness Testing in Football*, 1–136. www.bangsbosport.com (last accessed August 15, 2015).

Bangsbo, J. and Mohr, M. (2014). *Individual Training in Football*, 1–128. www.bangsbo sport.com (last accessed August 15, 2015).

Bradley, P.S., Sheldon, W., Wooster, B., Olsen, P., Boanas, P. and Krustrup, P. (2009). High-intensity running in English FA Premier League soccer matches. *Journal of Sports Sciences*, *27*(2), 159–168.

Carling, C., Le Gall, F. and Dupont, G. (2012). Analysis of repeated high-intensity running performance in professional soccer. *Journal of Sports Sciences*, *30*(4), 325–336.

Castagna, C., Impellizzeri, F., Cecchini, E., Rampinini, E. and Alvarez, J.C.B. (2009). Effects of intermittent-endurance fitness on match performance in young male soccer players. *Journal of Strength and Conditioning Research/National Strength and Conditioning Association*, *23*(7), 1954–1959.

Castagna, C., Impellizzeri, F.M., Chamari, K., Carlomagno, D. and Rampinini, E. (2006). Aerobic fitness and yo-yo continuous and intermittent tests performances in soccer players: a correlation study. *Journal of Strength and Conditioning Research/National Strength and Conditioning Association*, *20*(2), 320–325.

Castagna, C., Impellizzeri, F.M., Chaouachi, A. and Manzi, V. (2013). Preseason variations in aerobic fitness and performance in elite-standard soccer players: a team study. *Journal of Strength and Conditioning Research/National Strength and Conditioning Association*, *27*(11), 2959–2965.

Castagna, C., Manzi, V., Impellizzeri, F., Weston, M. and Barbero Alvarez, J.C. (2010). Relationship between endurance field tests and match performance in young soccer players. *Journal of Strength and Conditioning Research/National Strength and Conditioning Association*, *24*(12), 3227–3233.

Christensen, P. M., Krustrup, P., Gunnarsson, T. P., Kiilerich, K., Nybo, L. and Bangsbo, J. (2011). VO2 kinetics and performance in soccer players after intense training and inactivity. *Medicine and Science in Sports and Exercise*, *43*(9), 1716–1724.

Fanchini, M., Castagna, C., Coutts, A. J., Schena, F., McCall, A. and Impellizzeri, F. M. (2014). Are the Yo-Yo intermittent recovery test levels 1 and 2 both useful? Reliability, responsiveness and interchangeability in young soccer players. *Journal of Sports Sciences*, *32*(20), 1950–1957.

Ferrari Bravo, D., Impellizzeri, F. M., Rampinini, E., Castagna, C., Bishop, D. and Wisloff, U. (2008). Sprint vs. interval training in football. *International Journal of Sports Medicine*, *29*(8), 668–674.

Hader, K., Mendez-Villanueva, A., Ahmaidi, S., Williams, B. K. and Buchheit, M. (2014). Changes of direction during high-intensity intermittent runs: neuromuscular and metabolic responses. *BMC Sports Science, Medicine and Rehabilitation*, *6*(1), 2.

Halson, S. L. (2014). Monitoring Training Load to Understand Fatigue in Athletes. *Sports Medicine (Auckland, NZ)*.

Hill-Haas, S. V., Coutts, A. J., Rowsell, G. J. and Dawson, B. T. (2009). Generic versus small-sided game training in soccer. *International Journal of Sports Medicine*, *30*(9), 636–642.

Impellizzeri, F. M., Rampinini, E., Maffiuletti, N. A., Castagna, C., Bizzini, M. and Wisløff, U. (2008). Effects of aerobic training on the exercise-induced decline in short-passing ability in junior soccer players. *Applied Physiology, Nutrition, and Metabolism = Physiologie Appliquée, Nutrition Et Métabolisme*, *33*(6), 1192–1198.

Ingebrigtsen, J., Bendiksen, M., Randers, M. B., Castagna, C., Krustrup, P. and Holtermann, A. (2012). Yo-Yo IR2 testing of elite and sub-elite soccer players: performance, heart rate response and correlations to other interval tests. *Journal of Sports Sciences*, *30*(13), 1337–1345.

Ingebrigtsen, J., Brochmann, M., Castagna, C., Bradley, P. S., Ade, J., Krustrup, P. and Holtermann, A. (2014). Relationships between field performance tests in high-level soccer players. *Journal of Strength and Conditioning Research/National Strength and Conditioning Association*, *28*(4), 942–949.

Ingebrigtsen, J., Shalfawi, S. A. I., Tønnessen, E., Krustrup, P. and Holtermann, A. (2013). Performance effects of 6 weeks of aerobic production training in junior elite soccer players. *Journal of Strength and Conditioning Research/National Strength and Conditioning Association*, *27*(7), 1861–1867.

Karakoç, B., Akalan, C., Alemdaroğlu, U. and Arslan, E. (2012). The relationship between the yo-yo tests, anaerobic performance and aerobic performance in young soccer players. *Journal of Human Kinetics*, *35*, 81–88.

Krustrup, P., Mohr, M., Amstrup, T., Rysgaard, T., Johansen, J., Steensberg, A., Pedersen, P.K. and Bangsbo, J. (2003). The yo-yo intermittent recovery test: physiological response, reliability, and validity. *Medicine and Science in Sports and Exercise*, *35*(4), 697–705.

Krustrup, P., Mohr, M., Ellingsgaard, H. and Bangsbo, J. (2005). Physical demands during an elite female soccer game: importance of training status. *Medicine and Science in Sports and Exercise*, *37*(7), 1242–1248.

Krustrup, P., Mohr, M., Nybo, L., Jensen, J. M., Nielsen, J. J. and Bangsbo, J. (2006). The Yo-Yo IR2 test: physiological response, reliability, and application to elite soccer. *Medicine and Science in Sports and Exercise*, *38*(9), 1666–1673.

Krustrup, P., Ortenblad, N., Nielsen, J., Nybo, L., Gunnarsson, T. P., Iaia, F. M., Madsen, K., Stephens, F., Greenhaff, P. and Bangsbo, J. (2011). Maximal voluntary contraction force, SR function and glycogen resynthesis during the first 72 h after a high-level competitive soccer game. *European Journal of Applied Physiology*, *111*(12), 2987–2995.

McGawley, K. and Andersson, P.-I. (2013). The order of concurrent training does not affect soccer-related performance adaptations. *International Journal of Sports Medicine*, *34*(11), 983–990.

McGawley, K. and Bishop, D. J. (2014). Oxygen uptake during repeated-sprint exercise. *Journal of Science and Medicine in Sport/Sports Medicine Australia, 18*(2), 214–218.

Martínez-Lagunas, V. and Hartmann, U. (2014). Validity of the Yo-Yo Intermittent Recovery Test Level 1 for Direct Measurement or Indirect Estimation of Maximal Oxygen Uptake Among Female Soccer Players. *International Journal of Sports Physiology and Performance, 9,* 825–831.

Mohr, M. and Krustrup, P. (2014). Yo-Yo intermittent recovery test performances within an entire football league during a full season. *Journal of Sports Sciences*, *32*(4), 315–327.

Mohr, M., Krustrup, P. and Bangsbo, J. (2003). Match performance of high-standard soccer players with special reference to development of fatigue. *Journal of Sports Sciences*, *21*(7), 519–528.

Mujika, I. (2010). Intense training: the key to optimal performance before and during the taper. *Scandinavian Journal of Medicine and Science in Sports*, 20 Suppl. 2, 24–31.

Nakamura, D., Suzuki, T., Yasumatsu, M. and Akimoto, T. (2012). Moderate running and plyometric training during off-season did not show a significant difference on soccer-related high-intensity performances compared with no-training controls. *Journal of Strength and Conditioning Research/National Strength and Conditioning Association*, *26*(12), 3392–3397.

Rampinini, E., Coutts, A. J., Castagna, C., Sassi, R. and Impellizzeri, F. M. (2007). Variation in top level soccer match performance. *International Journal of Sports Medicine*, *28*(12), 1018–1024.

Rampinini, E., Sassi, A., Azzalin, A., Castagna, C., Menaspà, P., Carlomagno, D. and Impellizzeri, F. M. (2010). Physiological determinants of Yo-Yo intermittent recovery tests in male soccer players. *European Journal of Applied Physiology*, *108*(2), 401–409.

Rebelo, A., Brito, J., Seabra, A., Oliveira, J. and Krustrup, P. (2014). Physical match performance of youth football players in relation to physical capacity. *European Journal of Sport Science, 14 Suppl. 1*, S148–156.

Reilly, T. and Williams, A. M. (2003). *Science and Soccer*. Psychology Press.

Thomassen, M., Christensen, P. M., Gunnarsson, T. P., Nybo, L. and Bangsbo, J. (2010). Effect of 2-wk intensified training and inactivity on muscle Na+-K+ pump expression, phospholemman (FXYD1) phosphorylation, and performance in soccer players. *Journal of Applied Physiology (Bethesda, Md.: 1985)*, *108*(4), 898–905.

Wong, P., Chaouachi, A., Chamari, K., Dellal, A. and Wisloff, U. (2010). Effect of pre-season concurrent muscular strength and high-intensity interval training in professional soccer players. *Journal of Strength and Conditioning Research/National Strength and Conditioning Association*, *24*(3), 653–660.

3 Fitness coaching in an elite soccer team

With special focus on individual-based approaches

F. Marcello Iaia and Richard Hawkins

Contemporary issues in the working environment

Working in a world-class soccer environment, or, more specifically, training elite soccer players is one of the most intriguing and exciting aspects of applied sports sciences. Over the past few years, in many elite clubs, the role of the fitness coach has however been subjected to a substantial and radical evolution, shifting from exercising with the players to a more global position in charge of supervising and managing the multiple processes behind the team's performance.

With the rapid advances in technologies, that have accompanied this period of evolution, there has been a clear tendency toward utilizing extensive data to drive statistical and quantitative analysis and explanatory and predictive models to enhance decision making and direct actions to optimally prepare players for competition. This obviously implies a bigger complexity to the whole operational process and the implementation of larger backroom staffs in order to handle all the support activities. The increase in staff has direct implications on the group dynamics and requires clear definition of roles, efficient communication and streamlined procedures to ensure the increased intelligence is appropriately utilized by the coaching department; this is the role of modern-day performance managers and department heads, successfully transferring the relevant knowledge, attained via the complex web of operations, to the coaches.

Role of fitness training

Recent research in sports science has shown how fitness performance in team sports does not rely solely on the physical components, but it's affected greatly by the technical, tactical and psychological qualities (Bradley et al., 2011). Ingredients such as decision making, skills with the ball and motivation nowadays play a vital role in determining the success of an elite team. As a result, fitness coaching, rather than being purely focused on training the fitness aspects by themselves, should be part of an efficient holistic approach where the conditioning features are developed simultaneously, in combination with all the other areas. This is an ideal, but not all practices will achieve the desired multiple objectives, outcomes consistently having to be evaluated against the key performance indicators set by the club.

A key requirement for elite clubs to enhance the potential for success is to have as many players as possible available both for training and games. Recent Champions League events have shown the importance of this, since squads which lacked players failed to get through to the final stages of the competition. Thus, at the elite level, the primary purpose of fitness training is not pushing the boundaries of human performance and sustaining the highest work rates, but it is more oriented toward keeping the players injury free and making them capable of playing competitive games every three to four days for most of the season throughout their whole career. Based on this premise, it should be apparent that the physical development of players in their formative years takes on a far greater importance and the foundations developed from a young age will often determine the robustness a player has on entering the elite stage which in turn will impact potential success.

Ultimately, philosophies adopted by clubs will vary in emphasis depending upon many factors such as player needs, club aims and coach experience. However, the bedrocks of success remain: the suggested performance triad (Figure 3.1) encompasses the majority of areas addressed by performance managers, all strategies and processes designed to influence one or more of these areas. Despite the advances in sports science knowledge and the increase in the number of strategies designed to assist players maximize their potential, there remains some fundamental components that, if addressed appropriately, can significantly influence the desired outcome. These areas include planning, monitoring and individual training.

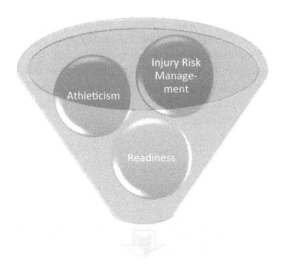

Elite Performance

Figure 3.1 Performance triad underpinning key objectives

Planning

Many factors need to be considered when designing a program and it is the evaluation of such practices combined with the relevant experiences accumulated over years of practice, in addition to the rigor of applied research findings that help formulate strategic processes adopted by performance managers and fitness coaches.

The planning of field-based training for elite soccer players addresses both the short- and the long-term needs of individual players and the team as a whole. The long-term strategy includes the selection of those team activities and individual player requirements which hold a high priority and are in need of development and/or maintenance throughout the season/s, whereas the short-term strategy represents the way multiple components are scheduled and delivered from game to game. In practice, the weekly planning is dictated by the number and type of games as well as by the current fitness status of the players and their respective characteristics. Although it is logical to expect that there exists flexibility and different weekly templates are tailored to the requirements of each specific situation, it is also fundamental to have some science-based procedural guidelines that need to be taken into account when creating a training plan (Figure 3.2).

It is well documented that the muscle contractile properties as well as various physiological parameters taxed during a match may require up to 72 hours to be completely restored (Jacobs et al., 1982; Andersson et al., 2008). Furthermore, it has been observed that two matches in a week do not allow a recovery of sufficient duration (Mohr et al., 2015) to maintain a low injury rate (Dupont et al., 2010) and when extended over a six-week period can also lead to impaired sprint and high-intensity intermittent performance as well as diminished stress and recovery indices (Rollo et al., 2014). It should be abundantly clear then that appropriate load management following games and leading into subsequent games is a critical process that should be supported by monitoring the stress imposed on players and its subsequent impact on a range of player biological systems (e.g. physiological, psychological, neuro-muscular, structural/functional).

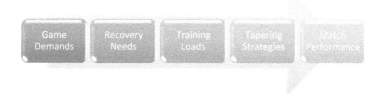

Figure 3.2 Game-to-game plan overview

Managing individuals in a team-oriented sport is critical to optimizing performance. Experience has shown us that the two most critical days in the planning process are 48 hours post-game (G+2) and 48 hours pre-game (G-2). Negative relationships have indeed been noticed between a few training load parameters taken in the session 48 hours after the game and some indices of technical/tactical efficiency measured during the subsequent game. In particular, high speed running accounted for 63 and 68 percent of the total variance observed in successful passes and ball possession percentage, respectively (data not published).

Appropriate tracking of player load is critical to optimal player management since elevated workload over periods of time, in particular exercises with pronounced musculoskeletal components (Barnett, 2006), may contribute to potentially long-term debilitating effects associated with overtraining and increased occurrence of injury events (Nimmo and Ekblom, 2007). This is consistent with recent findings indicating how sessions that can be recovered from within 36 hours (acute fatigue) are more advantageous than those leading to functional/non-functional overreaching (Meeusen et al., 2013). Also, unpublished data from our group seems to support such theory as high weekly training load negatively affected the technical/tactical performance during games. Thus, during the season the key principle is to ensure a balance is reached between training–performance adaptation, adequate rest and optimal readiness.

Once a player has recovered, the following days should be focused on managing the type and quantity of training: sessions based on soccer-related endurance, strength, speed or individual specific fitness attributes are usually performed depending on the time available prior to the next game. Training is implemented to maximize physiological adaptation when possible while minimizing injury risk. Although the lead into games has an element of tapering from a physical standpoint, there may well be situations when players carry out either team- or individual-based surrogates of high-quality field-based work. Appropriate monitoring is a key determinant of the workload applied.

Load monitoring and individual training

The main objective of team training should be developing technical and tactical skills at team level as well as some general conditioning components common to all players, while any additional specific fitness requirements for individuals can be delivered at different times according to the players' needs. The type and amount of training performed is dictated by the game and recovery demands, but usually tend to be primarily designed for those core players who play the majority of the games, with the rest of the squad carrying out supplementary drills during the session.

In general practice there is an extensive use of small-sided games and drills containing technical/tactical elements associated with match play to simultaneously enhance the physical and technical development of players. However, it is pivotal to ensure that the training stimulus is sufficient to promote the desired physiological adaptations related to the physical component of match performance. Appropriate monitoring is required to establish this and in situations where the necessary demands are not achieved there is quite likely a need for a more individualized approach to the training process.

Adequate monitoring methods enables the identification of the energy systems typically attained with certain drills to take place that may well impose specific technical/tactical demands on players and concurrently train desired components of physiology. This enables the staff to be better informed about the appropriateness of conditioning drills to select for overloading specific physical and physiological aspects of playing soccer while also taking into account recent loads incurred via training and matches.

Careful manipulation of training load and exercise selection play a key role in facilitating the maintenance of specific physiological parameters throughout the playing season, while at the same time raising the general levels of athletic abilities through a long-term development plan.

The use of specific methods to prepare elite players for match play requires a higher complexity in the quantification of the workload (Figure 3.3). With the advances in technology that have been made available to practitioners the extent of load evaluation routinely encompasses measures of internal stress, using heart rate and subjective exertion ratings, and external stress, utilizing global positioning systems and accelerometer derived indices. The external measures have enhanced the ability of practitioners to evaluate practice in more detail, manage risk more appropriately and attain a greater understanding of the movement demands to optimize conditioning drills.

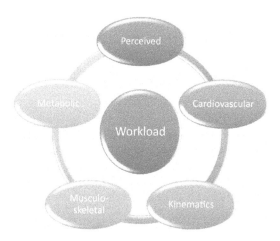

Figure 3.3 Workload parameters during training and rehab

Intense game periods

To optimize an individual-based approach to training, match performance has first to be measured and its details and characteristics understood. While the total loads typically reported in the literature yield a global overview of the physiological strain imposed on the players during competition, much of the detailed information regarding the specific physical demands each player is exposed to is not provided. A more appropriate model is to research in depth what occurs during the most critical phases of the game (Mohr et al., 2003; Krustrup et al., 2006), which better describes the players' individual physiological requirements and offers more qualitative information that can be effectively utilized in the design of field-based conditioning drills. Unfortunately, the mechanisms taxed during the intense periods are still poorly understood and warrants further investigation. Recent unpublished analyses from our group have indeed demonstrated that the nature of the most demanding phases do not include solely repeated intense runs above a certain speed, as classically assumed, but encompass also single supra-maximal/all-out efforts lasting several seconds, continuous prolonged moderate/high-intensity bouts (Figure 3.4), as well as acyclic sequences constituted by repetitive and unexpected low- to high-quality changes in velocity.

Due to the high number of games that elite players have, the time available for performing physical training is usually very limited. Therefore, in addition to incorporating the main conditioning components into the technical/tactical drills, it becomes also essential that any time a player has the possibility to carry out some intense fitness work, a very high-quality, individual specific session is delivered, maximal gains being desired. The focus of field-based training from a fitness perspective is predominantly aimed at producing the appropriate stressors to ensure the energy systems of players adapt and are best equipped to withstand the competitive demands of the game. Once the specific metabolic and mechanical requirements that a player is exposed to during the crucial periods of the match have been comprehensively examined, the approach is to create personalized drills that trigger the physiological mechanisms understood to be a limiting factor to the targeted performance if, as a result of the monitoring implemented, it is established that the holistic training performed does not fulfill the desired objectives. Hence, the prescription of the type and amount of exercise stimulus during fitness training should be adequate for the intended physiological adaptations and tailored to the technical/tactical needs of each player (Mohr and Iaia, 2014). Besides being an effective and time-efficient strategy for maximizing performance enhancement, the delivery of field-based conditioning within a technical/tactical context has direct implication also on injury prevention as it exposes the players' muscles to the position specific movements and high-intensity work patterns typical of those encountered during the fatiguing actions of the game (Figure 3.5). Many adaptive responses in some key physiological mechanisms regulating repetitive high-speed exercise are indeed more linked to the intensity of the stimulus rather than to its volume (Iaia et al., 2008, 2015),

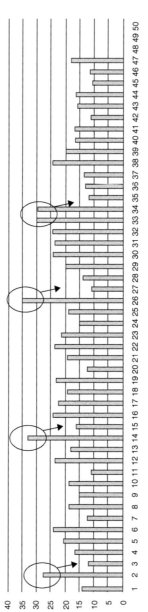

Avg pmet (W/kg) per min

Figure 3.4 Work rate profile of an elite player during half of a competitive game

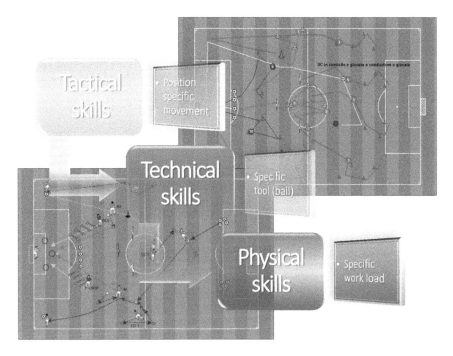

Figure 3.5 Example of individual specific technical/tactical and fitness drills

hence high-speed actions are generally incorporated into any additional work performed.

Conclusions

In an elite soccer environment, the approach to the performance management of the training process is constituted by three main stages (Figure 3.6); the first involves the collection of data, the second includes the analysis and interpretation of the data and the third aspect revolves around the effective delivery of an action plan, generated by amalgamating relevant information from the derived data, previous experience and intuition; a mix of art and science.

In this ever advancing scientific field, basic training principles still need to be adhered to: simply by planning effectively, managing load appropriately and prescribing individual-based training specifically to individual needs and match demands, risk management strategies can be optimized and performance potential enhanced. The end product is a squad of players capable of repeatedly performing all-out efforts in a game with an ability to recover quickly, both within the game and also after the game, the development of both being fundamental to the strategic aims of the fitness coach, maximizing player availability throughout the season.

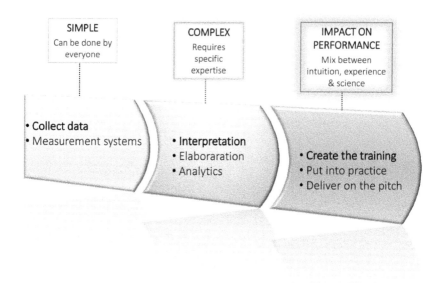

Figure 3.6 Outline of management stages of the performance training process

References

Andersson, H., Raastad, T., Nilsson, J., Paulsen, G., Garthe, I. and Kadi, F. (2008). Neuromuscular fatigue and recovery in elite female soccer: effects of active recovery. *Medicine and Science in Sports and Exercise*, *40*, 372–380.

Barnett, A. (2006). Using recovery modalities between training sessions in elite athletes: does it help? *Sports Medicine*, *36*, 781–796.

Bradley, P. S., Carling, C., Archer, D., Roberts, J., Dodds, A., Di, M. M., Paul, D., Diaz, A. G., Peart, D. and Krustrup, P. (2011). The effect of playing formation on high-intensity running and technical profiles in English FA Premier League soccer matches. *Journal of Sports Sciences*, *29*, 821–830.

Dupont, G., Nedelec, M., McCall, A., McCormack, D., Berthoin, S. and Wisloff, U. (2010). Effect of 2 soccer matches in a week on physical performance and injury rate. *American Journal of Sports Medicine*, *38*, 1752–1758.

Iaia, F. M., Fiorenza, M., Perri, E., Alberti, G., Millet, G. P. and Bangsbo, J. (2015). The Effect of Two Speed Endurance Training Regimes on Performance of Soccer Players. *PLoS.One.*, 10, e0138096.

Iaia, F. M., Thomassen, M., Kolding, H., Gunnarsson, T., Wendell, J., Rostgaard, T., Nordsborg, N., Krustrup, P., Nybo, L., Hellsten, Y. and Bangsbo, J. (2008). Reduced volume but increased training intensity elevates muscle Na+-K+ pump alpha1-subunit and NHE1 expression as well as short-term work capacity in humans. *American Journal of Physiology – Regulatory, Integrative and Comparative Physiology*, *294*, R966–R974.

Jacobs, I., Westlin, N., Karlsson, J., Rasmusson, M. and Houghton, B. (1982). Muscle glycogen and diet in elite soccer players. *European Journal of Applied Physiology and Occupational Physiology*, *48*, 297–302.

Krustrup, P., Mohr, M., Steensberg, A., Bencke, J., Kjaer, M. and Bangsbo, J. (2006). Muscle and blood metabolites during a soccer game: implications for sprint performance. *Medicine and Science in Sports and Exercise*, *38*, 1165–1174.

Meeusen, R., Duclos, M., Foster, C., Fry, A., Gleeson, M., Nieman, D., Raglin, J., Rietjens, G., Steinacker, J. and Urhausen, A. (2013). Prevention, diagnosis, and treatment of the overtraining syndrome: joint consensus statement of the European College of Sport Science and the American College of Sports Medicine. *Medicine and Science in Sports and Exercise*, *45*, 186–205.

Mohr, M., Draganidis, D., Chatzinikolaou, A., Barbero-Alvarez, J. C., Castagna, C., Douroudos, I., Avloniti, A., Margeli, A., Papassotiriou, I., Flouris, A. D., Jamurtas, A. Z., Krustrup, P. and Fatouros, I. G. (2016). Muscle damage, inflammatory, immune and performance responses to three football games in 1 week in competitive male players. *European Journal of Applied Physiology*, *116*(1), 179–193.

Mohr, M. and Iaia, F. M. (2014). Physiological basis of fatigue resistance training in competitive football. *Sports Science Exchange*, *27*(126), 1–9.

Mohr, M., Krustrup, P. and Bangsbo, J. (2003). Match performance of high-standard soccer players with special reference to development of fatigue. *Journal of Sports Sciences*, *21*, 519–528.

Nimmo, M. A. and Ekblom, B. (2007). Fatigue and illness in athletes. *Journal of Sports Sciences, 25 Suppl. 1*, S93–102.

Rollo, I., Impellizzeri, F. M., Zago, M. and Iaia, F. M. (2014). Effects of 1 versus 2 games a week on physical and subjective scores of subelite soccer players. *International Journal of Sports Physiology and Performance*, *9*, 425–431.

4 Soccer referee training and performance

Carlo Castagna

Introduction

Soccer refereeing has been the subject of many papers in the last decade, which has enabled the publication of two narrative reviews of the physiological demands of matches and associated fitness requirements (Castagna et al., 2007; Weston et al., 2012). The evidence provided showed that relative physiological match demands are similar to those reported in gender- and competition-level-matched soccer players, despite major reported differences in age and training background (Castagna et al., 2007; Weston et al., 2012). First-division matches were shown to tax the cardiovascular system of field referees (FRs) to 80–90 percent of their individual maximal heart rate (HR), with reported blood lactate concentrations $[La]_b$ up to 12 mmol·l^{-1} (Krustrup and Bangsbo, 2001). The FRs' match-related external load considered as distance accumulated during the game in arbitrarily chosen speed categories was reported to differ from that of players at the same competitive level (Weston et al., 2011). In fact, FRs were shown to cover a significantly greater total distance, accumulating similar distances at high intensity (HI) as officiated players in Premier League matches (Weston et al., 2011). There were also differences in sprint activity, with players accumulating significantly greater sprint distances than FRs. Interestingly, the FRs' match activities performed at high intensity were significantly correlated with those of the teams playing in those matches (Weston et al., 2007).

Large to very-large relationships between direct and indirect variables informing aerobic fitness and relevant match activities in the high-intensity domain were reported (Castagna et al., 2007; Weston et al., 2009), thereby supporting the relevance of aerobic fitness for the development of FR fitness at elite level. Despite the relevance of aerobic fitness for FR performance, the published literature provides little information on the aerobic make-up of elite-level FRs and assistant referees (ARs) assessed in a laboratory set-up under controlled conditions compared to field testing (Castagna et al., 2007; Krustrup and Bangsbo, 2001).

Given the link between the players' match activity and the FRs' external load, and the evidence provided for selective differences in match-related high-intensity activities, training methods for developing repeat sprint ability (RSA) and intermittent HI ability were proposed for the development of players' and referees' match activity (Castagna et al., 2007; Weston et al., 2012). However, given the complexity of match-related physical performance, it is deemed that elite FRs and ARs should train in agility and strength, and use appropriate evidence-based strategies to also prevent injuries (Weston et al., 2012).

ARs monitor the offside line, covering opposite halves of the pitch on diagonally opposing touchlines, thereby accumulating 5–7 km, of which 20–30 percent is performed with sideways running (Krustrup et al., 2002). In the only descriptive paper addressing match-related physiological demands of ARs, significant association was reported between match-related total distance covered and match-related percent HR_{max} with VO_{2max} (Krustrup et al., 2002). In this paper very-large associations between RSA and match-related HI running and distance from the offside line in ARs were reported. During matches, ARs are reported to have significantly less (70–80 percent HR_{max}) stress on their cardiovascular system (Helsen and Bultynck, 2004; Krustrup et al., 2002). With movement restricted to half the touchline (–50 m), selective agility is required on the part of elite ARs (Castagna et al., 2011). In this regard, the relevant involvement of sideways running suggested the use of specific field tests for change of direction (COD) ability and specific endurance in elite ARs (Castagna et al., 2011, 2012).

Like players, elite FRs and ARs have a congested fixture schedule during the competitive season, with national and international matches all year round (Weston et al., 2012), suggesting objective monitoring of activity stress to optimize training dose response (Costa et al., 2013). In what follows, scientific and empirical evidence will be provided on the current methodological principles informing elite FR and AR training.

Agility training

FR and AR ability to provide high- to maximal-intensity CODs in response to match demands is considered a logical training construct, requiring suitable and effective training strategies (Castagna et al., 2011; Weston et al., 2012). The use of match-related COD paradigms may be a viable strategy for developing the agility of match officials, provided that COD ability development is reported to be task specific (Castagna et al., 2011; Weston et al., 2012). Unpublished data showed that during Italian Serie A matches, most CODs are between 30 and 60° (–68 percent), with only –4 percent of reported CODs in the 150–180° range. Despite the preliminary interest in this unpublished evidence, further information needs to be gathered on the combination of CODs that makes up a discrete bout of agility during matches in FRs. In this regard, qualitative match analysis and time–motion analyses would be of great interest for developing effective specific agility drills for elite referees. Consideration for planned team or player's compartment match simulations (i.e. open match or small-sided games) with FR involvement may be considered as a possibility for specific agility training in elite referees (integrated training). However, reactive COD drills should be also considered, as the integrated training (i.e. match simulation with players) may not be easy to implement in regular training. As a general rule, agility and COD drills should not last more than 10–15 s per bout (Castagna et al., 2011; Weston, et al., 2012). As such, consideration should be given to repeated COD and repeated agility training, possibly using the construct currently considered for RSA training (agility endurance ability or repeated agility ability) (Wong del et al., 2012, 2015). In this regard, training drills should involve sprints of 3–8 s with recovery time no longer than 30 s (Bishop et al., 2011; Castagna et al., 2007; Weston et al., 2012).

Long-sprint ability

The increasing incidence of attack and counter-attack actions in team tactics has produced an increasing involvement of elite ARs in long sprints in order to keep up with play. This suggests a logical interest in long-sprint ability (LSA) training in elite soccer FRs.

Preliminary unpublished studies investigating LSA in FRs has shown that a long sprint can involve up to 90 percent of the individual maximal anaerobic capacity evaluated with a 30-s all-out running test on a non-motorized treadmill (Woodway Force, Milwaukee, USA). It could be speculated that in order to cope with this crucial aspect of the game (i.e. repeated long sprints interspersed with active recovery of medium-to-high intensity), LSA training should be included in the physiological development of elite FRs. Future descriptive and training studies addressing this interesting issue are warranted. In the absence of population-specific studies, LSA training can be tackled using the evidence provided by the speed endurance studies currently published (Iaia and Bangsbo, 2010).

Intermittent high-intensity aerobic training

Soccer refereeing was considered as an intermittent high-intensity activity, with most of the energy provided through the aerobic pathway (Castagna et al., 2007; Weston et al., 2012). As a result, aerobic fitness should be considered a prerequisite for successful refereeing. Unpublished data generated in connection with FIFA referees considered in the open list of candidates for the FIFA World Cup 2014 in Brazil showed VO_{2max} of 52±4.2 ml·kg^{-1}·min^{-1} with a maximal aerobic speed of 16.3±0.94 km·h^{-1} (n=52). Using the ventilatory threshold (VT) as a sign of the anaerobic threshold phenomenon, the average speed at VT was 14±1.0 km·h^{-1}. The selected candidates for the FIFA World Cup 2014 (n=32; age 37.9±years; height 180.3±5.5 cm; body mass 76±7 kg) showed similar VO_{2max} (52.6±4.6 ml·kg^{-1}·min^{-1} negligible change) to those on the original open list (n=52). The use of ROC curve analyses (n=154, open list FR+AR) revealed a cut-off value of 53 ml·kg^{-1}·min^{-1} for FRs. This may mean that an FR should have a VO_{2max} higher than 53 ml·kg^{-1}·min^{-1} to officiate at elite level. Peak [La]$_b$ at exhaustion was 10±2.3 mmol·l^{-1} in the open-list FR candidates, practically no difference from that of the corresponding ARs (10.4±2.3 mmol·l^{-1}). These results may suggest that training specifics should not be found in the classic aerobic fitness domain. Aerobic performance has been proposed as a better indicator of match-related physical performance in FRs, with consensus on the value of the Yo-Yo

Soccer referee training and performance 43

ReD-Test.2 (ReD-Test, 12 Laps)

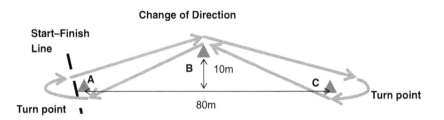

Total Distance = (41.23m x 4) x12 = 164.92x12 = **1979m**

Figure 4.1 Field set-up of the ReD-Test (Referee Diagonal Test). The referee must cover 1979m consisting in running over A–B–C–B–C–B–A–B–A and so on

intermittent recovery test level 1 as an ecologically valid test for FRs across the competitive levels (Castagna et al., 2007; Weston et al., 2012). This test provided a methodological change in fitness training paradigms for elite FRs, who turned from mainly continuous running training sessions to intermittent HI sessions with an important neuromuscular component to pass Yo-Yo IR1 national and international governing bodies' test limits (Krustrup and Bangsbo, 2001; Weston et al., 2004). However, the speeds reached during matches are higher than those reached during Yo-Yo IR1 and the required running biomechanics is different, suggesting the introduction of new field tests to evaluate specific endurance in FRs under field conditions. In this regard, an endurance field test was proposed involving "diagonal" coverage as observed in FRs during matches, to be performed with shuttle runs of alternating length (i.e. 80 and 40 m) with the aim of simulating attack and counter-attacks actions. The test, named DT2 (diagonal test 2), possess logical validity and very-large association (r from 0.72 to 0.85) with match-related HI variables (unpublished data, Figure. 4.1).

Repeat sprint ability (RSA)

The ability to maintain short-sprint performance over time with limited performance impairment despite incomplete recovery time (passive or active 10–30 s) was considered as a relevant component of FR and AR fitness (Castagna et al., 2007; Krustrup et al., 2002; Weston et al., 2012). The RSA literature reported evidence of an indirect effect of high-intensity aerobic training and anaerobic capacity training on enhancing recovery performance and buffer capacity respectively (Bishop et al., 2011; Taylor et al., 2015). It could be speculated that RSA training using match COD paradigms may be effective for FR and AR fitness development. Evidence from soccer players showed that, using RSA test drills, Yo-Yo IR1 performance can be significantly improved (Ferrari Bravo et al., 2008). Training

regimens involving LSA were shown to promote improvement in RSA performance, suggesting the complementary nature of RSA and LSA (Ingebrigtsen
et al., 2013). Due to lack of specific evidence on RSA and LSA training in soccer
refereeing, future training studies are warranted.

Injury prevention

The scientific evidence has shown that FR injury rates are similar to those for
players when considering non-contact events (Weston et al., 2012). Due to the
limited number of referees considered for elite level (n=20–25) and the congested
fixture schedule during a season, injury should be avoided as much as possible
by referees' associations in order to allow the necessary availability of officials.
FIFA F-MARC (FIFA Medical Assessment and Research Centre) recently developed a training protocol for injury prevention in FR and AR called 11+ Referee.
In order to promote adherence, 11+ Referee was conceived as a warm-up routine.
11+ Referee comprises exercises to promote balance, core stability and functional
strength of lower limbs and torso, with an emphasis on movement efficiency. 11+
Referee has been included in the teaching material of all FIFA Referee Assis-
tance Programs (RAP) and since 2013 has been used by the Technical Department (Settore Tecnico AIA) of the Italian Football Referees Association (AIA) to
prevent injury in Italian FRs and ARs. The data so far collected are encouraging in
terms of protocol compliance, adherence and injury rate decrement. Further studies involving randomized controlled trials in relation to FIFA's 11+ Referee are
warranted to provide strong evidence regarding this population-specific protocol
(Bizzini et al., 2013; Weston, 2014).

Training load control and regulation

The complex, multi-component nature of FR and AR performance requires the
simultaneous consideration of different training methods often included in the
same training session (Castagna et al., 2007; Weston et al., 2012). In elite-level
FR and AR training sessions, injury prevention intervention in sequences of HI
endurance, RSA or agility may be considered (Castagna et al., 2007; Weston et al.,
2012). This results in a multitude of metabolic demands that may complicate the
detection of the overall internal training load (Impellizzeri et al., 2004). The use
of advanced HR monitors may give a viable option for mainly aerobic training
sessions (Castagna et al., 2011). However, in the case of agility, RSA, LSA and
strength training, HR monitoring may be of limited interest. Furthermore, the
use of HR-based methods to define FR and AR internal training load requires
the accurate evaluation of individual maximal HR for percentage of HR_{max} or of
HR reserve training (Zavorsky, 2000). A wealth of knowledge of the use of psy-
chophysiological scales is currently available in the scientific community (Foster
et al., 2001; Impellizzeri et al., 2004). This approach enables a valid and reliable
estimation of athletes' internal load, overcoming the limitation that HR monitoring can present when different training regimens are incorporated in a single

session (Impellizzeri et al., 2004). In this regard, the session-RPE method using the CR10 Börg Scale is currently quite popular in FR and AR internal training load estimation (Costa et al., 2013). Familiarization on the part of FRs, ARs and fitness coaches with the use of session RPE is necessary to produce valid results. In this regard, experienced (i.e. 12±8.65 years) FR and AR fitness coaches (n=52) were shown to *a priori* overestimate low-to-medium and medium-to-high intensity training sessions proposed for elite FRs (unpublished study). In light of the relevance of internal training load evaluation in elite FRs and ARs, further studies are warranted using psychometric scales and HR variability to track post-match and training recovery (Weston et al., 2012).

Future studies

Fitness training for soccer referees is considered a relevant part of the development of match officials (Castagna et al., 2007; Weston et al., 2012). However, the strategies currently used are settled mainly as indirect evidence of effectiveness from soccer players descriptive and training studies. As a result, population-specific training studies are warranted. Furthermore, despite the consensus on the necessity of fitness training in soccer refereeing, there is still no strong scientific evidence of the effect of better FR and AR fitness on the quality of refereeing decisions during games. Furthermore, the assertion that "the closer the FR is to the incident, the better the decision" has to be further tested with suitable research designs. Given the importance of ARs in matches, further evidence should be gathered to improve knowledge of the key fitness determinants of elite AR performance. At the moment, descriptive evidence suggests that RSA and agility are the main components of the physical performance of ARs. Endurance has been shown to be relevant to the match-related physical performance of ARs, and for this reason the Assistant Referees Intermittent Endurance Test (ARIET) was proposed and used by national and international governing bodies for testing the specific endurance of ARs. The ARIET protocol involves intermittent (5-s recovery between bouts) forward (20-m) and sideways (12.5-m) shuttle runs performed at progressive speeds to exhaustion, and it was reported to possess criterion validity with VO_{2max} (Castagna et al., 2012). Given the resulting interest in ARIET, further studies examining the link between field-test performance and match activities (i.e. ecological validity) in elite ARs are warranted. Given that there are 1 million match officials active in soccer, more research should be devoted to non-elite FR and AR performance and to talent detection, selection and development.

Conclusions

Modern soccer, with its documented increase in match intensity, requires FRs and ARs to be able to cope with the increased match tempo. Physical fitness must be based on sound population-specific training interventions. In this regard, more research investment should be devoted to the performance of soccer officials than in recent years. Elite-level officials should be tested using ecologically valid tests with evidence-based cut-offs in the selection of FRs and ARs. Investments in AR and FR development should be at club level for the good of the game.

References

Bishop, D., Girard, O. and Mendez-Villanueva, A. (2011). Repeated-sprint ability – part II: recommendations for training. *Sports Medicine*, *41*(9), 741–756.

Bizzini, M., Junge, A. and Dvorak, J. (2013). Implementation of the FIFA 11+ football warm up program: how to approach and convince the Football associations to invest in prevention. *British Journal of Sports Medicine*, *47*(12), 803–806.

Castagna, C., Abt, G. and D'Ottavio, S. (2007). Physiological aspects of soccer refereeing performance and training. *Sports Medicine*, *37*(7), 625–646.

Castagna, C., Bendiksen, M., Impellizzeri, F. M. and Krustrup, P. (2012). Reliability, sensitivity and validity of the assistant referee intermittent endurance test (ARIET) – a modified Yo-Yo IE2 test for elite soccer assistant referees. [validation studies]. *Journal of Sports Sciences*, *30*(8), 767–775.

Castagna, C., Impellizzeri, F. M., Bizzini, M., Weston, M. and Manzi, V. (2011). Applicability of a change of direction ability field test in soccer assistant referees. [research support, non-US government validation studies]. *Journal of strength and conditioning research/National Strength and Conditioning Association*, *25*(3), 860–866.

Castagna, C., Impellizzeri, F. M., Chaouachi, A., Bordon, C. and Manzi, V. (2011). Effect of training intensity distribution on aerobic fitness variables in elite soccer players: a case study. *Journal of strength and conditioning research/National Strength and Conditioning Association*, *25*(1), 66–71.

Costa, E. C., Vieira, C. M., Moreira, A., Ugrinowitsch, C., Castagna, C. and Aoki, M. S. (2013). Monitoring external and internal loads of Brazilian soccer referees during official matches. *Journal of Sports Science and Medicine*, *12*(3), 559–564.

Ferrari Bravo, D., Impellizzeri, F. M., Rampinini, E., Castagna, C., Bishop, D. and Wisloff, U. (2008). Sprint vs. interval training in football. [comparative study randomized controlled trial]. *International Journal of Sports Medicine*, *29*(8), 668–674.

Foster, C., Florhaug, J. A., Franklin, J., Gottschall, L., Hrovatin, L. A., Parker, S., Doleshal, P. and Dodge, C. (2001). A new approach to monitoring exercise training. *Journal of Strength and Conditioning Research*, *15*(1), 109–115.

Helsen, W. and Bultynck, J. B. (2004). Physical and perceptual–cognitive demands of top-class refereeing in association football. [clinical trial]. *Journal of Sports Sciences*, *22*(2), 179–189.

Iaia, F. M. and Bangsbo, J. (2010). Speed endurance training is a powerful stimulus for physiological adaptations and performance improvements of athletes. [research support, non-US government review]. *Scandinavian Journal of Medicine and Science in Sports*, *20 Suppl. 2*, 11–23.

Impellizzeri, F. M., Rampinini, E., Coutts, A. J., Sassi, A. and Marcora, S. M. (2004). Use of RPE-based training load in soccer. *Medicine and Science in Sports and Exercise*, *36*(6), 1042–1047.

Ingebrigtsen, J., Shalfawi, S. A., Tonnessen, E., Krustrup, P. and Holtermann, A. (2013). Performance effects of 6 weeks of aerobic production training in junior elite soccer players. *Journal of Strength and Conditioning Research/National Strength and Conditioning Association*, *27*(7), 1861–1867.

Krustrup, P. and Bangsbo, J. (2001). Physiological demands of top-class soccer refereeing in relation to physical capacity: effect of intense intermittent exercise training. *Journal of Sports Sciences*, *19*(11), 881–891.

Krustrup, P., Mohr, M. and Bangsbo, J. (2002). Activity profile and physiological demands of top-class soccer assistant refereeing in relation to training status. *Journal of Sports Sciences*, *20*(11), 861–871.

Taylor, J., Macpherson, T., Spears, I. and Weston, M. (2015). The effects of repeated-sprint training on field-based fitness measures: a meta-analysis of controlled and non-controlled trials. *Sports Medicine*, *45*(6), 881–891.

Weston, M. (2014). Match performances of soccer referees: the role of sports science. *Movement and Sport Sciences – Science and Motricité* (87), 113–117.

Weston, M., Castagna, C., Helsen, W. and Impellizzeri, F. (2009). Relationships among field-test measures and physical match performance in elite-standard soccer referees. *Journal of Sports Sciences*, *27*(11), 1177–1184.

Weston, M., Castagna, C., Impellizzeri, F. M., Bizzini, M., Williams, A. M. and Gregson, W. (2012). Science and medicine applied to soccer refereeing: an update. *Sports Medicine*, *42*(7), 615–631.

Weston, M., Castagna, C., Impellizzeri, F. M., Rampinini, E. and Abt, G. (2007). Analysis of physical match performance in English Premier League soccer referees with particular reference to first half and player work rates. *Journal of Science and Medicine in Sport/Sports Medicine Australia*, *10*(6), 390–397.

Weston, M., Drust, B. and Gregson, W. (2011). Intensities of exercise during match-play in FA Premier League referees and players. *Journal of Sports Sciences*, *29*(5), 527–532.

Weston, M., Helsen, W., MacMahon, C. and Kirkendall, D. (2004). The impact of specific high-intensity training sessions on football referees' fitness levels. *The American Journal of Sports Medicine*, *32*(1 Suppl.), 54S–61S.

Wong del, P., Chan, G. S. and Smith, A. W. (2012). Repeated-sprint and change-of-direction abilities in physically active individuals and soccer players: training and testing implications. *Journal of Strength and Conditioning Research/National Strength and Conditioning Association*, *26*(9), 2324–2330.

Wong del, P., Hjelde, G. H., Cheng, C. F. and Ngo, J. K. (2015). Use of the RSA/RCOD Index to Identify Training Priority in Soccer Players. *Journal of Strength and Conditioning Research/National Strength and Conditioning Association*, *29*(10), 2787–2793.

Zavorsky, G. S. (2000). Evidence and possible mechanisms of altered maximum heart rate with endurance training and tapering. *Sports Medicine*, *29*(1), 13–26.

5 Ball kicking dynamics in football codes

New insight for coaching cues

Hiroyuki Nunome, Hironari Shinkai, Koichiro Inoue, Takahito Iga and Kevin Ball

Introduction

Kicking is the defining action of many football codes (Lees et al., 2010). To date, this skill has been the most widely studied one from a biomechanical perspective and much practical advice exists on how to kick the ball to achieve better performance outcomes.

On the field, coaches often advise players on swinging the kick leg and how to handle the ball action during the ball impact transient. Experienced coaches have also recognized the importance of the support leg action in improving kick performance, in particular for novice players. Further, coaches have explored ways to minimize the performance decline in kicking toward the end of the match due to fatigue. However, there has been limited evidence to support this instruction from a biomechanical perspective.

There are a large number of studies documenting the dynamics of the kicking leg action (Dörge et al., 2002; Nunome et al., 2002, 2006b; Apriantono et al., 2006). Recently, there have been a number of studies focusing on the support leg action (Nunome and Ikegami, 2005; Inoue et al., 2014) and ball impact transient (Tsaousidis and Zatsiorsky, 1996; Shinkai et al., 2009; Ball et al., 2013). It has been revealed by these recent works that some coaching cues have scientific support and likely work to fine-tune the kicking technique but others seem to be inaccurate while others warrant further investigation.

The aims of the current paper are to overview the latest kicking studies to better develop our understanding of the ball kicking motion and to shed some light on the veracity of some practical coaching instructions currently used.

Ball contact time

Is it possible to change ball impact time?

Practically, there are several instructions for kicking the ball with power in which the importance of a good follow through has been stressed (O'Challagan, 2010). Barfield (2000) suggested that one primary objective of the follow through is to keep the foot on touch with the ball as long as possible. Coaches, players and even researchers have believed that skilled players are capable of pushing the ball longer than less skilled players thereby increasing the resultant ball velocity. This coaching cue has a sound theoretical underpinning because the final momentum of the ball is determined by the amount of impulse applied to the ball. If players can apply more impulse to the ball by lengthening ball contact time, the ball will gain more momentum. Before recent technological advancement that has allowed for examining the ball impact transient, it has been treated as something of a 'black box' and thus the information regarding the interaction between the ball and foot has been very limited.

Tsaousidis and Zatsiorsky (1996) performed the first study that demonstrated the behavior of the ball and foot during the ball impact transient using a high enough sampling speed (4000 frames/s). However, in their study, the uncommon kicking technique (toe kicking) was used, rather than the more frequently used full instep kick. Also the study had several limitations in the mechanical models used for the foot and the ball. From these conditions, the study reported substantially longer contact times (16 ms) than that of the instep kicking.

Shinkai et al. (2009) clearly illustrated the nature of foot–ball interaction of the instep soccer kick using ultrahigh-speed cameras operating at 5,000 frames/s. The change in foot velocity, ball velocity and the pattern of ball deformation during ball impact (Figure 5.1) suggests interesting aspects of ball impact dynamics

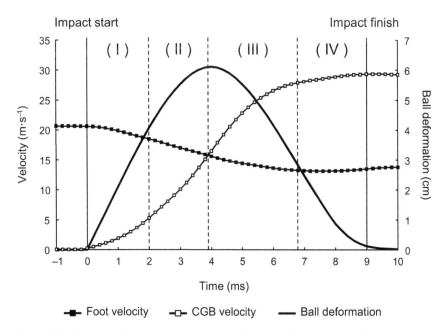

Figure 5.1 Change of the linear velocity of the foot, the linear velocity of ball center of gravity and ball deformation during soccer ball impact. The ball impact transient is divided into four phases

Source: modified from Shinkai et al. (2009).

during full instep kicking thereby providing new insight for practical instructions. As shown, until the end of phase II, foot velocity always exceeds that of the ball. However, in phase III, ball velocity begins to exceed that of the foot after the peak ball deformation. In this phase, the ball is reforming on the foot thereby contributing to the increase of ball velocity up to its approximate (95 percent) launching velocity. A quite similar phenomenon was confirmed in other football codes. Ball et al. (2013) reported comparable feature for the ball–foot interaction in the punt kicking typically used for Australian rules and the rugby codes.

The phenomenon that most likely explains this finding is that players in any skill levels are incapable of controlling the ball recoiling on the foot. In fact, we found a moderate, negative relationship between the ball contact time and resultant ball velocity in contrast to the coaching use.

Experimental validation

To confirm the relationship between ball contact time and resultant ball velocity more precisely, we made an attempt to mimic the soccer ball impact under controlled conditions. In the study of Iga et al. (2013), a regular soccer ball was directly fired from a launching machine at a force platform fixed vertically on a pedestal with five different velocities. The sagittal motion of the ball was captured at an ultrahigh sampling speed (5,000 frames/s) and from the combination of ball impact force and video footage, ball contact time and resultant ball velocity was computed.

As shown in Figure 5.2, the ball contact time systematically decreased as the ball velocity increased, which is conflicting with the practical advice to 'push the ball as

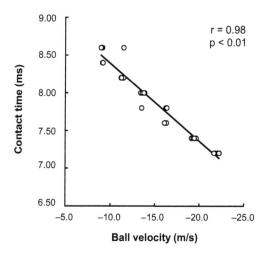

Figure 5.2 Relationship between the velocity of a ball fired from a soccer machine towards a force platform and the contact time while the ball contacts with the force platform

Source: modified from Iga et al. (2013).

long as possible' to increase time on the ball. This result confirmed that lengthening contact time during ball impact will not lead to faster ball velocity in soccer ball kicking.

The nature of the ball impact dynamics has produced a dilemma between what players try to do and phenomena actually happening on the foot during ball impact. However, this needs to be carefully interpreted from two sides: practical and scientific perspectives. While from a scientific point of view, increasing contact time will actually decrease performance, the coaching cue 'push the ball as long as possible' might still be an easy, clear target toward improving their kicking technique, in particular for novice players. It might also manifest other favorable technical components in the kick while not actually achieving what the cue is stating. To illustrate another example here, follow through is an often emphasized cue in Australian football. However, once the ball has left the foot, the performer cannot influence the outcome. Thus, while the follow through itself cannot influence performance, follow through cues work to produce better technique before and/or during ball contact such as straightening up to the target and remaining more upright.

Kick through the ball

Leg swing kinematics through the ball impact phase has been recognized as a difficult phase to adequately capture. Many studies, even in several textbooks have shown an apparent reduction in angular and/or linear velocity of the kicking leg immediately before ball impact (Barfield, 1995; Lees, 1996; Lees and Nolan, 1998; Dörge et al., 2002). This nature of the leg swing formed our initial general understanding of the kicking leg motion. However, this slowing down prior to ball contact was in contrast to a common coaching cue to 'kick through the ball' (LA84 Foundation, 1995; National Soccer Coaches Association of America, 2012), which might suggest increasing or maintaining velocity.

In our attempt to address this conflict, the soccer full instep kicking kinematics were captured using advanced technology, which included high-speed motion capture (1,000 Hz) and a new filtering procedure (time-frequency filtering) allowed changing of the cut-off frequency along the time-series (Nunome et al., 2006a). This was important as the lead-up to impact is relatively low frequency while impact itself is a high frequency event which cannot be appropriately handled using traditional smoothing techniques with a low constant cut-off frequency of 6–18 Hz (Andersen et al., 1999; Dörge et al., 2002; Nunome et al., 2002; Teixeira, 1999). Results from this study showed that shank angular velocity changes (Figure 5.3) were very different from those reported previously. In fact, the shank was still angularly accelerating toward ball impact (Figure 5.3 left panel). In contrast, the kinematic data processed using a conventional procedure (re-sampled to 250 Hz and smoothed using a conventional filter with a low, constant cut-off frequency of 10 Hz), created a descending nature of the shank angular velocity. This was a very important finding, as this was the very pattern generally seen in the previous studies, but when a more appropriate smoothing procedure was employed, this pattern did not exist. It can be assumed that sudden deceleration caused by ball impact would produce errors in its derivative parameters in the

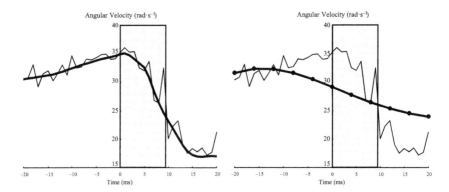

Figure 5.3 Comparison of changes of angular velocity of the shank through ball impact
from two different filtering and sampling schemas. In the left panel, high-speed
sampled data smoothed by a time–frequency filter is shown. In the right panel,
raw data was re-sampled and then smoothed by a conventional filter is shown

Source: modified from Nunome et al. (2006a).

last few frames before ball impact and this would be amplified if smoothing was
attempted through impact. However, most ball kicking studies have failed to
acknowledge this type of potential error, and it is often unclear how displacement
coordinates were smoothed (Isokawa and Lees, 1988; Rodano and Tavana, 1993;
Lees, 1996; Lees and Nolan, 1998).

Our attempt succeeded in illustrating 'true' or at least 'more representative'
nature of the leg swing. Thus, the finding seems to provide evidence that strongly
supports the coach's perspective for kicking and that 'kicking through the ball'
might indeed be a cue that has direct application to kicking performance.

Support leg action

While much is known about the kicking leg action, support leg action has received
insufficient interest from the researchers until recently. Experienced coaches commonly recognize the importance of the support leg action, having developed this
knowledge through years of coaching kicking (National Soccer Coaches Association of America, 2012). A big question, however, still remains as to how the support leg helps the kicking leg action.

From the point of view of dynamics, the support leg is the only body part that
receives external force (ground reaction force) up until ball contact, with this force

reaching over twice the kicker's body weight (Kellis et al., 2004; Katis and Kellis, 2010). Hence, the support leg has an important role during kicking: to resist this large external force in order to stabilize the body and to transfer mechanical energy to the proximal segment of the kick leg, thereby contributing to a proximal–distal sequential motion of the swing leg in indirect ways via the motion-dependent interaction moment (Putnam, 1991; Nunome and Ikegami, 2005).

Inoue et al. (2014) was the first study which demonstrated 3D dynamics of the support leg during instep kicking. Moments and angular velocities of the support leg were computed using inverse dynamics. In most joints of the support leg, the moments were not associated with or counteracting the joint motions. As the ankle joint never exhibited positive power throughout kicking, it can be interpreted that this joint works exclusively for absorbing the large external force from the ground. However, immediately before ball impact the knee extension motions came to be associated with the knee extension joint moments, thereby producing a distinctive positive power (Figure 5.4).

In general, the magnitude of the kick leg muscle moment systematically decreases as the angular velocity increases. Thus, the knee muscle moment was mostly inhibited during the final phase of kicking due to the high angular velocity of the shank. It is possible that, as the angular velocity of the lower leg has reached the inherent

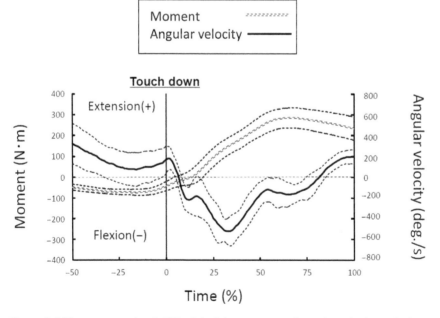

Figure 5.4 The average value (±SD) of the joint moment and angular velocity at the knee joint of the support leg: extension/flexion. The time of 0 percent and 100 percent correspond to the moment of "touch down" and "ball impact" respectively

Source: modified from Inoue et al. (2014).

force – velocity limitation of the knee extensor muscles immediately before ball impact, it becomes incapable of generating any concentric force. In contrast, the motion-dependent interaction moment increased rapidly in magnitude during the final phase of kicking (Nunome et al., 2006b). It is clear that the interaction moment dominates the acceleration of the shank immediately before ball impact.

This influence of the interactive moment on the kick leg has implications for the support leg, as it can generate these moments. As described before, muscles of the kicking leg are exposed to high velocity conditions but those of the support leg are in an almost static condition so it is possible to generate a large moment regardless of the kicking leg swing speed. Using the procedure of Putnam (1991), Nunome and Ikegami (2005) demonstrated that linear upward acceleration of the hip joint on the kicking leg side induces a motion-dependent interaction moment

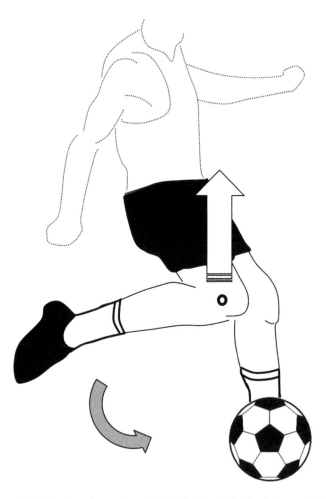

Figure 5.5 Typical shank configuration at the beginning of the final phase of kicking

for accelerating the lower leg swing during the final phase of kicking. Therefore, the positive power due to the knee extension moment on the support leg most likely serves to lift the body and contribute to the linear upward acceleration of the kick leg hip joint.

As shown in Figure 5.5, the kick leg shank is almost horizontal in the final phase of kicking. It is evident that to lift the whole body upward is the most effective way to induce a counter-clockwise rotation of the kick leg shank without using muscle moments about the knee joint. Thus, practically, in order to achieve a fluent action of the motion-dependent interaction moment acting on the kicking leg, lifting the whole body upward using support leg knee extension during the final phase of the kick would be an effective action. These findings support the thinking of experienced coaches that the support leg is important in kicking.

Fatigue effect

Typically, players find it difficult to retain leg muscle strength during a game, due to muscle fatigue. It can be assumed that an induced leg muscle fatigue somehow disturbs maximal kicking performance by reducing the ability to produce force and also leads to a less coordinated kicking motion, thereby making players more susceptible to injury (Rahnama et al., 2003). The effect of fatigue on the kicking action has received scant attention and only one study has focused on the influence of fatigue on kinematics (Lees and Davies, 1988).

Apriantono et al. (2006) reported the first study that investigated the effect of fatigue on the kicking leg kinetics. Muscle fatigue was induced by repeated knee extension and flexion on a weight-training machine, at a self-chosen pace. The loads were set at 50 percent body weight for the knee extensors and 40 percent body weight for the knee flexors. Participants were requested to perform three sets of knee extension and flexion bouts alternately without rest. In each bout, they were instructed to repeat the task as many times as possible until exhaustion.

Before and immediately after the fatigue protocol, all participants performed five maximal instep kicks with their kicking motion video-recorded by two high-speed cameras to reconstruct 3D coordinates of the kicking leg. Muscle fatigue reduced the toe velocity of the kicking leg significantly and also had a significant negative effect not only on the magnitude of the muscle moment but also on the magnitude of the motion-dependent interaction moment (Figure 5.6). The motion-dependent interaction moment has been widely accepted as an index of segmental coordination, which forms a typical 'whiplash' motion exhibited in kicking. Dörge et al. (2002) reported that a faster swing of the preferred leg can most likely be attributed to a greater amount of positive work done on the lower leg due to the interactive moment, indicating the preferred leg possesses a better intersegmental pattern. As shown in Figure 5.6, it is assumed that the motion-dependent interaction moment in the non-fatigue condition helps to increase and/or maintain the lower leg angular velocity during the final phase of kicking. One interpretation is that fatigue interfered with the effective action of the motion-dependent

Before fatigue   After fatigue

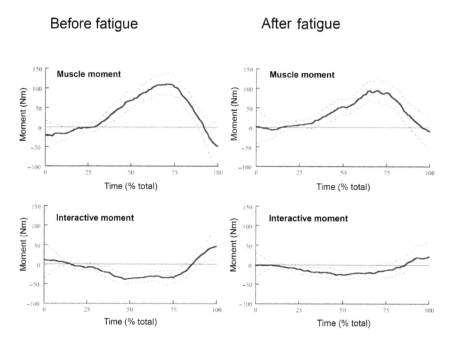

Figure 5.6 Changes in muscle moment and interactive moment acting on shank during soccer instep kicking with fatigue (right panel) and non-fatigue (left panel)

Source: modified from Apriantono et al. (2006).

interactive moment during lower leg extension due to a poorer segmental coordination. In turn, players come to rely more on the kick leg knee muscle moment to compensate for the fatigue-induced reduction leg swing velocity at ball impact. These findings provide useful insight into what kind of change actually happened on the kicking motion when fatigued.

Conclusion

A series of our studies have succeeded in providing novel insight for practical coaching cues. Supportive evidence was obtained for 'kick through the ball' while contradictory results existed for 'push the ball as long as possible.' Also, it has been illustrated that lifting the whole body upward by support leg motion would be an effective action to accelerate the kicking leg during the final phase of kicking. Finally, it has been demonstrated that fatigue interferes with the effective action of the interactive moment during lower leg extension due to a poorer segmental coordination and the player's kicking, which come to rely more on the muscle moment to compensate the reduced leg swing velocity at ball impact.

References

All links last accessed August 15, 2015, unless otherwise indicated.

Apriantono, T., Nunome, H., Ikegami, Y. and Sano, S. (2006). The effect of muscle fatigue on instep kicking kinetics and kinematics in association football. *Journal of Sports Sciences*, *24*, 951–960.

Ball, K., Ingleton, C., Peacock, P. and Nunome, H. (2013). Ball impact dynamics in the punt kick. In *e-Proceedings of the 31st Conference of the International Society of Biomechanics in Sports*. Taipei: National Taiwan Normal University.

Barfield, W.R. (1995). Effects of selected kinamatic and kinetic variables on instep kicking with dominant and nondominant limbs. *Journal of Human Movement*, *29*, 251–272.

Barfield, W.R. (2000). Biomechanics of kicking. In W. Garret and D. Kirkendall (eds.): *Exercise and Sports Science* (pp. 551–562). Philadelphia: Lippincott Williams & Wilkins.

Dörge, H.C., Anderson, T.B., Sørensen, H. and Simonsen, E.B. (2002). Biomechanical differences in soccer kicking with the preferred and the non-preferred leg. *Journal of Sports Sciences*, *20*(4), 293–299.

Iga, T. et al. (2013). Basic mechanical analysis of soccer ball impact. In *e-Proceedings of the 31st Conference of the International Society of Biomechanics in Sports*. Taipei: National Taiwan Normal University.

Inoue, K., Nunome, H., Sterzing, T., Shinkai, H. and Ikegami, Y. (2014). Dynamics of the support leg in soccer instep kicking. *Journal of Sports Sciences*, *32*, 1023–1032.

Isokawa, M. and Lees, A. (1988). A biomechanical analysis of the instep kick motion in soccer. In T. Reilly et al. (eds.): *Science and football* (pp. 449–455). London: E & FN Spon.

Katis, A. and Kellis, E. (2010). Three-dimensional kinematics and ground reaction forces during the instep and outstep soccer kicks in pubertal players. *Journal of Sports Sciences*, *28*, 1233–1241.

Kellis, E., Katis, A. and Gissis, I. (2004). Knee biomechanics of the support leg in soccer kicks from three angle of approach. *Medicine and Science in Sports and Exercise*, *36*(6), 1017–1028.

LA84 Foundation. (1995). *Soccer coaching manual.* Los Angeles. http://library.la84. org/3ce/CoachingManuals /LA84soccer.pdf

Lees, A. (1996). Biomechanics applied to soccer skills. In T. Reilly et al. (eds.): *Science and Football* (pp. 123–134). London: E & FN Spon.

Lees, A. and Davies, T. (1988). The effects of fatigue on soccer kick kinematics. *Journal of Sports Sciences*, *8*, 156–157.

Lees, A. and Nolan, L. (1998). The biomechanics of soccer: A review. *Journal of Sports Sciences*, *16*, 211–234.

Lees, A., Asai, T., Andersen, T.B., Nunome, H. and Sterzing, T. (2010). The biomechanics of kicking in soccer: A review. *Journal of Sports Sciences*, *28*, 805–817.

Levanon, J. and Dapena, J. (1998). Comparison of the kinematics of the full-instep and pass kicks in soccer. *Medicine and Science in Sports and Exercise*, *30*, 917–927.

National Soccer Coaches Association of America (2012). *Section 4: Basic Skills – Receiving, Passing and Shooting.* www.nscaa.com/education/resources/fundamentals/ basic-skills-receiving-passing-shooting

Nunome, H., Asai, T., Ikegami, Y. and Sakurai, S. (2002). Three-dimensional kinetic analysis of side-foot and instep soccer kicks. *Medicine and Science in Sports and Exercise*, *34*, 2028–2036.

Nunome, H. and Ikegami, Y. (2005). The effect of hip linear motion on lower leg angular velocity during soccer instep kicking. In *Proceedings of the XXIIIrd Symposium of the International Society of Biomechanics in Sports* (pp. 770–772). Beijing: People Sports Press.

Nunome, H., Lake, M., Georgakis, A. and Stergioulas, L. K. (2006a). Impact phase kinematics of instep kicking in soccer. *Journal of Sports Sciences, 24*, 11–22.

Nunome, H., Ikegami, Y., Kozakai, R., Apriantono, T. and Sano, S. (2006b). Segmental dynamics of soccer instep kicking with the preferred and nonpreferred leg. *Journal of Sports Sciences, 24*, 529–541.

O'Challagan, J. (2010). *How to kick a soccer ball. The Complete Soccer Guide.* www.completesoccerguide.com/how-to-kick-a-soccer-ball

Putnam, C.A. (1991). A segment interaction analysis of proximalto-distal sequential segment motion patterns. *Medicine and Science in Sports and Exercise, 23*, 130–144.

Rahnama, N., Reilly, T., Lees, A. and Graham-Smith, P. (2003). Muscle fatigue induced by exercise simulating the work rate of competitive soccer. *Journal of Sports Sciences, 21*, 933–942.

Rodano, R. and Tavana, R. (1993). Three dimensional analysis of the instep kick in professional soccer players. In T. Reilly et al. (eds.): *Science and Football II* (pp. 357–361). London: E & FN Spon.

Shinkai, H., Nunome, H., Isokawa, M. and Ikegami, Y. (2009). Ball impact dynamics of instep soccer kicking. *Medicine and Science in Sports and Exercise, 41*, 889–897.

Tsaousidis, N. and Zatsiorsky, V. (1996). Two types of ball–effector interaction and their relative contribution to soccer kicking. *Human Movement Science, 15*, 861–876.

Physiology

6 Soccer Fitness

Prevention and treatment of lifestyle diseases

Peter Krustrup

Introduction

It is now well established that physical activity is a cornerstone in the non-pharmacological prevention and treatment of lifestyle diseases (Pedersen and Saltin, 2006), and there is increasing evidence that sports participation has the potential to improve the health of nations (Khan et al., 2012). A very recent systematic review by Oja and colleagues investigating the available evidence on the health benefits of different sport disciplines for adults concluded that the "best evidence was found for soccer and running. These can especially improve cardiovascular and metabolic health" (Oja et al., 2015). This conclusion was based on more than 80 scientific articles published since 2009 describing the physiological demands of small-sided soccer training along with the fitness and health benefits of regular low-volume Soccer Fitness (football fitness) training for untrained individuals across the lifespan (Krustrup et al., 2009, 2010a, 2013, 2014; Bangsbo et al., 2015). The present chapter will provide an overview of the existing literature and a description of the relationship between the training elements of Soccer Fitness, the training-induced effects of Soccer Fitness on cardiovascular, metabolic and musculoskeletal fitness, and the potential of Soccer Fitness for the prevention and treatment of lifestyle diseases (see Figure 6.1).

Soccer fitness – cardiovascular demands and training effects

The average heart rate during Soccer Fitness training sessions lasting 45–60 min has been shown to be 80–90 percent of individual maximal heart rate (HRmax) in untrained women and men (Krustrup et al., 2009; Randers et al., 2010b; Bangsbo et al., 2015), which is actually similar to values obtained for elite soccer players during match play (Andersson et al., 2010). Such high average heart rates are elicited during Soccer Fitness irrespective of age, social status or skill level, with no influence of the number of players as long as the pitch size is adjusted (1v1 to 7v7 with ~80 m^2 per player) (Randers et al., 2012, 2014). It has also been observed that the heart rate fluctuates up and down between 70 and 100 percent HRmax during Soccer Fitness training, with 10–50 percent of the time in the highest HR zone above 90 percent HRmax both for untrained healthy women and men

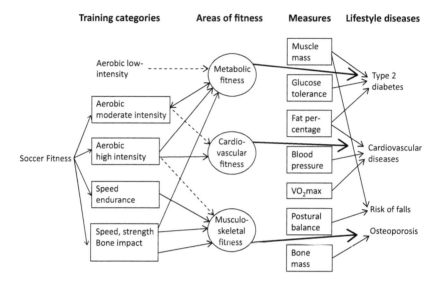

Figure 6.1 Holistic model describing that Soccer Fitness is a form of training that combines aerobic moderate and high intensity aerobic training with elements of speed endurance, speed, strength and bone impact training, and it is therefore an effective form of training for improving cardiovascular fitness, metabolic fitness and musculoskeletal fitness. These broad-spectrum favorable fitness effects make Soccer Fitness a powerful tool for broad-spectrum prevention and treatment of lifestyle diseases

Source: modified from Krustrup et al. (2010).

aged 18–80 (Krustrup et al., 2009; Randers et al., 2010b, 2014; De Sousa et al., 2014; Andersen et al., 2014a) and also for patient groups with hypertension, type 2 diabetes mellitus and prostate cancer (Krustrup et al., 2013; Andersen et al., 2014b; Uth et al., 2014). These observations make it clear that Soccer Fitness is a combination of endurance training and high-intensity interval training (HIIT) for basically everyone who takes to the soccer pitch (see Figure 6.1).

It is well established that HIIT training is an effective training type for elevating maximal oxygen uptake and improve cardiovascular function (Helgerud et al. 2007; Aspenes et al., 2011), and multiple randomized controlled trials (RCTs) have shown that this is also the case for Soccer Fitness. A recent systematic review and meta-analysis concluded that the average increase in VO_{2max} after a short-term Soccer Fitness training intervention was 3.51 ml/min/kg, with three- to four-month effects ranging from 5 to 20 percent, and that there were greater effects from Soccer Fitness than from interventions involving jogging or strength training (Milanović et al., 2015a, 2015b). In accordance with this finding, an RCT with 68 weeks of Soccer Fitness and jogging training revealed considerable cardiac adaptations after 16 and 68 weeks of training with greater effects from Soccer

Fitness than from continuous moderate-intensity training (Krustrup et al., 2010b). Interestingly, Soccer Fitness has also been shown to result in large and systematic reductions of blood pressure in hypertensive men and women that compare favorably with effects of beta-blockers and other commonly used antihypertensive medications (Hayashino et al., 2012). Thus, 12–16 weeks of Soccer Fitness training sessions of 2x1 hour/week lowered systolic and diastolic blood pressure by 12/8, 8/8 and 11/9 mmHg in three training studies with hypertensive and type 2 diabetic men (Knoepfli-Lenzin et al., 2010; Krustrup et al., 2013; Schmidt et al., 2013), while 15 weeks of Soccer Fitness training sessions of 3x1 hour/week resulted in a 12/6 mmHg drop in blood pressure in hypertensive women (Mohr et al., 2014).

Soccer fitness – metabolic demands and training effects

The metabolic demands and energy utilization are very high during Soccer Fitness, with a constantly high aerobic energy turnover amounting to an average of 70 percent VO_{2max} and periods with high anaerobic energy turnover (Castagna et al., 2007; Krustrup et al., 2009; Randers et al., 2010b). Actually, it has been estimated that the average energy turnover is 750 and 600 kcal per hour of training for untrained men and women, respectively (Krustrup et al., 2009, 2010b, 2010c). It is characteristic that all the metabolic energy systems are used during Soccer Fitness for participant groups across the lifespan, including carbohydrate and fat oxidation as well as lactate production and creatine phosphate utilization (Krustrup et al., 2010c; Randers et al., 2010b; Andersen et al., 2014a). It is also evident that most muscle groups are active during Soccer Fitness due to the very diverse movement pattern (see section below) and that all striated muscle fiber types are recruited during Soccer Fitness as well as during elite soccer, as revealed by high glycogen utilization in red slow-twitch fibers (Type I) and white fast-twitch fibers (Type IIa and IIx) (Krustrup et al., 2010c; Mujika et al., 2013).

Soccer fitness's combination of HIIT and endurance training, along with utilization of all energy systems and fiber types, has been shown to have marked and broad-spectrum effects on metabolic fitness (see Figure 6.1). Many training studies have shown that Soccer Fitness results in positive changes in body composition in healthy untrained men and women, with 1–3 kg less fat and 1–2.5 kg more muscle mass after just 12–16 weeks of training (Krustrup et al., 2009; Randers et al., 2012; Connolly et al. 2014). Similar reductions in fat mass have been observed in middle-aged men with T2DM (Andersen et al., 2014b) and women with hypertension (Mohr et al., 2014), and the fat loss was as high as 3.4 kg for 48–68-year-old Brazilian women and men with type 2 diabetes when using a 12-week intervention combining Soccer Fitness and a calorie-restricted diet (De Sousa et al., 2014). In several studies, but not all, short-term Soccer Fitness training has also resulted in positive alterations in blood lipid profile exemplified by 0.2–0.5 mM reductions in LDL cholesterol values in untrained young men, homeless men, hypertensive women and type 2 diabetics along with 0.2–0.4 mM reductions in triglycerides in the two latter studies (Krustrup et al., 2009; Randers et al., 2012; Mohr et al.,

2014; De Sousa et al., 2014). It has also been evidenced that Soccer Fitness training over 12–24 weeks for healthy untrained as well as patient groups results in a 7–24 percent increase in the number of capillaries around the type 1 and type 2 fibers (Krustrup et al., 2009, 2010b; Andersen et al., 2014b), a 10–14 percent increase in oxidative enzyme activity (Krustrup et al., 2010b) and improved fat oxidation during everyday activities (Krustrup et al., 2009). Furthermore, there is clear evidence that a combination of Soccer Fitness and diet manipulation can result in marked benefits in glucose tolerance after only 12 weeks (De Sousa et al., 2014, 2016) and also preliminary results indicate lower resting blood glucose levels in middle-aged men with type 2 diabetes after 24 weeks of Soccer Fitness (Andersen et al., 2014b), but further studies are required to elucidate the effects of Soccer Fitness per se (unaltered diet) on glucose tolerance and insulin sensitivity.

Soccer fitness – musculoskeletal demands and training effects

Movement analyses by GPS tracking and video recordings have clearly show that Soccer Fitness constitutes intense, versatile interval training with multiple repetitions of orthodox and unorthodox movements, altogether providing a high and multifaceted stimulus to muscles and bones (Krustrup et al., 2010a, 2010b; Randers et al., 2010a, 2010b; Helge et al., 2014a, 2014b; Krustrup and Bangsbo, 2015) (see Figure 6.1). A one-hour Soccer Fitness 7v7 session for untrained men involved 886 locomotor activities at various speeds, of which 98 were high-intensity runs, 16 were sprints and 59 were backwards and sideways runs (Krustrup et al., 2010b), with corresponding values for untrained women with no prior soccer experience of 954, 101, 15 and 46, respectively (Randers et al., 2010b). Additionally, it has been observed that Soccer Fitness involves multiple so-called specific intense actions, totaling an average of 192 for the untrained women during a 1-h 7v7 session, with 66 turns, 28 stops, 40 shots and passes, 17 dribbles, 21 shoulder contacts and 17 foot tackles (Pedersen et al., 2009). Interestingly, the same movement pattern was seen for 1-h Soccer Fitness sessions with 2, 4, 6 and 8 untrained women and men (Randers et al., 2010b), for homeless men playing 4v4 asphalt soccer (Helge et al., 2014b) and untrained young men playing 5v5 on sand, asphalt and artificial turf (Brito et al., 2012), with the only difference that 1v1, 2v2, 3v3 and 4v4 sessions involve even more sideways/backwards running bouts and more short high-intensity runs. A recent study using GPS tracking of a 45-min Soccer Fitness session for elderly men with prostate cancer has also shown that, despite the total distance of about half that observed in young men (2.65 km), the players performed as many as 194 accelerations, 296 decelerations and 100 running bouts (Uth et al., 2015a). Altogether, these findings emphasize that it is easy to organize Soccer Fitness sessions for participants across the lifespan with high player involvement and high and multifaceted musculoskeletal demands.

A number of recent investigations have shown that Soccer Fitness provides a marked osteogenic response, as evidenced by training-induced increases in circulating levels of the bone formation marker osteocalcin in untrained young women (37 percent, 16 weeks, Jackman et al., 2013), 25–65-year-old female hospital workers (21 percent, 12 weeks, Barene et al., 2014), hypertensive women (37 percent, 15 weeks, Mohr et al., 2015), homeless men (27 percent, 12 weeks, Helge et al., 2014a), elderly untrained men (45 percent, 16 weeks, Helge et al., 2014b) and elderly prostate cancer patients undergoing anti-androgen treatment (34 percent, 12 weeks, Uth et al., 2015a). Accordingly, Soccer Fitness interventions have caused improvements in bone mineral content (BMC) and bone mineral density (BMD) in young, middle-aged and elderly participants, with greater effects from Soccer Fitness than from swimming, continuous running and interval running (Helge et al., 2010; Krustrup et al., 2010a; Mohr et al., 2015). Thus, tibia BMD and leg BMC increased by 2–3 percent in untrained healthy women and men as well as hypertensive women after 12–16 weeks with 2–3 1-h Soccer Fitness sessions (Helge et al., 2010; Krustrup et al., 2010a; Mohr et al., 2015), and several studies have shown that BMD increases in clinically important sites such as the femoral shaft, femoral neck and hip, by 1–2 percent over 12–16 weeks in hypertensive women and elderly men (Mohr et al., 2015; Helge et al., 2014b; Uth et al., 2015a), but even more with medium-term and long-term Soccer Fitness interventions, with increases of 2–5 percent in elderly healthy men (52 weeks, Helge et al., 2014a) and elderly prostate cancer patients (32 weeks, Uth et al., 2015b). Interestingly, the study by Uth et al. (2015a) revealed a significant correlation ($r=0.65$) between the number of decelerations during training and the 12-week increase in leg BMC, supporting a link between the movement pattern and the training-induced skeletal effects (see Figure 6.1). Studies on Soccer Fitness have also shown marked effects on muscular function, including postural balance, muscle strength and functional capacity. Improvements in postural balance after 12–16 weeks of Soccer Fitness have been observed in untrained young men (Krustrup et al., 2009; Jakobsen et al., 2011), untrained young women (Krustrup et al., 2010b) and homeless men (Helge et al., 2014b), but not in elderly healthy men and elderly prostate cancer patients over 12–52-week intervention periods (Andersen et al., 2014a; Uth et al., 2015a, 2015b), which may be due to lack of sensitivity of the applied balance test, as the elderly men had several other measureable improvements in functional capacity. Thus, despite the lack of testosterone due to the antiandrogen treatment, the elderly men with prostate cancer had an increase in muscle mass of 0.7 kg and an increase in leg muscle strength of 15 percent compared to controls after 12 weeks of Soccer Fitness and 8–15 percent improvements in jump performance, sit-to-stand performance and stair climbing after 32 weeks, and the healthy elderly men had a 29 percent increase in sit-to-stand performance after 16 weeks of Soccer Fitness (Andersen et al., 2014a). To sum up, Soccer Fitness is an effective form of training for improving musculoskeletal fitness and, due to the combined favorable effects on bone mineralization, postural balance and muscle function, appears to be a relevant tool for the prevention of falls and bone fractures.

Implementation of soccer fitness

Soccer is by far the most popular sport in the world, with an estimated 400 million people playing regularly in sports clubs or on an unorganized basis, but there is a potential for even higher global participation. Soccer Fitness is a new type of soccer that can attract new participant groups, as it focuses on soccer training among friends in small groups rather than on competition (Bennike et al., 2014). Apart from its broad-spectrum fitness and health effects, investigations of Soccer Fitness have also shown that it is considered fun, enjoyable and motivating, and that it develops social capital, networking and general well-being (Ottesen et al., 2010; Bruun et al., 2014; Nielsen et al., 2014). The focus on team-mates, opponents and on the small-sided soccer game itself has also been shown to increase flow and to lower perceived exertion during Soccer Fitness, despite the high physical demands (Elbe et al., 2010; Krustrup et al., 2010a). These elements – including flow during training, motivational factors and the development of social capital – are very important for regular participation in and long-term adherence to sport (Elbe et al., 2016).

The concept of Soccer Fitness was developed in collaboration between researchers at Copenhagen University and the Danish FA in 2007–2010 and introduced in 2011. The concept has now been implemented in as many as 250 Danish soccer clubs (~15 percent) and the vision is to reach a total of 600 clubs (35 percent) over the next five-year period. A majority of the participants are untrained women aged 30–50, but also middle-aged and elderly men and women, along with different types of teams, including patient groups with hypertension and prostate cancer and teams of unemployed men and women in job training programs (Bennike et al., 2014). In spring 2015, the Soccer Fitness concept was introduced nationwide in the small country of the Faroe Islands with great success. Indeed, as many as 1.5 percent of the population started up before the summer, including 6 percent of all Faroese women aged 30–50, with the number of female members of the Faroese FA doubling in 9 months. In 2015, the FC Prostate study was expanded into the FC Prostate Community project, where patients are recruited from six hospitals across Denmark to play soccer in soccer clubs in close proximity to the hospitals (Bruun et al., 2014), and there is also an ongoing project in the Prevention Centers in the Municipality of Copenhagen, where ball games are now used as part of a 12-week training regime offered to 40–80-year-old patients with lifestyle diseases and many of these participants are encouraged to continue physical activity by playing Soccer Fitness in local soccer clubs. Without doubt, there is great potential in this project, and it will be interesting to monitor the extent to which this concept is implemented in the Nordic countries as well as in the rest of the world.

Conclusions

Soccer fitness is a new type of soccer developed for untrained individuals across the lifespan aiming at improving fitness and health of all participants, irrespective of gender, socioeconomic status, skills and prior experience. The Soccer Fitness concept involves regular small-sided outdoor or indoor soccer training among friends, using warm-up and 3v3 to 7v7 drills and no competitive games. Soccer fitness is a form of training that combines aerobic moderate and high intensity aerobic training with elements of speed endurance, speed, strength and bone impact training, and it is therefore an effective form of training for improving cardiovascular fitness, metabolic fitness and musculoskeletal fitness. It is now evident that these broad-spectrum fitness effects make Soccer Fitness a strong tool for the prevention and treatment of lifestyle diseases. Altogether, the available scientific publications provide evidence that Soccer Fitness is an intense, versatile, enjoyable and social all-in-one training type that combines high-intensity cardio, endurance and strength training and has great potential for preventing and treating lifestyle diseases as well as rehabilitating cancer patients undergoing anti-hormone treatment.

References

Andersen, T. R., Schmidt, J. F., Nielsen, J. J., Randers, M. B., Sundstrup, E., Jakobsen, M. D, Andersen, L. L., Suetta, C., Aagaard, P., Bangsbo, J. and Krustrup, P. (2014a). The effect of football or strength training on functional ability and physical performance in elderly untrained men. *Scandinavian Journal of Medicine and Science in Sports*, *24*(S1), 76–85.

Andersen, T. R., Schmidt, J. F., Thomassen, M., Hornstrup, T., Frandsen, U., Randers, M. B., Hansen, P. R., Krustrup, P. and Bangsbo, J. (2014b). A preliminary study: effects of football training on glucose control, body composition, and performance in men with type 2 diabetes. *Scandinavian Journal of Medicine and Science in Sports*, *24*(S1), 43–56.

Andersson, H. A., Randers, M. B., Heiner-Møller, A., Krustrup, P. and Mohr, M. (2010). Elite female soccer players perform more high-intensity running when playing in international games compared with domestic league games. *Journal of Strength and Conditioning Research*, *24*(4), 912–919.

Aspenes, S. T., Nauman, J., Nilsen, T. I., Vatten, L. J. and Wisløff, U. (2011). Physical activity as a long-term predictor of peak oxygen uptake: the HUNT Study. *Medicine and Science in Sports and Exercise*, *43*(9), 1675–1679.

Bangsbo, J., Hansen, P. R., Dvorak, J. and Krustrup, P. (2015). Recreational football for disease prevention and treatment in untrained men: a narrative review examining cardiovascular health, lipid profile, body composition, muscle strength and functional capacity. *British Journal of Sports Medicine, 49*(9), 568–576.

Barene, S., Krustrup, P., Jackman, S. R., Brekke, O. L. and Holtermann, A. (2014). Do soccer and Zumba exercise improve fitness and indicators of health among female hospital employees? A 12-week RCT. *Scandinavian Journal of Medicine and Science in Sports*, *24*(6), 990–999.

Bennike, S., Wikman, J. M. and Ottesen, L. S. (2014). Football Fitness – a new version of football? A concept for adult players in Danish football clubs. *Scandinavian Journal of Medicine and Science in Sports*, *24*(S1), 138–146.

Brito, J., Krustrup, P. and Rebelo, A. (2012). The influence of the playing surface on the exercise intensity of small-sided recreational soccer games. *Human Movement Science, 31*(4), 946–956.

Bruun, D. M., Krustrup, P., Hornstrup, T., Uth, J., Brasso, K., Rørth, M., Christensen, J. F. and Midtgaard, J. (2014). "All boys and men can play football": a qualitative investigation of recreational football in prostate cancer patients. *Scandinavian Journal of Medicine and Science Sports*, *24*(S1), 113–121.

Castagna, C., Belardinelli, R., Impellizzeri, F. M., Abt, G. A., Coutts, A. J. and D'Ottavio, S. (2007). Cardiovascular responses during recreational 5-a-side indoor-soccer. *Journal of Science and Medicine in Sport, 10*(2), 89–95.

Connolly, L. J., Scott, S., Mohr, M., Ermidis, G., Julian, R., Bangsbo, J., Jackman, S. R., Bowtell, J. L., Davies, R. C., Hopkins, S. J., Seymour, R., Knapp, K. M., Krustrup, P. and Fulford, J. (2014). Effects of small-volume soccer and vibration training on body composition, aerobic fitness, and muscular PCr kinetics for inactive women aged 20–45. *Journal of Sport and Health Science, 3*(4), 284–292.

De Sousa, M. V., Fukui, R., Krustrup, P., Pereira, R. M., Silva, P. R., Rodrigues, A. C., de Andrade, J. L., Hernandez, A. J. and da Silva, M. E. (2014). Positive effects of football on fitness, lipid profile, and insulin resistance in Brazilian patients with type 2 diabetes. *Scandinavian Journal of Medicine and Science in Sports, 24*(S1), 57–65.

De Sousa, M. V., Fukui, R., Krustrup, P., Dagogo-Jack, S. and Rossi da Silva, M. E. (2016). Combination of recreational soccer and caloric restricted diet reduces markers of protein catabolism and cardiovascular risk in patients with Type 2 Diabetes. *Journal of Nutrition, Health and Aging.* In press.

Elbe, A. M., Barene, S., Strahler, K., Holtermann, A. and Krustrup, P. (2016). Experiencing flow in a work place physical activity intervention: A longitudinal comparison between football and Zumba. *Women in Sport and Physical Activity Journal, 24,* 70–77.

Elbe, A. M., Strahler, K., Krustrup, P., Wikman, J. and Stelter, R. (2010). Experiencing flow in different types of physical activity intervention programs: three randomized studies. *Scandinavian Journal of Medicine and Science in Sports, 20*(S1), 111–117.

Hayashino, Y., Jackson, J. L., Fukumori, N., Nakamura, F. and Fukumori, N. (2012). Effects of supervised exercise on lipid profiles and blood pressure control in people with type 2 diabetes mellitus: a meta-analysis of randomized controlled trials. *Diabetes Research Clinical Practice, 98,* 349–360.

Helge, E. W., Aagaard, P., Jakobsen, M. D., Sundstrup, E., Randers, M. B., Karlsson, M. K. and Krustrup, P. (2010). Recreational football training decreases risk factors for bone fractures in untrained premenopausal women. *Scandinavian Journal of Medicine and Science in Sports, 20*(S1), 31–39.

Helge, E. W., Andersen, T. R., Schmidt, J. F., Jørgensen, N. R., Hornstrup, T., Krustrup, P. and Bangsbo, J. (2014a). Recreational football improves bone mineral density and bone turnover marker profile in elderly men. *Scandinavian Journal of Medicine and Science in Sports, 24*(S1), 98–104.

Helge, E. W., Randers, M. B., Hornstrup, T., Nielsen, J. J., Blackwell, J., Jackman, S. R. and Krustrup, P. (2014b). Street football is a feasible health-enhancing activity for homeless men – bone marker profile and balance improved. *Scandinavian Journal of Medicine and Science in Sports, 24*(S1), 122–129.

Helgerud, J., Høydal, K., Wang, E., Karlsen, T., Berg, P., Bjerkaas, M., Simonsen, T., Helgesen, C., Hjorth, N., Bach, R. and Hoff, J. (2007). Aerobic high-intensity intervals improve VO_{2max} more than moderate training. *Medicine and Science in Sports and Exercise, 39*(4), 665–771.

Jackman, S. R., Scott, S., Randers, M. B., Orntoft, C., Blackwell, J., Zar, A., Helge, E. W., Mohr, M. and Krustrup, P. (2013). Musculoskeletal health profile for elite female footballers versus untrained young women before and after 16 weeks of football training. *Journal of Sports Sciences, 31*(13), 1468–1474.

Jakobsen, M. D., Sundstrup, E., Krustrup, P. and Aagaard, P. (2011). The effect of recreational soccer training and running on postural balance in untrained men. *European Journal of Applied Physiology, 111*(3), 521–530.

Khan, K. M., Thompson, A. M., Blair, S. N., Sallis, J. F., Powell, K. E., Bull, F. C. and Bauman, A. E. (2012). Sport and exercise as contributors to the health of nations. *The Lancet, 380*(9836), 59–64.

Knoepfli-Lenzin, C., Sennhauser, C., Toigo, M., Boutellier, U., Bangsbo, J., Krustrup, P., Junge, A. and Dvorak, J. (2010). Effects of a 12-week intervention period with football and running for habitually active men with mild hypertension. *Scandinavian Journal of Medicine and Science in Sports*, *20*(S1), 72–79.

Krustrup, P., Aagaard, P., Nybo, L., Petersen, J., Mohr, M. and Bangsbo, J. (2010a). Recreational football as a health promoting activity: a topical review. *Scandinavian Journal of Medicine and Science in Sports*, *20*(S1), 1–13.

Krustrup, P. and Bangsbo, J. (2015). Recreational football is effective in the treatment of non-communicable diseases. *British Journal of Sports Medicine*, *49*(22), 1426–1427.

Krustrup, P., Christensen, J. F., Randers, M. B., Pedersen, H., Sundstrup, E., Jakobsen, M. D., Krustrup, B. R., Nielsen, J. J., Suetta, C., Nybo, L. and Bangsbo, J. (2010b). Muscle adaptations and performance enhancements of soccer training for untrained men. *European Journal of Applied Physiology*, *108*(6), 1247–1258.

Krustrup, P., Hansen, P. R., Andersen, L. J., Jakobsen, M. D., Sundstrup, E., Randers, M. B., Christiansen, L., Helge, E. W., Pedersen, M. T., Søgaard, P., Junge, A., Dvorak, J., Aagaard, P. and Bangsbo, J. (2010d). Long-term musculoskeletal and cardiac health effects of recreational football and running for premenopausal women. *Scandinavian Journal of Medicine and Science in Sports*, *20*(S1), 58–65.

Krustrup, P., Hansen, P. R., Randers, M. B., Nybo, L., Martone, D., Andersen, L. J., Bune, L. T., Junge, A. and Bangsbo, J. (2010c). Beneficial effects of recreational football on the cardiovascular risk profile in untrained premenopausal women. *Scandinavian Journal of Medicine and Science in Sports*, *20*(S1), 40–49.

Krustrup, P., Hansen, P. R., Nielsen, C. M., Larsen, M. N., Randers, M. B., Manniche, V., Hansen, L., Dvorak, J. and Bangsbo, J. (2014). Cardiovascular adaptations to a 10-wk small-sided school football intervention for 9–10-year-old children. *Scandinavian Journal of Medicine and Science in Sports*, *24*(S1), 4–9.

Krustrup, P., Nielsen, J. J., Krustrup, B. R., Christensen, J. F., Pedersen, H., Randers, M. B., Aagaard, P., Petersen, A. M., Nybo, L. and Bangsbo, J. (2009). Recreational soccer is an effective health promoting activity for untrained men. *British Journal of Sports Medicine*, *43*(11), 825–831.

Krustrup, P., Randers, M. B., Andersen, L. J., Jackman, S. R., Bangsbo, J. and Hansen, P. R. (2013). Soccer improves fitness and attenuates cardiovascular risk factors in hypertensive men. *Medicine and Science in Sports and Exercise*, *45*(3), 553–560.

Milanović, Z., Pantelić, S., Čović, N., Sporiš, G. and Krustrup, P. (2015a). Is recreational soccer effective for improving VO_{2max}? A systematic review and meta-analysis. *Sports Medicine*, *45*(9), 1339–1353.

Milanović, Z., Pantelić, S., Sporiš, G., Mohr, M. and Krustrup, P. (2015b). Health-related physical fitness in healthy untrained men: Effects on VO_{2max}, jump performance and flexibility of soccer and moderate-intensity continuous running. *PLoS One 10*(8), e0135319.

Mohr, M., Helge, E. W., Petersen, L. F., Lindenskov, A., Weihe, P., Mortensen, J., Jørgensen, N. R. and Krustrup, P. (2015). Effects of soccer vs swim training on bone formation in sedentary middle-aged women. *European Journal of Applied Physiology*, *115*(12), 2671–2679.

Mohr, M., Lindenskov, A., Holm, P. M., Nielsen, H. P., Mortensen, J., Weihe, P. and Krustrup, P. (2014). Football training improves cardiovascular health profile in sedentary, premenopausal hypertensive women. *Scandinavian Journal of Medicine and Science in Sports*, *24*(S1), 36–42.

Mujika, I., Halson, S., Argus, C. and Krustrup, P. (2013). Recovery from training and matches. In: A. Mark Williams (ed.): *Science and Soccer. Developing Elite Performers*, pp. 68–81. London: Routledge.

Nielsen, G., Wikman, J. M., Jensen, C. J., Schmidt, J. F., Gliemann, L. and Andersen, T. R. (2014). *Scandinavian Journal of Medicine and Science in Sports*, *24*(S1), 66–75.

Oja, P., Titze, S., Kokko, S., Kujala, U. M., Heinonen, A., Kelly, P., Koski, P. and Foster, C. (2015). Health benefits of different sport disciplines for adults: systematic review of observational and intervention studies with meta-analysis. *British Journal of Sports Medicine*, *49*, 434–440.

Ottesen, L., Jeppesen, R. S. and Krustrup, B. R. (2010). The development of social capital through football and running: studying an intervention program for inactive women. *Scandinavian Journal of Medicine and Science in Sports*, *20*(S1), 118–131.

Pedersen, B. K. and Saltin, B. (2006). Evidence for prescribing exercise as therapy in chronic disease. *Scandinavian Journal of Medicine and Science in Sports*, *16*(S1), 3–63.

Pedersen, M. T., Randers, M. B., Skotte, J. H. and Krustrup, P. (2009). Recreational soccer can improve the reflex response to sudden trunk loading among untrained women. *Journal of Strength and Conditioning Research*, *23*(9), 2621–2626.

Randers, M. B., Nielsen, J. J., Bangsbo, J. and Krustrup, P. (2014). Physiological response and activity profile in recreational small-sided football: no effect of the number of players. *Scandinavian Journal of Medicine and Science in Sports*, *24*(S1), 130–137.

Randers, M. B., Nielsen, J. J., Krustrup, B. R., Sundstrup, E., Jakobsen, M. D., Nybo, L., Dvorak, J., Bangsbo, J. and Krustrup, P. (2010a). Positive performance and health effects of a football training program over 12 weeks can be maintained over a 1-year period with reduced training frequency. *Scandinavian Journal of Medicine and Science in Sports*, *20*(S1), 80–89.

Randers, M. B., Nybo, L., Petersen, J., Nielsen, J. J., Christiansen, L., Bendiksen, M., Brito, J., Bangsbo, J. and Krustrup, P. (2010b). Activity profile and physiological response to football training for untrained males and females, elderly and youngsters: influence of the number of players. *Scandinavian Journal of Medicine and Science in Sports*, *20*(S1), 14–23.

Randers, M. B., Petersen, J., Andersen, L. J., Krustrup, B. R., Hornstrup, T., Nielsen, J. J., Nordentoft, M. and Krustrup, P. (2012). Short-term Street Soccer Improves Fitness and Cardiovascular Health of Homeless Men. *European Journal of Applied Physiology*, *112*(6), 2097–2106.

Schmidt, J. F., Andersen, T. R., Horton, J., Brix, J., Tarnow, L., Krustrup, P., Andersen, L. J., Bangsbo, J. and Hansen, P. R. (2013). Soccer Training Improves Cardiac Function in Men with Type 2 Diabetes. *Medicine and Science in Sports and Exercise*, *45*(12), 2223–2233.

Uth, J., Hornstrup, T., Christensen, J. F., Christensen, K. B., Jørgensen, N. R., Helge, E. W., Schmidt, J. F., Brasso, K., Helge, J. W., Jakobsen, M. D., Andersen, L. L., Rørth, M., Midtgaard, J. and Krustrup, P. (2015a). Football training in men with prostate cancer undergoing androgen deprivation therapy: activity profile and short-term skeletal and postural balance adaptations. *European Journal of Applied Physiology*, *116*(3), 471–480.

Uth, J., Hornstrup, T., Christensen, J. F., Christensen, K. B., Jørgensen, N. R., Schmidt, J. F., Brasso, K., Jakobsen, M. D., Sundstrup, E., Andersen, L. L., Rørth, M., Midtgaard, J., Krustrup, P. and Helge, E. W. (2015b). Efficacy of recreational football on bone health, body composition, and physical functioning in men with prostate cancer undergoing androgen deprivation therapy: 32-week follow-up of the FC prostate randomised controlled trial. *Osteoporosis International* , *27*(4), 1507–1518.

Uth, J., Hornstrup, T., Schmidt, J. F., Christensen, J. F., Frandsen, C., Christensen, K. B., Helge, E. W., Brasso, K., Rørth, M., Midtgaard, J. and Krustrup, P. (2014). Football training improves lean body mass in men with prostate cancer undergoing androgen deprivation therapy. *Scandinavian Journal of Medicine and Science in Sports*, *24*(S1), 105–112.

7 The health benefits of rugby-specific small-sided games for sedentary populations

Rob Duffield, Nicholas G. Allen and Amy E. Mendham

Introduction

A physically inactive lifestyle, coupled with excess calorie intake can lead to increased adiposity and decreased lean muscle mass (Lakka and Laaksonen, 2007). It has been suggested that these changes in fat–muscle-mass ratio are associated with altering chronic systemic inflammatory and glucose regulatory mechanisms (Egan and Zierath, 2013; Ouchi et al., 2011). Cross-sectional investigations have reported an inverse relationship between aerobic fitness with levels of chronic systemic inflammation (Panagiotakos et al., 2005). Accordingly, a primary prevention strategy involves engagement in exercise to promote changes in aerobic fitness and body composition to restore the pro- and anti-inflammatory balance (Ouchi et al., 2011). Furthermore, an improved systemic inflammatory state, as evidenced by a reduction in pro-inflammatory cytokines, may have direct influences on glycemic control and positive repercussions within skeletal muscle through improved anti-inflammatory mechanisms (Ouchi et al., 2011).

Historically, research has focused on the health benefits from continuous, aerobic-based exercise training (Egan and Zierath, 2013). Such exercise stimuli involve lower-body, concentric muscular contractions with the focus on reducing fat mass, and improving cardiovascular function, glucose regulation and mitochondrial biogenesis (Goodyear and Kahn, 1998; Hawley and Lessard, 2008). However, recent exercise prescription recommendations suggest incorporating varied intensities within a single exercise bout, i.e. high-intensity intervals interspersed with low-intensity movements (Garber et al., 2011), which lends credence to the use of football-based exercise modes.

It has been suggested that football-specific (soccer) Small-Sided Games (SSG) training can provide comparable or better improvements than aerobic training in body composition, aerobic capacity, capillary density and fiber type, which are all known to influence glucose regulation (Andersen et al., 2014; Krustrup et al., 2013; Serpiello et al., 2014). Recently, the application of SSG from alternate football codes has gained interest (Mendham et al., 2012, 2015a, 2015b). Rugby is the predominant football code in many regions of the world and may have the capacity to induce systemic inflammatory and glucose regulatory adaptations in inactive populations. Consequently, SSGs may provide therapeutic strategies for the prevention of non-communicable diseases in sedentary populations.

Systemic inflammatory adaptations

As highlighted in Table 7.1, a diversity of studies shows that exercise training from a range of modes can improve the chronic inflammatory state in otherwise healthy populations. Given that systemic inflammation is somewhat mediated by the ratio of adiposity to lean muscle mass, the extent to which exercise alters body composition may have a bearing on chronic inflammatory cytokine concentrations (Visser et al., 2002). Such findings highlight a potential role for SSG training in sedentary populations; particularly given the improved lean-mass and reduced fat mass observed following SSG training in a variety of populations (Bangsbo, Hansen, Dvorak and Krustrup, 2015; Mendham, Duffield, Marino and Coutts, 2014).

Typically, systemic concentrations of adipocyte derived cytokines (i.e. IL-6 and TNF-α) stimulate an acute-phase response through the hepatic secretion of CRP (Gleeson et al., 2011). The increase in leptin during states of inflammation suggests a role within the cytokine network, alongside corollary increases in other pro-inflammatory cytokines (Fernández-Riejos et al., 2010). Mendham et al. (2014) reported that rugby SSG training increased fat-free mass and decreased fat mass and pro-inflammatory markers (CRP, IL-6 and leptin). However, other findings are inconsistent regarding the effects of exercise training on inflammatory markers and the relationship with fat mass (Table 7.1). Consequently, a myriad of other mechanisms, including increased lean muscle mass (Visser et al., 2002), glucose regulation (Silha et al., 2003), and/or changes in other pro-inflammatory cytokines (Fernández-Riejos et al., 2010) and disease state (You et al., 2013) may be implicated in changes in resting concentrations of pro-inflammatory cytokines.

Glucose regulatory adaptations

In relation to improved post-training glucose control, Mendham et al. (2015a) showed eight weeks of either rugby SSG or cycle ergometry (CYC) training induced similar improvements in HbA1c, although this is not a consistent finding in other exercise modes (Donges et al., 2010). Further, 12 weeks of SSG (soccer) training did not change fasting glucose and insulin concentrations (Randers et al., 2010). An explanation for these findings may relate to the normoglycemic nature of the participants limiting the effect of exercise training. Regardless, to maintain normal glucose tolerance in response to an exogenous glucose load, increased insulin secretion to compensate for decreased insulin sensitivity is required (Unwin et al., 2002). Consequently, SSG training in sedentary men is an effective method to improve glucose control and reduce estimated insulin sensitivity in response to a standard glucose load (Mendham et al., 2015a).

The mitochondria regulate cellular glucose uptake and provide energy balance, thus, positive mitochondrial adaptations to exercise are hypothesized as a method to improve glucose tolerance. Given skeletal muscle is sensitive to glucose concentrations (Goodyear and Kahn, 1998), the resultant SSG-induced increase in lean muscle mass may have additional benefits (Mendham et al., 2015a). Improvements in insulin sensitivity and glucose uptake are facilitated by

Table 7.1 Chronic systemic inflammatory responses to various exercise training modes in non-disease populations

Author	Year	Participants	Intervention	Duration	Inflammatory outcomes	Other outcomes
Mendham et al.	2014	Sedentary middle-aged men (n=33)	Cycling vs rugby SSGs vs control	3 × pw, 8 weeks	Only SSG ↓ IL-6 Both modes ↓ CRP	Only SSG ↑ FFM & ↓ leptin. Both modes ↑ aerobic power and ↓ BF SSG ↓ SBP & DBP
Andersen et al.	2010	Untrained middle-aged men (n=25)	Football SSGs vs control	2 × pw, 12 weeks	No change in CRP	Aerobic training ↓ BF, no change in leptin or adiponectin
Arikawa et al.	2011	Sedentary women (n=319)	Moderate intensity aerobic vs control	5 × pw, 16 weeks	Aerobic training ↓ CRP	Aerobic training ↑ VO$_{2max}$ & ↓ BF
Church et al.	2010	Sedentary, middle-aged (n=162)	Aerobic; 60–80% VO$_{2max}$	3–5 × pw, 4 months	↓ CRP	Resistance training ↑ cholesterol; both groups ↑ HbA1c
Donges, Duffield and Drinkwater	2010	Sedentary adults (n=102)	Aerobic vs resistance	3 × pw, 10 weeks	No change in IL-6; resistance training greatest ↓ CRP	Aerobic training ↓ LDL-C
Martins et al.	2010	Adults aged >64 y (n=45)	Aerobic vs resistance vs control	3 × pw, 16 weeks, followed by 16 weeks' detraining	↓ CRP after 32 weeks (aerobic 51%, resistance 39%)	Resistance training ↓ SBP, triglycerides & insulin resistance; no change in BMI, LDL-C, HDL-C & waist circumference
Ogawa et al.	2010	Elderly women (n=21)	Low-intensity resistance training vs control	1 × pw, 12 weeks	Resistance training ↓ resting CRP, no change in IL-6 or TNF-α	Aerobic training ↓ BF, BM & waist circumference
Campbell et al.	2009	Postmenopausal, sedentary, overweight women (n=115)	Moderate intensity aerobic vs flexibility training	5 × pw aerobic exercise vs 1 × pw stretching, 12 months	Aerobic training ↓ resting CRP, no change in IL-6	

(Continued)

Table 7.1 (Continued)

Author	Year	Participants	Intervention	Duration	Inflammatory outcomes	Other outcomes
Campbell et al.	2008	Sedentary, middle-aged (n=202)	Aerobic, 60–85% MHR	6 x pw, 12 months	No change in CRP	Aerobic training ↑VO$_{2max}$, ↓ BF
Olson et al.	2007	Overweight, sedentary women (n=28)	Resistance vs control	2 x pw, 1 y	Resistance training ↓ CRP, no change in IL-6	Resistance training ↑ 1RM bench press, no change in lipid profile, SBP, DBP, BMI or BF
Stewart et al.	2007	Older (65–85yrs) and younger subjects (18–35 y) (n=50)	Combined aerobic & resistance vs active control	3 x pw, 12 weeks	Both age groups ↓ CRP; no effect on IL-6 or IL-1β	Both age groups ↑ VO$_{2max}$ & strength
Kohut et al.	2006	Healthy adults ≥ 64 y (n=87)	Aerobic vs strength/ flexibility training	3 x pw, 10 months	Aerobic training ↓ IL-6, TNF-α, CRP & IL-18	Aerobic training greater ↑ max METS
Rauramaa et al.	2004	Middle-aged men (n=140)	Moderate intensity aerobic vs control	3 x pw for 3 months, followed by 5 x pw for remainder of 6 y	No significant change in CRP	Aerobic training ↑ VT by 19.5%
Smith et al.	1999	Healthy adults (n=43)	Combined aerobic & resistance	2 x 70min sessions pw,6 months	↓CRP, TNF-α & IL-1α ↑ IL-4 & IL-10	

Notes: VO$_{2max}$ = Maximal oxygen consumption; CRP = C-reactive protein; TNF-α = Tumor necrosis factor alpha; IL = interleukin, SSG = Small sided games; FFM = Fat free mass; SBP = Systolic blood pressure; DBP = Diastolic blood pressure; BF = Body fat; BMI = Body mass index, LDL-C = Low density lipoprotein; HDL-C = High-density lipoprotein; BP = Blood pressure; MHR = Maximal heart rate; VT = Ventilitory threshold.

increased GLUT4 and Protein Kinase B (Akt) content which mediate insulin-induced glucose transport (Goodyear and Kahn, 1998). Mendham et al. (2015a) reported no corresponding increases in skeletal muscle GLUT4 or Akt protein content for either SSG or CYC training, despite favorable changes in response to an oral glucose tolerance test. A possible explanation for this result is that the improved insulin sensitivity may be more dependent on increased GLUT4 translocation to the cell surface, rather than increased total GLUT4 abundance per se (Goodyear and Kahn, 1998; Hawley and Lessard, 2008).

In addition to glucose signaling markers, both intermittent and continuous aerobic exercise are associated with the increased expression and activity of COX II and IV in sedentary adults (Hood et al., 2011). However, Mendham et al. (2015a) observed that adaptations noted in pulmonary VO_2 were not reciprocated by changes in total protein content of the mitochondrial complex (I-V) within skeletal muscle. In support, other studies have reported a similar lack of mitochondrial adaptations in inactive populations following a range of exercise training durations (i.e. 2–12 weeks) and modes (i.e. resistance, continuous cycling and concurrent resistance-aerobic exercise) (Skleryk et al., 2013). Accordingly, the absence of significant changes in the protein content of the mitochondrial complexes (I-V) may suggest that the predominant training adaptations were cardiovascular, and/or adaptations of mitochondrial functioning (Mendham et al., 2015a). Collectively, definitive conclusions regarding the effects of SSG on mitochondrial biogenesis in inactive populations are difficult, and thus their mechanistic role for improved glucose regulation remains equivocal.

Functional and body composition adaptations

Mendham et al. (2015a) reported rugby SSG training increased lean muscle mass and leg strength, compared to no changes following either CYC or inactive conditions. Previous interventions involving soccer SSG training reported increased maximal isometric hamstring strength and lean muscle mass (1.7 ± 0.4 kg), when compared to treadmill running. In contrast, CYC training is reported to induce minimal changes in lean muscle mass (i.e. -0.6kg and $+0.7$kg) within a sedentary cohort (Donges et al., 2010). These findings suggest SSG training provides sufficient eccentric loading to induce myofibrillar protein synthesis and skeletal muscle hypertrophy, especially compared to concentric-dominant contractions in CYC (Coffey and Hawley, 2007). Importantly, the increased leg strength and lean muscle mass indicates a potential advantage of SSG training over continuous, aerobic training to improve glucose metabolism regulation.

Training intensity is an important consideration for reversing risk-factors associated with metabolic abnormalities (Egan and Zierath, 2013). Previous SSG-based studies in middle-aged, inactive men report an increase in VO_{2max} by ~13 percent; similar to continuous training with similar intensities (65–85 percent HR_{max}) and training durations (6–16 weeks) (Krustrup et al., 2010). In particular, an increase in VO_{2max} reported for soccer SSG (7 percent) and continuous running (6 percent) occurred in the first four weeks of training, though only the SSG condition increased a further 6 percent from 4–12 weeks (Krustrup et al., 2010). Mendham et al. (2015a) reported sedentary, middle-age men increased sub-maximal VO_2 in both CYC and SSG conditions (19.1 percent CYC, 18.9 percent rugby-SSG). Accordingly, a similar improvement in aerobic capacity is obtained when training is matched for volume and intensity, and thus SSG represents an effective exercise mode to improve cardiovascular fitness.

Small-sided games training combines multiple fitness components to deliver glucose regulatory, inflammatory and body composition adaptations that are superior to both running and cycling (Krustrup et al., 2010). The superior physiological adaptations in the SSG conditions may be due to the metabolic effect of intermittent- over continuous-based modes in sedentary populations (Mendham et al., 2015b). Previously unpublished data (Figure 7.1) compares the oxidative responses of intermittent-sprint exercise (ISE) replicating rugby SSGs (Mendham et al., 2015b) to that of CYC. Eight sedentary middle-aged men completed ISE, CYC and control (CON) conditions, with all testing and dietary procedures standardized (Zhang et al. 2014). The ISE involved 4x11 min bouts of self-paced ISE separated by 2 min passive recovery. There were no differences between conditions in percentage of maximum heart rate (ISE 76 ±4; CYC 81 ±8 percent; P>0.05) or session-RPE (ISE 12.5 ±1.6; CYC 13.9 ±1.5 AU; P>0.05). Despite the expected fluctuation in VO_2 during ISE, both conditions showed comparable mean VO_2 (ISE 24.4 ±0.9; CYC 26.5 ±1.0 mL.kg^{-1}min^{-1}; P>0.05), and thus estimated energy expenditure. The 'mean' metabolic demands may be comparable between modes although, the high-intensity efforts in SSGs are likely to result in greater skeletal muscle recruitment (Mendham et al., 2015b). These mode specific

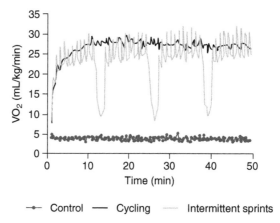

Figure 7.1 Oxygen consumption (VO_2; Cosmed K4b², Cosmed, Rome, Italy) during 50 min. of passive resting in a recumbent seated position (control), moderate-intensity continuous cycling (Monark 828E, Monark Exercise AB, Varburg, Sweden) at 80–85 percent of maximal heart rate and intermittent-sprint exercise designed to simulate the workload of rugby-specific small-sided games

characteristics may separate the glucose and inflammatory adaptations noted earlier, though further research is required to elucidate this hypothesis.

Conclusion

The differences in characteristics between SSG and CYC are likely to have positive effects on differential aspects of inflammatory and glucose regulation. While both modes seem appropriate to improve aerobic capacity, the distinct SSG training responses seem to confer greater benefits for body composition alteration, reduced chronic inflammation and insulin secretion to a glucose load. Consequently, SSG training can induce definitive improvements in functional outcomes (i.e. aerobic capacity and strength), clinical markers (i.e. inflammatory, glucose control and body composition), though the molecular mechanisms underlying such adaptations remain equivocal. Regardless, rugby and other football-based SSG can be considered evidenced-based exercise modes to prescribe to sedentary populations to promote improvements in physical health.

References

Andersen, L. J., Randers, M. B., Westh, K., Martone, D., Hansen, P. R., Junge, A., Dvorak, J., Bangsbo, J. and Krustrup, P. (2010). Football as a treatment for hypertension in untrained 30–55-year-old men: a prospective randomized study. *Scandinavian Journal of Medicine and Science in Sports*, *20*(suppl. 1), 98–102.

Andersen, T. R., Schmidt, J. F., Thomassen, M., Hornstrup, T., Frandsen, U., Randers, M. B., Hansen, P. R., Krustrup, P. and Bangsbo, J. (2014). A preliminary study: effects of football training on glucose control, body composition, and performance in men with type 2 diabetes. *Scandinavian Journal of Medicine and Science in Sports*, *24*(suppl. 1), 43–56.

Bangsbo, J., Hansen, P. R., Dvorak, J. and Krustrup, P. (2015). Recreational football for disease prevention and treatment in untrained men: a narrative review examining cardiovascular health, lipid profile, body composition, muscle strength and functional capacity. *British Journal of Sports Medicine*, *49*(9), 568–576.

Coffey, V. G. and Hawley, J. A. (2007). The molecular bases of training adaptation. *Sports Medicine*, *37*(9), 737–763.

Donges, C. E., Duffield, R. and Drinkwater, E. J. (2010). Effects of resistance or aerobic exercise training on interleukin-6, C-reactive protein, and body composition. *Medicine and Science in Sports and Exercise*, *42*(2), 304–313.

Egan, B. and Zierath, J. R. (2013). Exercise metabolism and the molecular regulation of skeletal muscle adaptation. *Cell Metabolism*, *17*(2), 162–184.

Fernández-Riejos, P., Najib, S., Santos-Alvarez, J., Martín-Romero, C., Pérez-Pérez, A., González-Yanes, C. and Sánchez-Margalet, V. (2010). Role of leptin in the activation of immune cells. *Mediators of Inflammation*, *2010*, 1–8.

Garber, C. E., Blissmer, B., Deschenes, M. R., Franklin, B. A., Lamonte, M. J., Lee, I. M., Nieman, D. C. and Swain, D. P. (2011). American College of Sports Medicine position stand. Quantity and quality of exercise for developing and maintaining cardiorespiratory, musculoskeletal, and neuromotor fitness in apparently healthy adults: guidance for prescribing exercise. *Medicine and Science in Sports and Exercise*, *43*(7), 1334–1359.

Gleeson, M., Bishop, N. C., Stensel, D. J., Lindley, M. R., Mastana, S. S. and Nimmo, M. A. (2011). The anti-inflammatory effects of exercise: mechanisms and implications for the prevention and treatment of disease. *Nature Reviews Immunology*, *11*(9), 607–615.

Goodyear, L. J. and Kahn, B. B. (1998). Exercise, glucose transport, and insulin sensitivity. *Annual Review of Medicine*, *49*(1), 235–261.

Hawley, J. A. and Lessard, S. J. (2008). Exercise training-induced improvements in insulin action. *Acta physiologica*, *192*(1), 127–135.

Hood, M. S., Little, J. P., Tarnopolsky, A., Myslik, F. and Gibala, M. J. (2011). Low-volume interval training improves muscle oxidative capacity in sedentary adults. *Medicine and Science in Sports and Exercise*, *43*(10), 1849–1856.

Krustrup, P., Christensen, J. F., Randers, M. B., Pedersen, H., Sundstrup, E., Jakobsen, M. D., Krustrup, B. R., Nielsen, J. J., Suetta, C., Nybo, L. and Bangsbo, J. (2010). Muscle adaptations and performance enhancements of soccer training for untrained men. *European Journal of Applied Physiology*, *108*(6), 1247–1258.

Krustrup, P., Randers, M. B., Andersen, L. J., Jackman, S. R., Bangsbo, J. and Hansen, P. R. (2013). Soccer improves fitness and attenuates cardiovascular risk factors in hypertensive men. *Medicine and Science in Sports and Exercise*, *45*(3), 553–560.

Lakka, T. A. and Laaksonen, D. E. (2007). Physical activity in prevention and treatment of the metabolic syndrome. *Applied Physiology, Nutrition, and Metabolism*, *32*(1), 76–88.

Mendham, A. E., Coutts, A. J. and Duffield, R. (2012). The acute effects of aerobic exercise and modified rugby on inflammation and glucose homeostasis within Indigenous Australians. *European Journal of Applied Physiology*, (112), 3787–3795.

Mendham, A. E., Duffield, R., Coutts, A. J., Marino, F., Boyko, A. and Bishop, D. J. (2015a). Rugby-specific small-sided games training is an effective alternative to stationary cycling at reducing clinical risk factors associated with the development of type 2 diabetes: a randomized, controlled trial. *PloS One*, *10*(6), e0127548.

Mendham, A. E., Duffield, R., Marino, F. and Coutts, A. J. (2014). Small-sided games training reduces CRP, IL-6 and leptin in sedentary, middle-aged men. *European Journal of Applied Physiology*, *114*(11), 2289–2297.

Mendham, A. E., Duffield, R., Marino, F. and Coutts, A. J. (2015b). Differences in the acute inflammatory and glucose regulatory responses between small-sided games and cycling in sedentary, middle-aged men. *Journal of Science and Medicine in Sport*, *18*(6), 712–719.

Ouchi, N., Parker, J. L., Lugus, J. J. and Walsh, K. (2011). Adipokines in inflammation and metabolic disease. *Nature Reviews Immunology*, *11*(2), 85–97.

Panagiotakos, D. B., Pitsavos, C., Chrysohoou, C., Kavouras, S. and Stefanadis, C. (2005). The associations between leisure-time physical activity and inflammatory and coagulation markers related to cardiovascular disease: the ATTICA Study. *Preventive Medicine*, *40*(4), 432–437.

Randers, M. B., Nielsen, J. J., Krustrup, B. R., Sundstrup, E., Jakobsen, M. D., Nybo, L., Dvorak, J., Bangsbo, J. and Krustrup, P. (2010). Positive performance and health effects of a football training program over 12 weeks can be maintained over a 1-year period with reduced training frequency. *Scandinavian Journal of Medicine and Science in Sports*, *20*(s1), 80–89.

Serpiello, F. R., McKenna, M. J., Coratella, G., Markworth, J. F., Tarperi, C., Bishop, D., Cameron-Smith, D. and Schena, F. (2014). Futsal and Continuous Exercise Induce Similar Changes in Specific Skeletal Muscle Signalling Proteins. *International Journal of Sports Medicine*, *35*(10), 863–870.

Silha, J. V., Krsek, M., Skrha, J. V., Sucharda, P., Nyomba, B. L. and Murphy, L. J. (2003). Plasma resistin, adiponectin and leptin levels in lean and obese subjects: correlations with insulin resistance. *European Journal of Endocrinology*, *149*(4), 331–335.

Skleryk, J. R., Karagounis, L. G., Hawley, J. A., Sharman, M. J., Laursen, P. B. and Watson, G. (2013). Two weeks of reduced-volume sprint interval or traditional exercise training does not improve metabolic functioning in sedentary obese men. *Diabetes, Obesity and Metabolism*, *15*(12), 1146–1153.

Unwin, N., Shaw, J., Zimmet, P. and Alberti, K. (2002). Impaired glucose tolerance and impaired fasting glycaemia: the current status on definition and intervention. *Diabetic Medicine*, *19*(9), 708–723.

Visser, M., Pahor, M., Taaffe, D. R., Goodpaster, B. H., Simonsick, E. M., Newman, A. B., Nevitt, M. and Harris, T. B. (2002). Relationship of interleukin-6 and tumor necrosis factor-a with muscle mass and muscle strength in elderly men and women the Health ABC Study. *Journals of Gerontology Series A: Biological and Medical Sciences*, *57*(5), 326–332.

You, T., Arsenis, N. C., Disanzo, B. L. and LaMonte, M. J. (2013). Effects of exercise training on chronic inflammation in obesity. *Sports Medicine*, *43*(4), 243–256.

Zhang, Y., Haddad, A., Su, S. W., Celler, B. G., Coutts, A. J., Duffield, R., Donges, C. E. and Nguyen, H. T. (2014). An equivalent circuit model for onset and offset exercise response. *Biomedical Engineering Online*, *13*(1), 145.

8 Recent research findings in Australian football

Application to other codes?

Brian Dawson

Introduction

Ever since 1987, when the first World Congress of Science and Football was held in Liverpool (UK), desired outcomes have been the translation of research findings into applied practice across all football codes. Recently, research in the various football codes and other team sports has increased greatly. Australian football is no exception, as research groups within the country have published (collectively) over 100 papers in the past three years on various game aspects. Broadly, these cover four main themes:

1 Altitude training (incorporating both actual altitude camps and hypoxic 'top up' repeat sprint training).
2 Recovery from training/games (incorporating methods like cold water immersion, plus effects on ensuing performance).
3 Game movement profiles (incorporating GPS/accelerometer data and match statistics/coach performance ratings).
4 Injury risk/prediction/management (incorporating multi season training/ game loads, player maturity and injury history analyses).

This chapter summarizes the important findings from Australian football research into these topics, and attempts to apply these results (where applicable) to the other football codes.

Altitude training

Always topical, altitude training has generally been investigated with regard to endurance performance enhancement (at sea level). However, interest in altitude training for team sports such as Australian football has recently grown; in 2012 the Australian Football League (AFL) commissioned a report into its use and efficacy from the Australian Institute of Sport (Saunders et al., 2012). These authors suggested that as Australian football requires good endurance and repeat sprint ability, altitude training could be advantageous, by boosting fitness levels and then allowing harder training phases to be programmed when back at sea level.

McLean et al. (2013a and 2013b) had AFL players participate in pre-season training camps for 18–19 days at Flagstaff (Arizona: ~2130 m) and Park City (Utah: ~2100 m). Of note, 2 km time trial performance was improved more (~1.5 percent) after altitude exposure than in sea-level controls doing the same training program; this improvement was also maintained four weeks later (after returning to sea level). Additionally, hemoglobin mass increased by ~3–4 percent after the camps (versus ~0.5 percent in controls), but had returned to baseline levels four weeks later. Collectively, these results suggest that altitude training camps can help build a greater pre-season fitness base, and that improved training quality may be possible on sea-level return (for ~4 weeks). However, the authors did report a large variability in the hemoglobin mass responses of individual players to the altitude exposure, including from one year to the next.

The potential additive effects of a 'cocktail' of altitude and heat exposure was investigated in AFL players by Buchheit et al. (2013). The altitude–heat group had ~14 h (each day) and ~4 h cycle training in simulated altitude (~2,500–3,000 m) across two weeks, with outdoor training sessions performed in ~32 °C for both the altitude–heat and normoxia–heat groups. Post-camp, both groups had similar improvements in the Yo-Yo Intermittent Recovery level 2 test, and in plasma volume and sweat Na^+ concentrations; the only noted difference was a greater hemoglobin mass in the altitude–heat group, which was maintained four weeks later. These findings again suggest that pre-season base fitness might be enhanced by exposure to altitude or heat (or a combination of both), but camp scheduling remains an issue for consideration, as in all of these studies, they were conducted some four months prior to the commencement of the 22 week AFL competition season.

One approach to this issue is to use hypoxic training to 'top up' the altitude exposure during the season (Saunders et al., 2012). Generally, simulated altitudes of 2,000–3,000 m are suggested for this purpose, as greater altitudes may compromise power outputs, especially in repeated sprint efforts (Goods et al., 2014). However, whether hypoxia is necessary to add further fitness benefits, to simply performing 'top up' training at sea level, requires more investigation. In addition to their normal training, Goods et al. (2015) had state league Australian footballers perform cycling repeat sprint 'top up' training for five weeks (three sessions per week) in the pre-season, with one group at simulated altitude (~3,000 m), another at sea level, plus a control group who did no extra training. 'Top up' training improved cycling (~5–14 percent) and running (~2 percent) repeat sprint test scores in both the hypoxia and sea-level groups, with no differences between them, showing that doing 'top up' training at simulated altitude did not improve training outcomes.

Application: altitude camps are expensive and difficult to plan/conduct, and for the football codes, which all involve a competitive season across several months, the cost–benefit ratio of a pre-season short-term fitness boost should be carefully considered. Similarly, using hypoxic 'top up' training during the season may not add additional benefits to simply performing the extra training at sea level.

Recovery

Sophisticated post-training/game recovery procedures are now commonplace in the football codes; it is now recognized that accelerated recovery from exertion is both possible and vital for optimizing next performance. Of the various recovery methods used, cold water immersion is both effective and preferred, based on recent AFL research. Elias et al. (2012) had AFL players use cold water immersion (14 min/12 °C), contrast water therapy (7 x 1 min in 38/12 °C, alternating) or a passive (control) recovery after a standardized intense training session across a three-week period. The session caused reductions in physical/psychological measures across the next 48 h, but muscle soreness and fatigue ratings were better, and repeat sprint ability test scores restored more quickly after cold water immersion than contrast water therapy or passive recovery (least effective). Banhert et al. (2013) followed an AFL squad across a full season: their novel approach was that players chose their preferred post-game recovery procedures. Players using (one or more of) cold water immersion (8 min in 6–11 °C), static stretching (10 min), lower body compression garments and doing no active recovery (neither bike or pool) had greater probability of reporting better (perceptual) recovery over the next week. Although no associations were found between recovery procedures and next game (coach ratings) or physical (weekly vertical jump measures) performance, the effects of improved perceived recovery should not be ignored or understated for elite performance.

Recovery markers, like heart rate variability, counter movement jump scores, exertion, fatigue and wellness scales and urine/saliva/blood measures have been used in Australian football, but which of these may be most effective (or necessary) at present remains unclear. Hunkin et al. (2014) recorded pre-game plasma creatine kinase levels across a full AFL season; while mean levels were elevated above pre-season baseline values (376 vs 78 U/L), there was only a very weak relationship with match performance ($r = -0.15/-0.16$; statistical data and coach game ratings). Interestingly, player age and experience were important moderating factors in these relationships; the authors suggested that using physiological markers such as creatine kinase might be most relevant in younger/less experienced players and those with lower aerobic capacities, to help optimize preparation and performance. Gastin et al. (2013) also reported that recovery from intense training sessions may be slower in AFL players with lower aerobic fitness; improving this capacity by programming high intensity 'top up' interval training was recommended.

Application: using cold water immersion and a combination of other recovery procedures (players choosing from selected options) is recommended for post-game recovery in the football codes. Although there are no compelling associations with recovery methods/markers and match performance, player perception of recovery is more important than any physical/physiological measure, and should be tracked. Potentially, younger/less experienced players and those with lower aerobic capacities may need more close monitoring, as more experienced players will usually cope better with accumulating training and game loads across a season.

Player movements

Player movements/actions within the football codes are somewhat specific, based on their particular rules, player numbers, ball shape and playing area dimensions. Therefore, although much information is now available (especially in Australian football, Rugby League/Union and soccer), the movements/actions of Australian footballers have little relevance to other football codes. What may be of value to other codes are potential links to game performance and analysis techniques, as investigated in recent research in Australian football.

Unsurprisingly, Mooney et al. (2011, 2013) found higher Yo-Yo Intermittent Recovery level 2 test scores were related to AFL players having more game ball possessions, and also a greater work rate and fatigue sparing effect across quarters one to four. The association with more ball possessions was stronger in midfielders (than set position players) and in more experienced players (50+ games). From a preparation/strategy standpoint, these results show that greater high intensity running ability and playing experience are valuable for gaining ball possession; this can also be interpreted to suggest that certain players train differently, depending on their team roles. Set position players may not require as much aerobic and high intensity running capacity as midfielders, and therefore might devote more training time to skill/technical/strategy aspects. These findings also (indirectly) emphasize the fitness/work rate 'gap' that exists between senior elite players and aspiring tyros (Brewer et al., 2010; Burgess et al., 2012a). These results provide supporting evidence for AFL new recruits to be trained differently to more experienced players, to better accommodate the large step up in training/game volume and intensity required, to reduce injury rates in these new players.

Sullivan et al. (2014) investigated the relationship between player movements, skill involvements and win/loss in one AFL team across 15 games, finding that in losses, players had higher activity (more high speed running), as identified in some soccer research (Di Salvo et al., 2009), and also reduced skill effectiveness. Further analysis also revealed greater activity and lower skill efficiency when quarter score margins were close (<9 points). Gronow et al. (2014) found that an AFL team across 14 games had more ball possession in winning quarters, but interestingly, a significant predictor of success was also greater movement time spent >14km/h without possession, suggesting that both higher speed offensive and defensive running (to make good position to both attack and defend) is important. Unsurprisingly, forwards had increased ball possession time, defenders more time without possession, with midfielders equally split in these terms.

Application: relationships between player movements and game performance require more research, but presently, player 'work rate' indicators have little association with game success. For the football codes, improving skill and effectiveness of actions, to increase ball possession time as much as possible, should be key strategy objectives. Within this overall theme, high intensity running without possession may be important for both more successful offensive and defensive actions. Younger players should also be carefully managed, as a considerable step up in training/game volume and intensity is common as they graduate from lower grades to elite competition.

Injury

Every football code has injuries reflecting their unique game demands, but in most (if not all) codes hamstring strains are the most common soft tissue (and non-contact) injury. In the AFL, there are ~6 hamstring strains per club per season, resulting in ~20 missed matches (Orchard et al., 2013). Understandably, research attention has been directed towards identifying specific risk factors for this injury. In the AFL, some of these are peculiar to game rules (player interchange rates: Orchard et al., 2012) and racial descent (increased risk in indigenous players: Taylor et al., 2011) but others broadly apply across all codes, such as increasing age, strength deficits, recent hamstring injury and prior calf and anterior cruciate ligament knee injury (Orchard et al., 2012, 2013). Using screening tests and specific 'prehabilitation' programs, such as eccentric strengthening exercises, should be routinely applied at elite levels in all codes.

Recognizing the injury difficulties often experienced by young recruits on entry into the AFL, some studies have concentrated on injury prediction themes. Burgess et al. (2012b) found AFL draft camp tests and final draft order, as well as under-18 game movement (speed/distance) data, had no predictive value for subsequent five-year injury risk. Chalmers et al. (2013) also studied elite under-18 players, finding lower 20-meter shuttle run scores were associated with greater risk of shin/ankle/foot injuries, and faster 5 meter and agility test times were linked with more knee and hip/groin/thigh injuries, respectively. However, whether these same associations are present in more experienced/older players is unknown. Nevertheless, recent findings show that first year AFL players have an injury incidence (per 1,000 game hours) 2.5 times greater than third-year players (Fortington et al., 2016). Close monitoring of younger players, particularly those less aerobically fit (and faster/more agile) remains vital, as lower injury rates are important for team success (Hägglund et al., 2013).

Given the presence of non-modifiable risk factors such as age and prior injury, it is well recognized that specific individual player monitoring is necessary to reduce injury in the football codes. This should extend to the accumulation of training/game loads across a season, as reported by Rogalski et al. (2013) and Colby et al. (2014). Tracking an AFL squad across a full season, these studies both found that cumulative loading values (measured by RPE/GPS/accelerometer data) across a rolling one–four-week period were more strongly associated with increased injury risk (rather than single training sessions/games), as was also large weekly changes in total load. Accurately determining residual fatigue in football players across a full season remains challenging for sports medicine/science staff and underscores the importance of player durability/resilience as highly valued individual characteristics.

Application: in all football codes, team success is enhanced if the best players are regularly available to play. In particular, reducing the incidence of soft tissue (non-contact) injuries such as hamstring strains is vital; screening tests and specific injury prevention exercise programs should be routinely used for this purpose. Careful monitoring of younger, less experienced squad members is also important, as they are more injury prone than more experienced players. Lastly, across a season lasting several months, weekly cumulative (training + games) loading of all players should be closely tracked, to reduce injury incidence and promote player durability.

References

Banhert, A., Norton, K. and Lock, P. (2013). Association between post game recovery protocols, physical and perceived recovery, and performance in elite Australian Football League players. *Journal of Science and Medicine in Sport, 16*, 151–156.

Brewer, C., Dawson, B., Heasman, J., Stewart, G. and Cormack, S. (2010). Movement pattern comparisons in elite (AFL) and sub-elite (WAFL) Australian football games using GPS. *Journal of Science and Medicine in Sport, 13*, 618–623.

Buchheit, M., Racinais, S., Bilsborough, J., Hocking, J., Mendez-Villanueva, A., Bourdon, P. C., Voss, S., Livingston, S., Christian, R., Périard, J., Cordy, J. and Coutts, A. J. (2013). Adding heat to the live-high train-low altitude model: a practical insight from professional football. *British Journal of Sports Medicine, 47*, i59–i69.

Burgess, D., Naughton, G. and Hopkins, W. (2012b). Draft-camp predictors of subsequent career success in the Australian Football League. *Journal of Science and Medicine in Sport, 15*, 561–567.

Burgess, D., Naughton, G. and Norton, K. (2012a). Quantifying the gap between under 18 and senior AFL football: 2003 and 2009. *International Journal of Sports Physiology and Performance, 7*, 53–58.

Chalmers, S., Magarey, M. E., Esterman, A., Speechley, M., Scase, E. and Heynen, M. (2013). The relationship between pre-season fitness testing and injury in elite junior Australian football players. *Journal of Science and Medicine in Sport, 16*, 307–311.

Colby, M., Dawson, B., Heasman, J., Rogalski, B. and Gabbett, T. (2014). Accelerometer and GPS-derived running loads and injury risk in elite Australian footballers. *Journal of Strength and Conditioning Research, 28*, 2244–2252.

Di Salvo, V., Gregson, W., Atkinson, G., Tordoff, P. and Drust, B. (2009). Analysis of high intensity activity in Premier League Soccer. *International Journal of Sports Medicine, 30*, 205–12.

Elias, G. P., Varley, M. C., Wyckelsma, V. L., McKenna, M. J., Minahan, C. L. and Aughey, R. J. (2012). Effects of water immersion on post training recovery in Australian footballers. *International Journal of Sports Physiology and Performance, 7*, 357–366.

Fortington, L., Berry, J. Buttifant, D., Ullah, S., Diamantopoulou, K. and Finch, C. F. (2016). Shorter time to first injury in first year professional football players: a cross-club comparison in the Australian Football League. *Journal of Science and Medicine in Sport, 19*(1), 18–23.

Gastin, P., Fahrner, B., Meyer, D., Robinson, D. and Cook, J. (2013). Influence of physical fitness, age, experience, and weekly training load on match performance in elite Australian football. *Journal of Strength and Conditioning Research, 27*, 1272–1279.

Goods, P., Dawson, B., Landers, G., Gore, C. and Peeling, P. (2014). Effect of different simulated altitudes on repeat-sprint performance in team-sport athletes. *International Journal of Sports Physiology and Performance, 9*, 857–862.

Goods, P., Dawson, B., Landers, G., Gore, C. and Peeling, P. (2015). No additional benefit of repeat-sprint training in hypoxia than in normoxia on sea-level repeat sprint ability. *Journal of Sports Science and Medicine, 14*(3), 681–688.

Gronow, D., Dawson, B., Heasman, J., Rogalski, B. and Peeling, P. (2014). Team movement patterns with and without ball possession in Australian Football League players. *International Journal of Performance Analysis in Sport*, *14*, 635–651.

Hägglund, M., Waldén, M., Magnusson, H., Kristenson, K., Bengtsson, H. and Ekstrand, J. (2013). Injuries affect team performance negatively in professional football: an 11-year follow-up of the UEFA Champions League injury study. *British Journal of Sports Medicine*, *47*, 738–742.

Hunkin, S., Fahrner, B. and Gastin, P. (2014). Creatine kinase and its relationship with match performance in elite Australian Rules football. *Journal of Science and Medicine in Sport*, *17*, 332–336.

McLean, B., Buttifant, D., Gore C., White, K. and Kemp, J. (2013a). Year-to-year variability in haemoglobin mass response to two altitude training camps. *British Journal of Sports Medicine*, *47*, i51–i58.

McLean, B., Buttifant, D., Gore, C., White, K. and Kemp, J. (2013b). Physiological and performance responses to a preseason altitude-training camp in elite team-sport athletes. *International Journal of Sports Physiology and Performance*, *8*, 391–399.

Mooney, M., O'Brien, B., Cormack, S., Coutts, A., Berry, J. and Young, W. (2011). The relationship between physical capacity and match performance in elite Australian football: A mediation approach. *Journal of Science and Medicine in Sport*, *14*, 447–452.

Mooney, M., Cormack, S., O'Brien, B. and Coutts, A. (2013). Do physical capacity and interchange rest periods influence match intensity profile in Australian football? *International Journal of Sports Physiology and Performance*, *8*, 165–172.

Orchard, J., Driscoll, T., Seward, H. and Orchard, J. (2012). Relationship between interchange usage and risk of hamstring injuries in the Australian Football League. *Journal of Science and Medicine in Sport*, *15*, 201–206.

Orchard, J., Seward, H. and Orchard J. (2013). Results of 2 decades of injury surveillance and public release of data in the Australian Football League. *American Journal of Sports Medicine*, *41*, 734–741.

Rogalski, B., Dawson, B., Heasman, J. and Gabbett, T. (2013). Training and game loads and injury risk in elite Australian footballers. *Journal of Science and Medicine in Sport*, *16*, 499–503.

Saunders, P., Garvican, L. and Gore, C. (2012). *Altitude training for AFL*. Report commissioned by the Australian Football League from the Australian Institute of Sport.

Sullivan, C., Bilsborough, J., Cianciosi, M., Hocking, J., Cordy, J. and Coutts, A. J. (2014). Match score affects activity profile and skill performance in professional Australian football players. *Journal of Science and Medicine in Sport*, *17*, 326–331.

Taylor, C., Pizzari, T., Ames, N., Orchard, J., Gabbe, B. and Cook, J. (2011). Groin pain and hip range of motion is different in Indigenous compared to non-indigenous young Australian football players. *Journal of Science and Medicine in Sport*, *14*, 283–286.

9 Physiology of women's soccer from competitive to recreational level

Magni Mohr

Introduction

The popularity of women's soccer has increased markedly during the last decade and is today globally one of the sporting activities that display the fastest growth rate. On a global basis there are now more than 30 million active players, and elite women's players are employed on either a professional or semi-professional basis. Moreover, recreational soccer participation appears to be dominated by women players. In Denmark and the Faroe Islands 75–85 percent of the participants in the Soccer Fitness concept are women (Bennike et al., 2014).

The increased focus on women's soccer has also accelerated scientific research investigating physical demands, fatigue development, recovery kinetics and physical capacity of competitive players (Bradley and Vescovi, 2015), as well as the effect of training on broad spectrum health status in untrained women (Krustrup et al., 2010a; Mohr et al., 2015b). This chapter provides a short overview of the physiology of women's soccer at elite and recreational level.

The present chapter also aims to provide a brief overview of the physiological demands of competitive women's soccer with the main focus on match activity analysis, physiological game responses, fatigue and recovery. Moreover, the impact of recreational soccer on different health components in sedentary women is provided.

Match analysis

The activity pattern during women's soccer match play along with the effect of factors such as the standard of competition, playing position and fatigue has been explored extensively (Mohr et al., 2008; Bradley et al., 2014a; Bradley and Vescovi, 2015). For example, the total game distance for elite women players is approximately 10 km, with 1.7 km completed as high intensity running, which often is defined as running >15 km·h^{-1} (Mohr et al., 2008). In a recent study we compared the work profile of female and male elite players during UEFA Champions League games, and large gender differences were observed in the high speed threshold (Bradley et al., 2014a). For example, males ran 23, 57, 89 and 139 percent longer at speed 18–21, 21–23, 23–25 and 25–27 km·h^{-1}, and covered fourfold more ground at the highest speed (>27 km·h^{-1}) compared to women. Thus, the differences between the genders appear to increase the higher the speed threshold, which is supported by earlier findings (Mohr et al., 2008). This questions the application of similar speed threshold between the genders, which is addressed in a recent review by Bradley and Vescovi (2015). World-class women players have been shown to complete 28 percent more high-speed running and 24 percent more sprinting than elite players on a lower competitive standard (Mohr et al., 2008). Moreover, international games tend to be more physically demanding than domestic games with more high intensity running especially for players in demanding roles (Andersson et al., 2010b). These findings demonstrate the importance of high intensity intermittent exercise in elite women's soccer.

Physiological loading and physical capacity

Cardiovascular loading is high during a competitive soccer game with average and peak heart rates being 87 and 97 percent HR$_{max}$ (Krustrup et al., 2005), while blood lactate levels increase approximately fivefold during a game (Krustrup et al., 2010). Most data on the physiological response to a women's soccer game are sampled from competitive games. However, due to the inter-game variability in soccer, simulated game protocols may add to the understanding of the physical demands. Recently, the Copenhagen Soccer Test for women (CSTw) was developed, and applied to elite soccer (Bendiksen et al., 2013). The test resulted in average heart rates of 85 percent HR$_{max}$ with 35 percent of the playing time being >90 percent HR$_{max}$, while blood lactate concentrations averaged at ~5 mM. Thus, the physiological responses to CSTw confirm that both aerobic and anaerobic energy systems are highly utilized during a women's soccer game. In contrast to males, no study so far has investigated muscle metabolic variables during a competitive soccer game in the women players. For example, fluctuations in muscle CP, lactate and glycogen during a game, as well as the glycogen resynthesizes in different muscle fiber types and subcellular compartments after a game would provide valuable data in relation to fatigue and recovery aspects in women's soccer.

Physical capacity is the most thoroughly researched area in women's soccer players. For example, maximal oxygen uptake values ranging from 49–58 ml·kg^{-1}·min^{-1} are reported, while Yo-Yo Intermittent Endurance test level 2 (Yo-Yo IE2) of~1800 m and 20 m sprint times of ~3.2 s are found on average (Krustrup et al., 2005; Bangsbo and Mohr, 2012). Similar to competitive males the Yo-Yo Intermittent Recovery, level 1 (Yo-Yo IR1) and the Yo-Yo IE2 test seem to predict physical match performance in women soccer (Krustrup et al., 2005; Bradley et al., 2014b). These and other test results demonstrate clearly that elite women soccer players have a markedly lower physical capacity compared to their male counterparts. However, similar inter-player variability as found in the men is present in women, where full backs and midfielders appear to display the highest fitness levels among playing positions (Bangsbo and Mohr, 2012). Finally, as in match activities large inter-player variability in physical capacity exists, this calls for a more individualized research approach for future studies.

Fatigue development

Decrements in high intensity running distance have been reported between and within halves in women's soccer games (Krustrup et al., 2005; Mohr et al., 2008; Bradley et al., 2014a) indicating an inability to maintain high-intensity activity over prolonged periods of time. Indeed in the study by Krustrup et al. (2005) a significant high-intensity running distance deficit was observed during the last 15-min interval of each half, and performance in these two game intervals was positively correlated to Yo-Yo IR1 test scores. These observations are supported by several studies demonstrating deteriorations in sprinting ability (Andersson et al., 2010a; Bendiksen et al., 2013), high intensity intermittent exercise performance (Krustrup et al., 2010) and counter-movement jump height, as well as peak knee extensor and flexor torque (Andersson et al., 2010a) after a game. In a study by Andersson et al. (2010a) in addition to performance responses, indicators of muscle damage, inflammation and oxidative stress were assessed after a soccer game. The studies show a marked and long-lasting fatigue response, where for example knee flexor performance was not back to baseline until more than 50 h post-game (Andersson et al., 2010a). Thus, these findings indicate a long recovery period of performance and physiological parameters as also observed in male players (Mohr et al., 2005, 2015a; Krustrup et al., 2011). Finally, similar to male players, temporary fatigue (Mohr et al., 2003) may also occur during a competitive soccer game in women players, which has been shown in match-analysis studies in well-trained elite players (Mohr et al., 2008; Andersson et al., 2010b).

In a recent study top-class men and women soccer players were compared in relation to match profile (Bradley et al., 2014b). No gender differences were found for technical events such as the number of ball touches, time in possession of the ball or total duels won. However, female players lost the ball more often and displayed lower pass completion rates than male players during the game. These findings demonstrate gender differences in technical performance of players competing at the highest competitive standard. However, it is unknown whether these differences were associated with inferior technical abilities of women players compared to men, and/or greater degree of fatigue development.

Recreational soccer

During the last decade solid evidence has emerged that recreational soccer appears to be a broad spectrum training method causing improved cardiovascular, metabolic and bone health (Krustrup et al., 2010a, 2010b). In relation to women, several studies have been conducted on health beneficial effects of participation in soccer training. It has been demonstrated that soccer training, consisting of small-sided games for women unfamiliar with the game, includes a high number of intense actions, has a high cardiovascular loading with heart rates >90 percent HR_{max} for 8–13 percent of the training time, while significant increases and decreases are observed in muscle lactate and glycogen, respectively (Randers et al., 2010). Thus, soccer training can be used as a complex training method in untrained women. In a recent study soccer training three times per week for a minimum of 15 weeks caused a reduction in mean arterial pressure of 8 mmHg with a concomitant decrement in fat mass, resting and submaximal heart rates, plasma triglycerides and total cholesterol, as well as increased lean body mass in a group of middle-aged moderately hypertensive women (Mohr et al., 2014). This finding is supported by others (Krustrup et al., 2010b; Connolly et al., 2014). In the study by Connolly et al. (2014) we studied the impact of small volume soccer training (15 min twice per week for 24 weeks), which was potent enough to induce a decrement in total fat content. Moreover, the study by Krustrup et al. (2010b) found that cardiac function improved by 25–50 percent after 16 weeks of soccer training, as evaluated by echocardiographical measures. Finally, soccer training organized as 1 h sessions twice per week increased VO_{2max} (Milanović et al., 2015), endurance performance and lowered cardiovascular loading during exercise (Mohr et al., 2014). Thus, cardiovascular heath can be improved in normotensive and hypertensive sedentary women.

Soccer training has also been demonstrated to improve glycemic control in sedentary premenopausal women (Krustrup et al., 2010b). Moreover, four weeks of recreational soccer increased maximal citrate synthase and 3-hydroxyacyl-CoA dehydrogenaseas activity in the vastus lateralis muscle in healthy untrained premenopausal women (Bangsbo et al., 2010). Recently, we also found significant increases in muscle oxidative capacity in both leg and arm muscle after 15 weeks with soccer training in middle-aged sedentary women (Nordsborg et al., 2015). Thus, soccer training improved muscle metabolic health in different muscle groups after 15 weeks of training.

Women are at risk of developing sarcopenia and osteoporosis, especially after the menopause, and it has been suggested that exercise training can counteract this development (Rizzoli et al., 2014). It has been shown in a cross-sectional study that elite women soccer national team players have markedly higher bone health than their age-matched untrained counterparts (Jackman et al., 2013). For example, total bone mineral density (BMD) and bone mineral content (BMC) was 13 percent higher and values for the legs were 25–30 percent higher in the soccer players. Moreover, 16 weeks of soccer training caused an elevation of 37 percent in resting plasma osteocalcin concentration, ~1.5 kg increase in lean body mass and a 30 percent improvement in balance in the untrained group (Jackman et al., 2013). These findings are supported by others (Helge et al., 2010; Barene et al., 2014). Thus, several of the factors reducing the risk of bone fractures can be improved with soccer training. Also in middle-aged women being close to the menopause soccer training has a high osteogenic stimulus. It was demonstrated recently that 15 weeks of soccer training significantly increased femur BMD and BMC with concomitant elevations (37–52 percent) in plasma markers of bone turnover such as osteocalcin, procollagen type I N propeptide and C-terminal telopeptide (Mohr et al., 2015b). Thus, soccer training seems to provide a powerful osteogenic stimulus to young and middle-aged women. It is however currently unknown whether postmenopausal women can obtain similar benefits.

Thus, soccer training for sedentary young and middle-aged women has a broad spectrum of health benefits, having an impact on cardiovascular, metabolic and musculoskeletal fitness and health profile.

Conclusion

Women's soccer is an intense intermittent activity where prolonged intermittent exercise is conjoined with brief intense runs and explosive movements. This activity pattern results in a high loading of the aerobic and anaerobic energy systems during a women's soccer game. Fatigue occurs during the end of the game, which is limiting physical performance during the first two to three days of recovery from a game. Compared to their male counterparts, top-class women players perform less running in the fastest speed categories and appear to be inferior in technical ability. It can furthermore be concluded that recreational soccer for women is a highly efficient training method to improve cardiovascular, metabolic and bone health. Beneficial broad spectrum effects suggest that soccer training may be applied as prevention and treatment of lifestyle diseases in women.

References

Andersen, L. J., Hansen, P. R., Søgaard, P., Madsen, J. K., Bech, J. and Krustrup, P. (2010). Improvement of systolic and diastolic heart function after physical training in sedentary women. *Scandinavian Journal of Medicine and Science in Sports*, *20*(suppl. 1), 50–57.

Andersson, H., Karlsen, A., Blomhoff, R., Raastad, T. and Kadi, F. (2010a). Active recovery training does not affect the antioxidant response to soccer games in elite female players. *British Journal of Nutrition*, *104*(10), 1492–1499.

Andersson, H., Randers, M. B., Heiner-Møller, A., Krustrup, P. and Mohr, M. (2010b). Elite female soccer players perform more high-intensity running when playing in international games compared with domestic league games. *The Journal of Strength Conditioning Research*, *24*(4), 912–919.

Bangsbo, J. and Mohr, M. (2012). *Fitness Testing in Football*. Bangsbosport, Copenhagen, Denmark.

Bangsbo, J., Nielsen, J. J., Mohr, M., Randers, M. B., Krustrup, B. R., Brito, J., Nybo, L. and Krustrup, P. (2010). Performance enhancements and muscular adaptations of a 16-week recreational football intervention for untrained women. *Scandinavian Journal of Medicine and Science in Sports*, *20*(suppl. 1), 24–30.

Barene, S., Krustrup, P., Brekke, O. L. and Holtermann, A. (2014). Soccer and Zumba as health-promoting activities among female hospital employees: a 40-weeks cluster randomised intervention study. *Journal of Sports Sciences*, *32*, 1539–1549.

Bendiksen, M., Pettersen, S. A., Ingebrigtsen, J., Randers, M. B., Brito, J., Mohr M., Bangsbo J. and Krustrup, P. (2013). Application of the Copenhagen Soccer Test in high-level women players – locomotor activities, physiological response and sprint performance. *Human Movement Science*, *32*(6), 1430–1442.

Bennike, S., Wikman, J. M. and Ottesen, L. S. (2014). Football Fitness – a new version of football? A concept for adult players in Danish football clubs. *Scandinavian Journal of Medicine and Science in Sports*, *24*(1), 138–146.

Bradley, P. S., Bendiksen, M., Dellal, A., Mohr, M., Wilkie, A., Datson, N., Orntoft, C., Zebis, M., Gomez-Diaz, A., Bangsbo, J. and Krustrup, P. (2014a). The application of the Yo-Yo intermittent endurance level 2 test to elite female soccer populations. *Scandinavian Journal of Medicine and Science in Sports*, *24*(1), 43–54.

Bradley, P. S., Dellal, A., Mohr, M., Castellano, J. and Wilkie, A. (2014b). Gender differences in match performance characteristics of soccer players competing in the UEFA Champions League. *Human Movement Science*, *33*, 159–171.

Bradley, P. S. and Vescovi, J. D. (2015). Velocity thresholds for women's soccer matches: sex specificity dictates high-speed running and sprinting thresholds – Female Athletes in Motion (FAiM). *International Journal of Sports Physiology and Performance*, *10*(1), 112–116.

Connolly, L. J., Scott, S., Mohr, M., Ermidis, G., Julian, R., Bangsbo, J., Jackman, S. R., Bowtell, J. L., Davis, R. C., Hopkins, S., Seymour, R., Knapp, K. M., Krustrup, P. and Fulford, J. (2014). Effects of small-volume soccer and vibration training on body composition, aerobic fitness, and muscular PCr kinetics for inactive women aged 20–45. *Journal of Sport and Health Science*, *3*(4), 284–292.

Helge, E. W., Aagaard, P., Jakobsen, M. D., Sundstrup, E., Randers, M. B., Karlsson, M. K. and Krustrup, P. (2010). Recreational football training decreases risk factors for bone fractures in untrained premenopausal women. *Scandinavian Journal of Medicine and Science in Sports*, *20*(suppl. 1), 31–39.

Jackman, S. R., Scott, S., Randers, M. B., Orntoft, C., Blackwell, J., Zar, A., Helge, E. W., Mohr, M. and Krustrup, P. (2013). Musculoskeletal health profile for elite female footballers versus untrained young women before and after 16 weeks of football training. *Journal of Sports Sciences*, *31*, 1468–1474.

Krustrup, P., Dvorak, J., Junge, A. and Bangsbo, J. (2010a). Executive summary: the health and fitness benefits of regular participation in small-sided football games. *Scandinavian Journal of Medicine and Science in Sports*, *20*(suppl. 1), 132–135.

Krustrup, P., Hansen, P. R., Andersen, L. J., Jakobsen, M. D., Sundstrup, E., Randers, M. B., Christiansen, L., Helge, E. W., Pedersen, M. T., Sogaard, P., Junge, A., Dvorak J., Aagaard, P. and Bangsbo, J. (2010b). Long-term musculoskeletal and cardiac health effects of recreational football and running for premenopausal women. *Scandinavian Journal of Medicine and Science in Sports*, *20*(suppl. 1), 58–71.

Krustrup, P., Mohr, M., Ellingsgaard, H. and Bangsbo, J. (2005). Physical demands during an elite female soccer game: importance of training status. *Medicine and Science in Sports and Exercise*, *37*(7), 1242–1248.

Krustrup, P., Ortenblad, N., Nielsen, J., Nybo, L., Gunnarsson, T. P., Iaia F. M. and Bangsbo, J. (2011). Maximal voluntary contraction force, SR function and glycogen resynthesis during the first 72 h after a high-level competitive soccer game. *European Journal of Applied Physiology*, *111*, 2987–2995.

Milanović, Z., Pantelić, S., Sporiš, G., Mohr, M. and Krustrup, P. (2015). Health-related physical fitness in healthy untrained men: effects on vo_{2max}, jump performance and flexibility of soccer and moderate-intensity continuous running. *PLoS One*, *10*(8), e0135319.

Mohr, M., Krustrup, P., Andersson, H., Kirkendal, D. and Bangsbo, J. (2008). Match activities of elite women soccer players at different performance levels. *Journal of Strength Conditioning Research*, *22*(2), 341–349.

Mohr, M., Krustrup, P. and Bangsbo, J. (2003). Match performance of high-standard soccer players with special reference to development of fatigue. *Journal of Sport Sciences*, *21*, 519–528.

Mohr, M., Krustrup, P. and Bangsbo, J. (2005). Fatigue in soccer: A brief review. *Journal of Sport Sciences*, *23*, 593–599.

Mohr, M., Lindenskov, A., Holm, P. M., Nielsen, H. P., Mortensen, J., Weihe, P. and Krustrup, P. (2014). Football training improves cardiovascular health profile in sedentary, premanopausal hypertensive women. *Scandinavian Journal of Medicine and Science in Sports*, *24*(suppl. 1), 36–42.

Mohr, M., Draganidis, D., Chatzinikolaou, A., Barbero-Álvarez, J. C., Castagna, C., Douroudos, I., Avloniti, A., Margeli, A., Papassotiriou, I., Flouris, A. D., Jamurtas, A. Z., Krustrup, P. and Fatouros, I. G. (2015a). Muscle damage, inflammatory, immune and performance responses to three football games in 1 week in competitive male players. *European Journal of Applied Physiology*. 10.1007/s00421–015–3245-2

Mohr, M., Helge, E. W., Petersen, L. F., Lindenskov, A., Weihe, P., Mortensen, J., Jørgensen, N. R. and Krustrup, P. (2015b). Effects of soccer vs swim training on bone formation in sedentary middle-aged women. *European Journal of Applied Physiology*, *115*(12), 2671–2679.

Nordsborg, N. B., Connolly, L., Weihe, P., Iuliano, E., Krustrup, P., Saltin, B. and Mohr, M. (2015). Oxidative capacity and glycogen content increase more in arm than leg muscle in sedentary women after intense training. *Journal of Applied Physiology*, *119*, 116–123.

Randers, M. B., Nybo, L., Petersen, J., Nielsen, J. J., Christiansen, L., Bendiksen, M., Brito, J., Bangsbo, J. and Krustrup, P. (2010). Activity profile and physiological response to football training for untrained males and females, elderly and youngsters: influence of the number of players. *Scandinavian Journal of Medicine and Science in Sports*, *20*(suppl. 1), 14–23.

Rizzoli, R., Bischoff-Ferrari, H., Dawson-Hughes, B. and Weaver, C. (2014). Nutrition and bone health in women after the menopause. *Women's Health*, *10*, 599–608.

10 Soccer in the heat

Impact on physiological responses, match-play characteristics and recovery

Lars Nybo, George Nassis and Sébastien Racinais

Introduction

Physiological responses to prolonged exercise are noticeably influenced by the environmental temperature and in hot conditions this may accelerate the development of fatigue and markedly impair exercise endurance (Gonzalez-Alonso et al., 1999; Nybo and Nielsen, 2001; Nybo et al., 2014). In contrast, rapid movements may benefit from the higher muscle tissue temperatures associated with exercise in hot environments (Asmussen and Bøje, 1945; Racinais and Oksa, 2010). Accelerations, sprints, jumps and all short-term performance parameters may therefore improve unless hyperthermia-induced fatigue offset the beneficial effect of the temperature associated increase in muscle contraction velocity (Drust et al., 2005; Girard et al., 2012). Since soccer is an intermittent sport with many short intense actions frequently repeated over a prolonged period, it implies that some parameters may benefit from an elevated environmental temperature while the accumulation of heat over time may deteriorate other performance parameters as fatigue develops (Maughan et al., 2010; Mohr et al., 2012; Ozgunen et al., 2010). In this review we will describe the heat-related issues of importance for physical and technical/cognitive performance in soccer and its associated influence on match-play characteristics. For each parameter we will briefly discuss the underlying physiological mechanisms and subsequently provide guidelines for preparing players and highlight the factors coaches and the medical staff should considerer before, during and after match play in the heat.

Prior to competitions/matches in the heat the most important intervention to optimize physical performance is to acclimatize to the environmental conditions (Bergeron et al., 2012; Racinais et al., 2015a) and based on our experience from several heat acclimatization studies and training camps with team sport players, we will provide brief practical recommendation and key point for the individual considerations that coaches, physical trainers and the medical staff should be aware of. In addition to acclimatization, the ability to cope with acute heat stress as well as recovering between matches may rely on relevant hydration and rehydration strategies. Total water loss and sweat sodium concentration display marked individual variation (Maughan et al., 2004) and while acclimatization improves the evaporative cooling capacity via increased sweat rates (Karlsen et al., 2015;

Taylor, 2014), it also elevates fluid losses and hence the importance of adequate and individualized hydration strategies to limit dehydration to levels that will not impair the players' performance capacity.

Physiological responses and their influence on running patterns during match play in the heat

The average exercise intensity during elite soccer matches conducted in cool to moderate temperatures corresponds to ~ 70 percent of the players' maximal oxygen uptake (Bangsbo et al., 2006) implying that players have a metabolic heat production of approximately 1,200 watt. Since the core temperature in such conditions usually stabilizes around 38.5°C (Mohr et al., 2004), it entails that heat dissipation to the environment via dry and evaporative heat loss mechanisms matches the individual players' metabolic heat production. When matches are conducted in hot environments the ability to dissipate heat via convective mechanisms (heat transfer to the surrounding air) is impaired and solar radiation may provide an additional heat load on the player and although the sweat rate increases markedly, it may not be sufficient to establish heat balance. In such conditions the players core temperature will increase continuously during each half (Ozgunen et al., 2010) and they will literally run into trouble unless they slow down and hence lower their metabolic heat production. Accordingly, in an experimental match conducted in 43°C dry heat (WBGT ~ 35°C) the total distance covered by the players was reduced by 7 percent compared to the prior control match conducted six days ahead in 21°C (WBGT ~ 17°C, see Figure 10.1 and Mohr et al., 2012). In this match we also observed a marked reduction in high-intensity running and these adjustments in total distances and intense running implied that the players maintained similar average heart rate (HR) in the hot match as observed for the prior control game and the plasma lactate levels were not different across the environmental conditions (Mohr et al., 2012). When a given submaximal exercise intensity is maintained in the heat the HR normally increases to compensate for reductions in stroke volume (Gonzalez-Alonso et al., 2008) and at intensities eliciting peak HR and maximally taxation of the aerobic capacity, anaerobic metabolism will increase to compensate for hyperthermia-induced impairments in maximal oxygen uptake (Gonzalez-Alonso et al., 2008; Nybo et al., 2001).

In agreement with the observations from experimental studies, analyses of all matches from the 2014 FIFA World Cup in Brazil revealed that high-intensity distance running declined as the environmental temperature increased (see Figure 10.1 and Nassis et al., 2015). This adjustment in work rate could be part of a behavioral modification strategy adopted by the experienced players to avoid excessive fatigue and ensure maintenance of other key performance indicators (e.g. technical skills and sprinting ability). The exact mechanisms underlying the conscious or unconscious lowering of exercise intensity during self-paced sport activities are not entirely clear (see Nybo et al., 2014 and Periard and Racinais, 2015 for discussion), however it is assumed that unless players reduce total running and especially the amount of high-intensity work, we would observe very

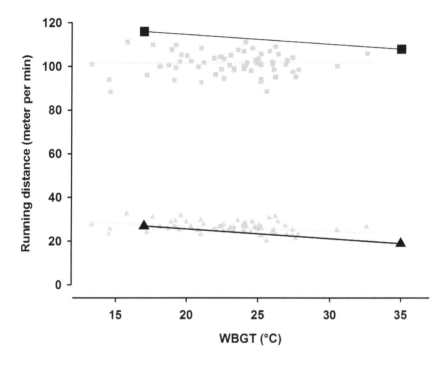

Figure 10.1 Total running distances (squares) and high intensity running (triangles) versus
wet bulb globe temperature (WBGT) for the 64 matches in the 2014 FIFA
World Cup (grey symbols) and for the experimental matches conducted by
Mohr et al. 2012 (black symbols). High intensity running in the competitive
matches was negatively correlated to WBGT in agreement with the significant
reduction observed in the experimental matches conducted with identical set-
up except for the different environmental temperature (17 vs 35°C WBGT).
Total running distance was also significantly reduced in the hot experimental
match (compared with the cool control), whereas for the 2014 FIFA world cup
matches, it appeared that the reduction in high intensity running was compensated for by increased distances at lower running speeds to maintain similar
total distances across the environmental settings

Sources: modified Mohr et al. (2012) and Nassis et al. (2015) with permission

high lactate levels and excessive fatigue already in the middle of the first half
(Nybo et al., 2014). However, when comparing the most intense 5-min period of
the game (usually observed in the first half) with the 5-min period immediately
following this period, it is clear that in cool conditions the players experience
some very intense periods where HR, lactate levels and plasma potassium concentrations are markedly elevated and with a subsequent recovery/fatigue period
where the exercise intensity is markedly lower (high-intensity running reduced to
~ one-quarter of the proceeding period (Mohr et al., 2005, 2012). In contrast, in
the heat the players cover less ground in the most intense period, but also experience less reduction in the subsequent period, indicating that excessive fatigue is

avoided by altering the individual players pacing strategy (Mohr et al., 2012). In acclimatized cyclists we also observe changes in the pacing strategy that allows time trials to be completed without excessive fatigue development early in the competitions/trials, whereas in experienced but unacclimatized cyclists the ability to adjust the intensity and complete time trials with an appropriate pacing strategy is lacking (Racinais et al., 2015b). This may emphasize the importance of adapting and learning how to cope with heat stress, not just to gain the physiological benefits from acclimatization but also for developing appropriate pacing strategies. For team sports such as soccer it is clear that the unique nature of each single game and how match play develops will influence the individual work patterns (Paul et al., 2015). However, as both teams (all players) are exposed to the same environmental conditions it appears that from the collective level to the individual physiological responses and changes in pacing (i.e. lowering of intensity to limit the cardiovascular stress (similar HR across conditions) and limit the development of hyperthermia) are comparable to those observed for individual sports (Periard and Racinais, 2015; Periard et al., 2014; Racinais et al., 2015). Thus, acclimatized athletes are capable of adjusting their effort and exercise intensity to the conditions they are exposed to.

While endurance parameters are impaired in the heat, sprinting performance is largely unaffected (Nassis et al., 2015; Ozgunen et al., 2010) or even slightly improved (Mohr et al., 2012) as the elevated muscle temperature benefits nerve conduction and peak muscle contraction velocities (Girard et al., 2012; Todd et al., 2005). Hyperthermia has been associated with central fatigue and impaired ability to sustain maximal muscle activation during prolonged contractions (Nybo and Nielsen, 2001), however, the average sprint in soccer usually lasts ~ 2 seconds (Bangsbo et al., 2006) and the central nervous system can readily produce the adequate neural output for this period of time as long as the maximal activations are interspersed by brief breaks (Nybo and Nielsen, 2001; Todd et al., 2005). Thus, when excessive hyperthermia and fatigue are prevented all brief actions are largely unaffected and this also included technical parameters relying on a combination of motors skill and cognitive performance (Mohr et al., 2012). Accordingly, in the latest World Cup the number of goals per match was not affected by the environmental conditions (Nassis et al., 2015) and passing success may even be slightly higher in the heat compared to cool conditions, presumably due to the reduced running distances and hence also less defensive running and increased space around each player (Mohr et al., 2012; Nassis et al., 2015). In summary, match characteristics are modified when games are conducted in the heat with less total and high-intensity running, while sprinting performance is maintained or slightly improved. Technical quality of the matches as signified by the better rate of successful passes and the similar goals scores are not impaired by the heat.

Countermeasures

This section provides brief recommendations to minimize the detrimental effects of heat on fatigue development and hence benefit soccer physical performance when playing in hot ambient conditions. Without these precautions, players will not be able to limit the detrimental effects of heat to the above described influences, but may experience marked fatigue and inability to even tolerate the heat and complete the match.

Heat acclimatization

Heat acclimatization is the most important intervention to adopt prior to competing in the heat to reduce the physiological strain and optimize performance (Racinais et al., 2015b). Consequently, players should train in the heat before any game or tournament in hot, ambient conditions in order to obtain the beneficial biological adaptations as signified by increased sweat rates, decreases in sweat sodium concentration, lower core temperature and heart rate at given exercise intensities (Taylor, 2014). Significant sudomotor and cardiovascular adaptations are observed after only few days of training in the heat (Karlsen et al., 2015; Racinais et al., 2012). However, even if improvement in heat tolerance and important physiological adaptations are obtained within very short time and practical limitations may allow teams to spend only few days in the heat prior to a match, it is recommended that the heat acclimatization period is at least five to six days and ideally prolonged to two weeks for optimal performance (Grantham et al., 2010; Racinais et al., 2015b).

Importantly, since we observe large individual differences in the early adaptive response, it is recommended to determine the acclimatization response for each player by recording, for example, the changes in hematocrit concentration after a heat-response test (Racinais et al., 2012, 2014). This index is of particular interest for coaches and team doctors as it may predict the ability of the individual player to cope with heat stress during a football match in hot ambient conditions (Racinais et al., 2012).

Heat acclimatization sessions should at least include 60 min per day and induce an additional increase in body core and skin temperatures, as well as stimulate sweating. Ideally, players should train in the same environment as the competition venue (e.g. tropical or desert environments, same time of day). However, when teams do not have the possibility to travel to the competition venue weeks in advance, other heat acclimation methods can be used. For example, physical training can be organized in hot rooms, with additional clothing or regular training may be combined with passive heat stress (Nielsen et al., 1997).

Hydration

Sufficient hydration prior to, during and in the recovery period is integral to athlete performance and safety during training and competition in the heat (Bergeron et al., 2012). Given the limited opportunity to drink during matches, players should be cautious to initiate games in a euhydrated state, while permissive dehydration is acceptable during matches and training (usually limiting dehydration to ~2 percent body weight deficit; Maughan et al., 2010; Mohr et al., 2012). This is generally achieved by ad libitum drinking during exercise, but securing adequate rehydration following each match and training bout by accounting for the elevated daily water and sodium (i.e. salt) requirements (Maughan et al., 2010; Sawka et al., 2007). From a general point of view, recovery hydration regimens should include sodium, carbohydrates and protein as the latter will also support fluid retention (James et al., 2013). For tournament lasting several days, coaches and team doctors can implement simple monitoring techniques such as daily assessments of body mass and urine-specific gravity. Individual strategies may also be refined on the basis of assessments of each player sweat rate and sweat sodium losses (Maughan et al., 2004).

Warming up or cooling down

Like most other athletes, soccer players typically warm up using moderate intensity, interspersed with higher intensity efforts, and followed by a few minutes of recovery before the game. The aim of the warm-up is generally to practice some skills and increase the muscle temperature to elevate the speed of metabolic reactions and nerve conduction velocity. However, warm-up can also induce a significant increase in core temperature that may limit heat-storage capacity and aerobic performance when playing in the heat (Gonzalez-Alonso et al., 1999). Consequently, it is advisable that the warm-up is modified to obtain both temperature-dependent (e.g. physiological preparation) and non-temperature-dependent (e.g. psychological preparation) benefits while limiting the increase in core temperature (Bishop, 2003a, 2003b).

This can notably be achieved by using cooling technique to minimize the rise in core and skin temperatures. Some of these techniques can be used before, during or after the warm-up as well as during the half-time break. Cooling methods include external e.g. application of iced garments, cooling vests towels, water immersion or fanning and internal methods e.g. ingestion of cold fluids or ice-slurry (Ross et al., 2013). A practical approach for games in hot-humid environments might be to use fans and commercially available ice or evaporative cooling vests to improve heat dissipation capacity without impairing muscle temperature. Alternatively, the intensity and duration of the warm-up may be reduced as less activity is required to achieve the physiological benefits (elevated muscle temperature). In any case, changes in the warm-up procedure and cooling methods should be tested and individualized during training to minimize disturbance of the athlete (Racinais et al., 2015b).

A role for the governing bodies and tournament organizers

Given that evaporation is the main source for heat dissipation when exercise is conducted at high ambient temperatures, evaporative heat loss should be maximized by minimizing the barriers between the skin and the environment. However, some game requirements such as protective garments may increase evaporative resistance and elevated the risk of excessive hyperthermia (Grundstein et al., 2012). Players should therefore aim for garments that maximize the evaporation of sweat, while balancing the protection of the skin from solar radiation. Furthermore, event organizers may minimize solar radiation by planning for large shaded areas and scheduling games at appropriate times of the day. Event organizers should also plan for cooling and rehydration facilities as this will allow players to recover following matches or at the half-time break. Also, additional breaks during matches for hydration opportunities will allow players to prevent excessive dehydration.

Recovery and health considerations

Heat-related illnesses are a major concern when competing in the heat and excessively high core and muscle temperatures have been considered as potential risk factors for the exercising athlete (O'Connor et al., 2010). The large number of 'unsuccessful starters' and medical encounters when marathons are held in hot environment signifies the potential risk of competing in the heat (Ely et al., 2007; Roberts, 2007). Analogously, soccer match play in the heat will challenge the players' ability to maintain homeostasis and if athletes are not adequately prepared, it will increase the risk of heat illnesses (O'Connor et al., 2010; Gisolfi and Robinson, 1969; Roberts, 2010). However, when well-trained subjects follow the acclimatization and hydration guidelines described above, exercise in the heat does not aggravate recovery (Nybo et al., 2013) and athletes commonly compete in the heat achieving very high core temperatures without experiencing other symptoms than the fatigue associated with such exercise (Pugh et al., 2002; Racinais et al., 2015b). Indeed, during the 2014 FIFA World Cup in Brazil there was no report of heat-related medical conditions (Dvorak and Junge, 2015). Soccer matches are associated with muscle damage, slow recovery of muscle glycogen and functional performance (Krustrup et al., 2011; Nielsen et al., 2012). However, neither indices of muscle damage nor the recovery of sprint or intermittent endurance performance are aggravated following match play in the heat (see Figure 10.2).

In conclusion, we support the position statements from athletic trainers (Binkley et al., 2002) and consensus statements from international expert panels (O'Connor et al., 2010; Racinais et al., 2015a), that medical doctors and event organizers should be extraordinary aware of potential heat illness symptoms and for safety reasons provide the set-up for treatment of overheating, excessive dehydration and other potential pathophysiological responses (Capacchione and Muldoon, 2009; Kerr et al., 2014; Sawka et al., 2011). However, if players are properly trained, acclimatized and remain adequately hydrated, soccer matches can be completed in the heat without jeopardizing the participants' health or aggravating recovery (Nybo et al., 2013). The environmental temperature will influence match-play characteristics and especially reduce high-intensity running. However, players are capable of adjusting their exercise effort and maintain other key performance indicators. Consequently, playing in the heat does not attenuate the technical quality of the game or influence the number of goals per match.

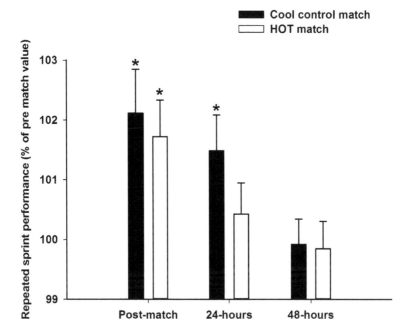

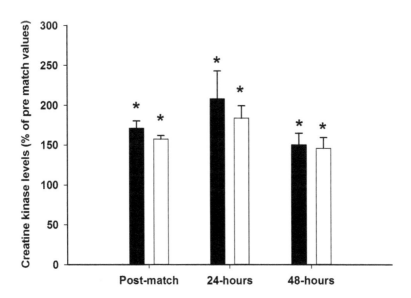

Figure 10.2 Recovery of functional sprint capacity (top panel) and creatine kinase (CK; lower panel) responses immediately post-match, 24 hours and 48 hours following experimental games conducted in either cool control settings (17 °C WBGT − 21 degree Celsius with 55 percent relative humidity) or in the heat (35 °C WBGT; 43 degree Celsius with 12 percent relative humidity). * Significantly elevated compared to pre-match value

Source: modified from Nybo et al. (2013) with permission.

References

Asmussen, E. and Bøje, O. (1945). Body temperature and capacity for work. *Acta Physiologica Scandinavica, 10*, 1–22.

Bangsbo, J., Mohr, M. and Krustrup, P. (2006). Physical and metabolic demands of training and match-play in the elite football player. *Journal of Sports Sciences, 24*, 665–674.

Bergeron, M., Bahr, R., Bartsch, P., Bourdon, L., Calbet, J., Carlsen, K. Castagna, O., González-Alonso, J., Lundby, C., Maughan, R. J., Millet, G., Mountjoy, M., Racinais, S., Rasmussen, P., Subudhi, A. W., Young, A. J., Soligard, T. and Engebretsen, L. (2012). International Olympic Committee consensus statement on thermoregulatory and altitude challenges for high-level athletes. *British Journal of Sports Medicine, 46*(11), 770–779.

Binkley, H. M., Beckett, J., Casa, D. J., Kleiner, D. M. and Plummer, P. E. (2002). National Athletic Trainers' Association position statement: exertional heat illnesses. *Journal of Athletic Training, 37*, 329–343.

Bishop, D. (2003a). Warm up I: potential mechanisms and the effects of passive warm up on exercise performance. *Sports Medicine, 33*, 439–454.

Bishop, D. (2003b). Warm up II: performance changes following active warm up and how to structure the warm up. *Sports Medicine, 33*, 483–498.

Capacchione, J. F. and Muldoon, S. M. (2009). The relationship between exertional heat illness, exertional rhabdomyolysis, and malignant hyperthermia. *Anesthesia and Analgesia Journal, 109*, 1065–1069.

Drust, B., Rasmussen, P., Mohr, M., Nielsen, B. and Nybo, L. (2005). Elevations in core and muscle temperature impairs repeated sprint performance. *Acta Physiologica Scandinavica, 183*, 181–190.

Dvorak, D. and Junge, A. (2015) Twenty years of the FIFA Medical Assessment and Research Centre: from 'Medicine for Football' to 'Football for Health'. *British Journal of Sports Medicine, 49*, 561–563.

Ely, M. R., Cheuvront, S. N., Roberts, W. O. and Montain, S. J. (2007). Impact of weather on marathon-running performance. *Medicine and Science in Sports and Exercise, 39*, 487–493.

Girard, O., Bishop, D. J. and Racinais, S. (2012). Hot conditions improve power output during repeated cycling sprints without modifying neuromuscular fatigue characteristics. *European Journal of Applied Physiology, 113*, 359–369.

Gisolfi, C. and Robinson, S. (1969). Relations between physical training, acclimatization, and heat tolerance. *Journal of Applied Physiology, 26*, 530–534.

Gonzalez-Alonso, J., Crandall, C. G. and Johnson, J. M. (2008). The cardiovascular challenge of exercising in the heat. *Journal of Physiology, 586*, 45–53.

Gonzalez-Alonso, J., Teller, C., Andersen, S., Jensen, F., Hyldig, T. and Nielsen, B. (1999). Influence of body temperature on the development of fatique during prolonged exercise in the heat. *Journal of Applied Physiology, 86*, 1032–1039.

Grantham, J., Cheung, S. S., Connes, P., Febbraio, M. A., Gaoua, N., Gonzalez-Alonso, J., Hue, O., Johnson, J. M., Maughan, R. J., Meeusen, R., Nybo, L., Racinais, S., Shirreffs, S. M. and Dvorak, J. (2010). Current knowledge on playing football in hot environments. *Scandinavian Journal of Medicine and Science in Sports, 20 suppl. 3*, 161–167.

Grundstein, A. J., Ramseyer, C., Zhao, F., Pesses, J. L., Akers, P., Qureshi, A., Becker, L., Knox, J. A. and Petro, M. (2012). A retrospective analysis of American football hyperthermia deaths in the United States. *International Journal of Biometeorology, 56*, 11–20.

James, L. J., Evans, G. H., Madin, J., Scott, D., Stepney, M., Harris, R., Stone, R. and Clayton, D. J. (2013). Effect of varying the concentrations of carbohydrate and milk protein in rehydration solutions ingested after exercise in the heat. *British Journal of Nutrition, 110*, 1285–1291.

Karlsen, A., Nybo, L., Norgaard, S. J., Jensen, M. V., Bonne, T. and Racinais, S. (2015). Time course of natural heat acclimatization in well-trained cyclists during a 2-week training camp in the heat. *Scandinavian Journal of Medicine and Science in Sports, 25 suppl. 1*, 240–249.

Kerr, Z. Y., Marshall, S. W., Comstock, R. D. and Casa, D. J. (2014). Implementing exertional heat illness prevention strategies in US high school football. *Medicine and Science in Sports and Exercise, 46*, 124–130.

Krustrup, P., Ortenblad, N., Nielsen, J., Nybo, L., Gunnarsson, T. P., Iaia, F. M., Madsen, K., Stephens, F., Greenhaff, P. and Bangsbo, J. (2011). Maximal voluntary contraction force, SR function and glycogen resynthesis during the first 72 h after a high-level competitive soccer game. *European Journal of Applied Physiology, 111*, 2987–2995.

Maughan, R. J., Merson, S. J., Broad, N. P. and Shirreffs, S. M. (2004). Fluid and electrolyte intake and loss in elite soccer players during training. *International Journal of Sport Nutrition and Exercise Metabolism, 14*, 333–346.

Maughan, R. J., Shirreffs, S. M., Ozgunen, K. T., Kurdak, S. S., Ersoz, G., Binnet, M. S. and Dvorak, J. (2010). Living, training and playing in the heat: challenges to the football player and strategies for coping with environmental extremes. *Scandinavian Journal of Medicine and Science in Sports, 20 suppl. 3*, 117–124.

Mohr, M., Krustrup, P. and Bangsbo, J. (2005). Fatigue in soccer: a brief review. *Journal of Sports Sciences, 23*, 593–599.

Mohr, M., Krustrup, P., Nybo, L., Nielsen, J. J. and Bangsbo, J. (2004). Muscle temperature and sprint performance during soccer matches – beneficial effect of re-warm-up at half-time. *Scandinavian Journal of Medicine and Science in Sports, 14*, 156–162.

Mohr, M., Nybo, L., Grantham, J. and Racinais, S. (2012). Physiological responses and physical performance during football in the heat. *PLoS.One, 7*, e39202.

Nassis, G. P., Brito, J., Dvorak, J., Chalabi, H. and Racinais, S. (2015). The association of environmental heat stress with performance: analysis of the 2014 FIFA World Cup Brazil. *British Journal of Sports Medicine, 49*, 609–613.

Nielsen, J., Krustrup, P., Nybo, L., Gunnarsson, T. P., Madsen, K., Schroder, H. D., Bangsbo, J. and Ortenblad, N. (2012). Skeletal muscle glycogen content and particle size of distinct subcellular localizations in the recovery period after a high-level soccer match. *European Journal of Applied Physiology, 112*(10), 3559–3567.

Nielsen, B., Strange, S., Christensen, N. J., Warberg, J. and Saltin, B. (1997). Acute and adaptive responses in human to exercise in a warm, humid environment. *Pflügers Archiv – European Journal of Physiology, 434*, 49–56.

Nybo, L., Girard, O., Mohr, M., Knez, W., Voss, S. and Racinais, S. (2013). Markers of muscle damage and performance recovery after exercise in the heat. *Medicine and Science in Sports and Exercise, 45*, 860–868.

Nybo, L., Jensen, T., Nielsen, B. and Gonzalez-Alonso, J. (2001). Effects of marked hyperthermia with and without dehydration on VO_2 kinetics during intense exercise. *Journal of Applied Physiology, 90*, 1057-1064.

Nybo, L. and Nielsen, B. (2001). Hyperthermia and central fatigue during prolonged exercise in humans. *Journal of Applied Physiology, 91*, 1055–1060.

Nybo, L., Rasmussen, P. and Sawka, M. N. (2014). Performance in the heat-physiological factors of importance for hyperthermia-induced fatigue. *Comprehensive Physiology, 4*, 657–689.

O'Connor, F. G., Casa, D. J., Bergeron, M. F., Carter, R., III, Deuster, P., Heled, Y., Kark, J., Leon, L., McDermott, B., O'Brien, K., Roberts, W. O. and Sawka, M. (2010). American

College of Sports Medicine Roundtable on exertional heat stroke – return to duty/return to play: conference proceedings. *Current Sports Medicine Reports*, 9, 314–321.

Ozgunen, K. T., Kurdak, S. S., Maughan, R. J., Zeren, C., Korkmaz, S., Yazici, Z., Ersöz, G., Shirreffs, S. M., Binnet, M. S. and Dvorak, J. (2010). Effect of hot environmental conditions on physical activity patterns and temperature response of football players. *Scandinavian Journal of Medicine and Science in Sports*, 20 suppl. 3, 140–147.

Paul, D.J., Bradley, P.S. and Nassis, G.P. (2015). Factors affecting match running performance of elite soccer players: shedding some light on the complexity. *International Journal of Sports Physiology and Performance*, 10, 516–519.

Periard, J.D. and Racinais, S. (2015). Self-paced exercise in hot and cool conditions is associated with the maintenance of %VO2peak within a narrow range. *Journal of Applied Physiology (1985)*, 118, 1258–1265.

Periard, J.D., Racinais, S., Knez, W.L., Herrera, C.P., Christian, R.J. and Girard, O. (2014). Thermal, physiological and perceptual strain mediate alterations in match-play tennis under heat stress. *British Journal of Sports Medicine*, 48 suppl. 1, i32–i38.

Pugh, L., Corbett, J. and Johnson, R. (2002). Rectal temperatures, weight losses, and sweat rates in marathon running. *Journal of Applied Physiology*, 23, 347–352.

Racinais, S., Alonso, J. M., Coutts, A. J., Flouris, A.D., Girard, O., Gonzalez-Alonso, J., Hausswirth, C., Jay, O., Lee, J. K., Mitchell, N., Nassis, G. P., Nybo, L., Pluim, B. M., Roelands, B., Sawka, M. N., Wingo, J. E. and Périard, J. D. (2015a). Consensus recommendations on training and competing in the heat. *Scandinavian Journal of Medicine and Science in Sports*, 25 suppl. 1, 6–19.

Racinais, S., Buchheit, M., Bilsborough, J., Bourdon, P.C., Cordy, J. and Coutts, A.J. (2014). Physiological and performance responses to a training camp in the heat in professional Australian football players. *International Journal of Sports Physiology and Performance*, 9, 598–603.

Racinais, S., Mohr, M., Buchheit, M., Voss, S.C., Gaoua, N., Grantham, J. and Nybo, L. (2012). Individual responses to short-term heat acclimatisation as predictors of football performance in a hot, dry environment. *British Journal of Sports Medicine*, 46, 810–815.

Racinais, S. and Oksa, J. (2010). Temperature and neuromuscular function. *Scandinavian Journal of Medicine and Science in Sports*, 20 suppl. 3, 1–18.

Racinais, S., Periard, J.D., Karlsen, A. and Nybo, L. (2015b). Effect of heat and heat acclimatization on cycling time trial performance and pacing. *Medicine and Science in Sports and Exercise*, 47, 601–606.

Roberts, W.O. (2007). Exercise-associated collapse care matrix in the marathon. *Sports Medicine*, 37, 431–433.

Roberts, W.O. (2010). Determining a "do not start" temperature for a marathon on the basis of adverse outcomes. *Medicine and Science in Sports and Exercise*, 42, 226–232.

Ross, M., Abbiss, C., Laursen, P., Martin, D. and Burke, L. (2013). Precooling methods and their effects on athletic performance: a systematic review and practical applications. *Sports Medicine*, 43, 207–225.

Sawka, M.N., Leon, L., Montain, S.J. and Sonna, L. (2011). Integrated physiological mechanisms of exercise performance, adaptation, and maladaptation to heat stress. *Comprehensive Physiology*, 1, 1883–1928.

Sawka, M.N., Burke, L.M., Eichner, E.R., Maughan, R.J., Montain, S.J. and Stachenfeld, N.S. (2007). American College of Sports Medicine position stand. Exercise and fluid replacement. *Medicine and Science in Sports and Exercise*, 39, 377–390.

Taylor, N.A. (2014). Human heat adaptation. *Comprehensive Physiology*, 4, 325–365.

Todd, G., Butler, J.E., Taylor, J.L. and Gandevia, S.C. (2005). Hyperthermia: a failure of the motor cortex and the muscle. *Journal of Physiology*, 563, 621–631.

Injuries

11 Epidemiology of rugby injuries

Colin Fuller

Introduction

Rugby union (Rugby) is played by women, girls, men and boys; however, men and schoolboys make up the majority of players. In 2014, there were 2.6 million registered and 4.5 million non-registered players playing the game of Rugby across the world (World Rugby, 2015a). The sport is played in 15-a-side (Rugby 15-s; forwards: 8; backs: 7) and 7-a-side (Rugby-7s; forwards: 3; backs: 4) formats of the game. Although both versions of Rugby are played on the same size pitch, the two versions of the game are different in terms of the size of players (Fuller et al., 2013a) and the skills required by players (Roberts et al., 2008) in the two formats. There are major national and regional competitions for Rugby in both the northern and southern hemispheres. World Cup competitions take place every four years in both Rugby-15s and Rugby-7s; in addition, Rugby-7s was recently accepted as an Olympic sport for Rio 2016.

Rugby is governed by five core values: integrity, passion, solidarity, discipline and respect. These values are important for the game, as the Foreword to the Laws of the Game (page 3) emphasizes the physical nature of the game and clearly recognizes the associated risks of injury (World Rugby, 2014):

> Rugby Union is a sport which involves physical contact. Any sport involving physical contact has inherent dangers. It is very important that players play the game in accordance with the Laws of the Game and be mindful of the safety of themselves and others.
>
> (World Rugby, 2014)

Consequently, World Rugby places a high priority on player welfare in all aspects of the game and routinely monitors and reports the incidence and nature of injuries at all international Rugby competitions (Fuller et al., 2008, 2010a, 2013b).

This chapter summarizes the incidence, severity, nature and causes of match injuries sustained at the senior men's international level of play in both Rugby-15s and Rugby-7s; the results presented are based on epidemiological studies carried out on behalf of World Rugby at the 2007 (Fuller et al., 2008) and 2011 (Fuller et al., 2013b) Rugby World Cups and the 2008 to 2014 Sevens World Series (World Rugby, 2015b).

Incidence of injuries

As for many sports, published epidemiological data for Rugby have been blighted over the years by variations in injury and exposure definitions and data collection and reporting methodologies. This issue was addressed in 2007 when the International Rugby Board facilitated the development of an international consensus statement on the reporting of epidemiology studies within Rugby (Fuller et al., 2007a). Subsequent to the preparation of this consensus statement, all significant published epidemiological studies for Rugby have followed these recommendations and guidelines (World Rugby, 2015b).

The overall incidence of injury in Rugby-15s is 86.5 injuries/1,000 player–match–hours. While there is no significant difference in the overall incidences of injury for forwards and backs, there are differences when specific playing positions are examined: forwards – all players: 84.5 injuries/1,000 player–match–hours, front row: 80.7 injuries/1,000 player–match–hours, second row: 64.5 injuries/1,000 player–match–hours, back row: 101.6 injuries/1,000 player–match–hours; backs – all players: 88.7 injuries/1,000 player–match–hours, halves: 82.0 injuries/1000 player–match–hours, inside backs: 97.6 injuries/1000 player–match–hours, outside backs: 87.2 injuries/1000 player–match–hours, respectively.

For Rugby-7s, the overall incidence of injury is 108.5 injuries/1000 player–match–hours with the incidence of injury for backs (119.5 injuries/1,000 player–match–hours), significantly higher than that for forwards (93.8 injuries/1,000 player–match–hours). Overall, the incidence of injuries sustained by Rugby-7s players is significantly higher than that for Rugby-15s players.

Severity of injuries

The mean severity of all injuries sustained by all players in Rugby-15s is 19.1 days (median severity: 6.5 days): the difference in the severity of injuries sustained by forwards (mean: 17.6 days; median: 6 days) and backs (mean: 20.8 days; median: 8.5 days) is small. There are, however, again some differences between specific playing positions: forwards: mean – front row: 15.7 days, second row: 16.2 days, back row: 19.9 days; median – front row: 5.5 days, second row: 8 days, back row: 6 days; backs: mean – halves: 23.1 days, inside backs: 26.9 days, outside backs: 14.9 days; median – halves: 8 days, inside backs: 9 days, outside backs: 7 days, respectively.

For Rugby-7s, the mean severity of all injuries sustained by all players is 44.9 days (median severity: 28 days): there is no significant difference in the severity of injuries sustained by forwards (mean: 42.2 days; median: 26 days) and backs (mean: 46.5 days; median: 29 days). The difference in injury severity between Rugby-7s and Rugby-15s is related to the differing nature of the injuries sustained in Rugby-7s compared to Rugby-15s (see section below on location and type of injury). Overall, the severity of injuries sustained by Rugby-7s players is significantly higher than that for Rugby-15s players.

Nature of injuries

Location

The distributions of injury locations observed for Rugby-7s and Rugby-15s are summarized in Table 11.1.

Table 11.1 Location of injuries sustained in Rugby 7-a-side (Rugby-7s) and Rugby-15s

Body location of injury	Proportion of injuries, %					
	Rugby-7s			Rugby-15s		
	Forwards	*Backs*	*All*	*Forwards*	*Backs*	*All*
Head/neck	29.5	14.4	19.4	18.8	10.9	15.0
Upper limb	20.5	15.6	17.2	15.6	24.6	20.1
Trunk	4.5	4.4	4.5	15.6	9.2	12.5
Lower limb	45.5	65.6	59.0	50.0	55.3	52.3

Injuries to the lower limbs predominate in both Rugby-7s (59.0 percent of injuries) and Rugby-15s (52.3 percent) but injuries to the head/neck for forwards and backs and injuries to the lower limb for backs are higher in Rugby-7s than Rugby-15s, which reflects the faster, more open nature of the game of Rugby-7s compared to Rugby-15s.

Type

The distributions of injury types sustained in Rugby-7s and Rugby-15s are summarized in Table 11.2.

Joint (non-bone)/ligament injuries (49.3 percent of injuries) predominate in Rugby-7s while muscle/tendon injuries (46.0 percent) predominate in Rugby-15s. A higher proportion of injuries sustained to the central nervous system in

Table 11.2 Type of injuries sustained in Rugby 7-a-side (Rugby-7s) and Rugby-15s

Type of injury	Proportion of injuries, %					
	Rugby-7s			Rugby-15s		
	Forwards	*Backs*	*All*	*Forwards*	*Backs*	*All*
Bone	11.4	8.9	9.7	9.0	6.0	7.6
CNS/PNS*	18.2	11.1	13.4	10.3	5.9	8.2
Joint/ligament	43.2	52.2	49.3	33.6	34.0	33.7
Muscle/tendon	22.7	25.6	24.6	42.2	50.3	46.0
Skin	2.3	2.2	2.2	0.6	1.3	1.0
Other	2.3	0.0	0.7	4.3	2.6	3.5

* C/PNS: central/peripheral nervous system

Rugby-7s compared to Rugby-15s, for both forwards and backs, reflects the higher incidence of head injuries and a high proportion of joint/ligament injuries sustained by backs in Rugby-7s reflects the high incidence of lower limb injuries in Rugby-7s.

Causes of injury

The majority of injuries sustained in both Rugby-7s (all players: 78.2 percent of injuries, forwards: 87.7 percent, backs: 72.5 percent) and Rugby-15s (all players: 78.6 percent, forwards: 81.9 percent, backs: 75.0 percent) occur during contact events, such as tackling, being tackled and collisions (Fuller et al., 2007b, 2010b; Quarrie and Hopkins, 2008). However, a high proportion of injuries are also sustained during non-contact events (Rugby-7s – all players: 21.3 percent of injuries, forwards: 11.8 percent, backs: 26.9 percent; Rugby-15s – all players: 21.3 percent, forwards: 18.3 percent, backs: 24.7 percent); see Table 11.3.

Although infrequent in number, cervical spine injuries have historically received the greatest attention in Rugby due to the potentially catastrophic consequences from such injuries. This type of injury is most likely to result from an arm tackle above shoulder height, a spear tackle in which the ball carrier is turned upside down during contact resulting in the tackled player's head forcefully hitting the ground or from an incorrect scrum engagement, respectively. The Laws of the Game have been changed in recent years in order to reduce the risks associated with these actions (World Rugby, 2014). Spear tackles and arm tackles above shoulder height are banned in the game with any player committing either of these actions being immediately red-carded by the referee and then severely punished post-game in terms of future match bans. For the scrum, the

Table 11.3 Match events leading to injuries sustained in Rugby 7-a-side (Rugby-7s) and Rugby-15s

Match events	Proportion of injuries, %					
	Rugby-7s			Rugby-15s		
	Forwards	*Backs*	*All*	*Forwards*	*Backs*	*All*
Collision	14.6	12.3	13.1	14.0	17.4	15.7
Kicking	0.0	0.9	0.5	0.0	2.8	1.4
Lineout	2.4	0.0	0.9	1.3	0.0	0.6
Maul	0.5	0.6	0.5	5.1	4.1	4.7
Ruck	10.7	5.6	7.5	12.0	6.4	9.3
Running	10.2	24.3	19.0	13.0	20.0	16.4
Scrum	2.4	0.0	0.9	8.3	0.0	4.4
Tackled	32.0	33.9	33.2	23.3	34.2	28.4
Tackling	22.8	19.0	20.4	19.1	12.9	16.0
Other	4.4	3.5	3.8	4.0	1.9	2.9

most vulnerable players (front row) must be specially trained and be sufficiently experienced before they are allowed to play in this position at the senior level, and the scrum engagement process has been modified to de-power the scrum engagement process.

More recently, World Rugby has focused on the risk of concussion injuries in Rugby. For this type of injury, World Rugby has invested in improving the on-pitch identification of concussion, and the post-match management and return-to-play criteria for concussed players.

Summary

Taking both the incidence and the severity of match injuries sustained in Rugby-7s and Rugby-15s into account, the overall risk of injury in Rugby-7s is around three times higher than that observed in Rugby-15s.

References

Fuller, C.W., Ashton, T., Brooks, J.H.M., Cancea, R.J., Hall, J. and Kemp, S.P. (2010b). Injury risks associated with tackling in rugby union. *British Journal of Sports Medicine*, *44*, 159–167.

Fuller, C.W., Brooks, J.H.M., Cancea, R.J., Hall, J. and Kemp, S.P. (2007b). Contact events in rugby union and their propensity to cause injury. *British Journal of Sports Medicine*, *41*, 862–867.

Fuller, C.W., Laborde, F., Leather, R.J. and Molloy, M.G. (2008). International Rugby Board Rugby World Cup 2007 injury surveillance study. *British Journal of Sports Medicine*, *42*, 452–459.

Fuller, C.W., Molloy, M.G., Bagate, C., Bahr, R., Brooks, J.H., Donson, H., Kemp, S.P.T., McCrory, P., McIntosh, A.S., Meeuwisse, W.H., Quarrie, K.L., Raftery, M. and Wiley, P. (2007a). Consensus statement on injury definitions and data collection procedures for studies of injuries in rugby union. *British Journal of Sports Medicine*, *41*, 328–331.

Fuller, C.W., Sheerin, K. and Targett, S. (2013b). Rugby World Cup 2011: International Rugby Board injury surveillance study. *British Journal of Sports Medicine*, *47*, 1184–1191.

Fuller, C.W., Taylor, A., Brooks, J.H.M. and Kemp, S.P. (2013a). Changes in the stature, body mass and age of English professional rugby players: a 10-year review. *Journal of Sports Science*, *31*, 795–802.

Fuller, C.W., Taylor, A. and Molloy, M.G. (2010a). Epidemiological study of injuries in international rugby sevens. *Clinical Journal of Sport Medicine*, *20*, 179–184.

Quarrie, K.L. and Hopkins, W.G. (2008). Tackle injuries in professional rugby union. *American Journal of Sports Medicine*, *36*, 1705–1716.

Roberts, S.P., Trewartha, G., Higgitt R.J., El-Abd, J. and Stokes, K.A. (2008). The physical demands of elite English rugby union. *Journal of Sports Science*, *26*, 825–833.

World Rugby (2014). *Laws of the Game: Rugby Union*. World Rugby, Dublin, 2014.

World Rugby (2015a). *Player numbers*. www.worldrugby.org (last accessed May 1, 2015).

World Rugby (2015b). *Surveillance Studies*. World Rugby, Dublin 2015. Available at: http://playerwelfare.worldrugby.org (last accessed May 1, 2015).

12 Prevention of contact and non-contact injuries in football/soccer

20 years of F-MARC

Mario Bizzini

Introduction

Soccer (football) is the most popular sport worldwide, with an estimated 300 million players and even more individuals involved at any levels (coaching refereeing, other). Playing soccer is also associated with a certain risk of injury. Injury prevention is one important task of the Medical Committee of the Fédération Internationale de Football Association (FIFA). This contribution summarizes more than 20 years of scientific and on-field work in injury prevention by FIFA, the governing body of soccer, and its Medical Assessment and Research Centre (F-MARC). The epidemiology of soccer injuries, injury mechanisms and risk factors will not be addressed in this contribution.

Why injury prevention?

From a medical perspective: with every injury the risk for a subsequent injury rises (especially in case of insufficient rehabilitation and retraining), and severe injuries (as anterior cruciate ligament and cartilage lesions) may increase the risk of osteoarthritis in the long term. From a player perspective: staying injury-free is crucial to train and perform at the highest possible personal level. From a coach's perspective, to have fewer injuries means to have most of the players at disposal for training and matches. Additionally, it has been found that elite teams with fewer injured players were better in terms of results and championship ranking. From a socioeconomic perspective, the overall amount of injuries causes a significant impact on the health-related costs (medical treatment, rehabilitation, sickness leave, etc.). As an example, in Switzerland (7.9 million inhabitants) the healthcare costs for injuries in amateur soccer were nearly US$170 million in 2010 (Bizzini et al., 2013).

Preventing contact injuries

Contact injuries account for a high percentage of all injuries, especially at international competitive level: approximately 50–60 percent of all traumatic injuries are caused by the actions of another player (usually an opponent), and 12–28 percent of all injuries by foul play (Junge and Dvorak, 2004).

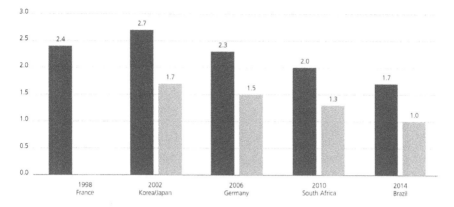

Figure 12.1 Number of injuries per match in FIFA World Cups 1998–2014 (all injuries
(grey bars); injuries expected to result in time loss (black bars)); *information
with regard to time loss was not documented during the 1998 FIFA World Cup

Source: with permission of F-MARC.

In 2006, and following several F-MARC research projects, the International
Football Association Board (IFAB) decided that any incident of elbow to the head
should be sanctioned with a red card and later, the same was decided for the
tackles from behind, and the two-footed tackles from the side. The consequent
application of these decisions helped in reducing the number of head and ankle
injuries caused by elbowing and dangerous tackles (Dvorak, 2009). Data from the
last male FIFA World Cups (2006, 2010, 2014) proved that the reinforcement of
the Laws of the Game and the subsequent stricter refereeing during the competitions were important in protecting the health of the players (Figure 12.1) (Junge
and Dvorak, 2015).

Preventing non-contact injuries

The percentage of non-contact injuries ranges from 26–59 percent (Junge and
Dvorak, 2004). Overuse injuries account for 9–34 percent of all injuries, but
probably these numbers underestimated the real prevalence, e.g. due to methodological problems with the injury definitions used in many studies (Bahr,
2009). Research also shows that about 20–30 percent of all injuries (mostly
non-contact) are re-injuries of the same type and location (Junge and Dvorak,
2004).

Jan Ekstrand was the first to publish a controlled trail on injury prevention
in soccer, showing that a multimodal intervention program comprising adapted
equipment, warm-up routine, prophylactic ankle taping, controlled rehabilitation, etc. was effective in reducing overall incidence of injuries by 75 percent
in male Swedish senior teams (Ekstrand et al., 1983). About 20 years later,

F-MARC and Astrid Junge duplicated this study introducing specific stabilization and coordination exercises for the trunk, ankle and knee joints in the multimodal program, and found an injury reduction of 21 percent in male Swiss amateur youth teams (Junge et al., 2002). Thereby, the basis was set for a working strategy for the years to come: non-contact injuries may be targeted with specific exercises or exercise-based programs, and F-MARC along with international collaborators intensified their work in the following years in developing and evaluating programs aimed at injury prevention, e.g. "The 11" and its advanced version "FIFA 11+."

About 30 publications on the effectiveness of injury prevention measures in soccer players can be found in the literature and F-MARC was actively involved in about half of these papers.

Summarizing these publications, between 20 and 50 percent all non-contact soccer injuries can be prevented with exercise-based prevention programs (Silvers-Granelli et al., 2015; Soligard et al., 2008). The best available evidence is for female adolescent players, whereas the impact of such programs in male players has been demonstrated only recently. Based on the current evidence, the key elements of effective injury prevention programs (at best, embedded in a warm-up format) are core stability/strength, neuromuscular control and balance, eccentric training (especially of the hamstrings), plyometric and agility. Research has further identified how compliance is a crucial factor in prevention: the regular, quasi 'routine' performance of such exercises is needed to maximize the protective effect of those programs (Silvers-Granelli et al., 2015; Soligard et al., 2010). Other areas have been investigated around the neuromuscular warm-up/injury prevention programs: related performance effects, delivery methods and implementation strategies. The "FIFA 11+" injury prevention program is the most studied program worldwide, with 25 publications in these areas (Bizzini and Dvorak, 2015) (Figure 12.2).

In one of the best available randomized controlled trials (RCTs) on the performance effects of "FIFA 11+," it was found that the neuromuscular control (quicker stabilization time of lower extremity and core) was significantly better in players after nine weeks of "FIFA 11+" practice (Impellizzeri et al., 2013). Several other studies have found better functional balance, agility, knee muscle strength ratios, core and hip muscle activation in female and male player after performing this program (Bizzini and Dvorak, 2015). Additionally, a pre-post study in Italian male amateur players, showed how "FIFA 11+" induces similar physiological responses as other published warm-ups (Bizzini et al., 2013). A recent RCT evaluated different delivery methods of "FIFA 11+," and found that a pre-season coaching workshop was more effective (than unsupervised delivery, additional on-field supervision) in terms of adherence and even reduced injury risk in teams performing this injury prevention program (Steffen et al., 2013).

It is important to note that there's a lack of publications in injury prevention particularly in children younger than 12 years of age and in professional soccer players.

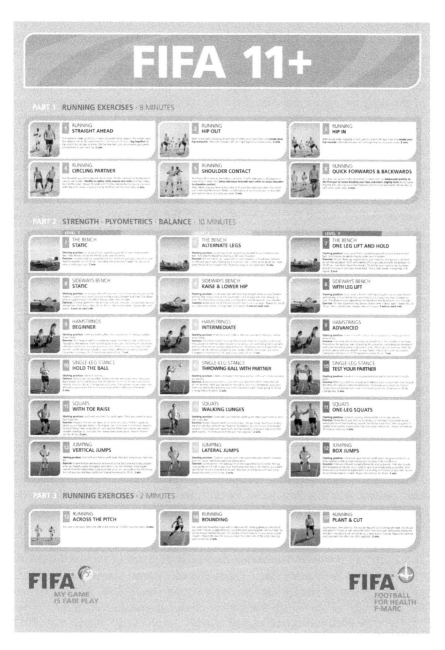

Figure 12.2 Official "FIFA 11+" poster (www.f-marc.com/11plus)

Source: with permission of F-MARC.

Dissemination and implementation of F-MARC programs

The first F-MARC injury prevention program "The 11" (ten evidence-based or best-practice exercises and the promotion of fair play) was implemented in two countrywide campaigns (Switzerland and New Zealand) in cooperation with the national accident insurance company and the national soccer association. The implementation of "The 11" in Swiss amateur soccer clubs and its effect on the injury rate were analyzed by an independent institute. Four years after the launch of the program, teams that included "The 11" as a part of their warm-up had 11.5 percent fewer match injuries and 25.3 percent fewer training injuries than teams that warmed-up as usual, and the insurance company also reported significant financial savings due to reduced medical-care costs (Junge et al., 2011). In New Zealand, the implementation of "The 11" resulted in 8.2 dollars in return of investment per each invested dollar in prevention for the national accident insurance company after eight years (Bizzini et al., 2013).

In 2009 FIFA started the dissemination of "FIFA 11+" in its 209 member associations (MAs). Based on the experience with the countrywide implementation in Switzerland and New Zealand, a guideline on how to implement the "FIFA 11+" injury prevention program at a larger scale in amateur soccer was developed. The implementation is conducted either in close cooperation with MAs or via FIFA coaching instructor courses (Bizzini et al., 2013). Although important results have been achieved and, for example, top MAs as Germany, Brazil and Japan have endorsed the program, a lot still remains to be done, especially in prioritizing 'injury prevention' in the overall enhancement of the health of soccer players within the MAs' responsibilities.

Prevention of sudden cardiac death

Considering the inherent risk of injury and sudden cardiac death (SCD) while competing, the health of soccer players and referees is of utmost importance. The prevention of SCD, a tragic event that might occur in presence of an underlying heart disease, in athletes is of utmost importance. A standardized Pre-Competition Medical Assessment (PCMA), focusing on the cardiovascular and musculoskeletal systems, was first introduced for all teams participating in the 2006 FIFA World Cup in Germany (Dvorak et al., 2009). Since then the PCMA has become mandatory for every player (male or female) and referee participating at a FIFA tournament at all levels (Bizzini et al., 2012). In recent years, F-MARC has also developed and promoted worldwide the "FIFA 11 Steps to Prevent SCD," the "FIFA Medical Emergency Bag," conducted educational courses on the practical management of sudden cardiac arrest on the soccer field, and emphasized the importance of immediate availability of an automated external defibrillator (AED) on the pitch during training and matches, respectively (Dvorak et al., 2013; Kramer et al., 2015). In 2014, FIFA, in cooperation with the Institute of Sports and Preventive Medicine in Saarbrücken, Germany, also established a worldwide Sudden Death Registry with the aim of documenting fatal events on the soccer fields (Scharhag et al., 2015).

Conclusions

Non-contact injuries in soccer can be prevented by 20 to 50 percent with specific injury prevention programs, whereas contact injuries may be prevented by enhanced fair play and stricter refereeing. Although there's still a lack of scientific studies in certain groups (i.e. children, professional players) and in different areas (i.e. influence of the playing surface, role of soccer shoes), the available evidence strongly supports the implementation of injury prevention programs on a large scale. Studies also showed performance benefits and even reduced health-related costs, if performing injury prevention programs. All involved associations and individuals, e.g. federations, clubs, coaches, players, fitness trainers, doctors, and physiotherapists, should endorse and promote injury prevention, thus keeping soccer a health-enhancing leisure activity.

References

Bahr, R. (2009). No injuries, but plenty of pain? On the methodology for recording overuse symptoms in sports. *British Journal of Sports Medicine*, *43*(13), 966–972.

Bizzini, M. and Dvorak, J. (2015). FIFA 11+: an effective programme to prevent football injuries in various player groups worldwide – a narrative review. *British Journal of Sports Medicine*, *49*(9), 577–579.

Bizzini, M., Impellizzeri, F. M., Dvorak, J., Bortolan, L., Schena, F., Modena, R. and Junge, A. (2013). Physiological and performance responses to the "FIFA 11+" (part 1): is it an appropriate warm-up? *Journal of Sports Sciences*, *31*(13), 1481–1490.

Bizzini, M., Junge, A. and Dvorak, J. (2013). Implementation of the FIFA 11+ football warm up program: how to approach and convince the Football associations to invest in prevention. *British Journal of Sports Medicine*, *47*(12), 803–806.

Bizzini, M., Schmied, C., Junge, A. and Dvorak, J. (2012). Precompetition medical assessment of referees and assistant referees selected for the 2010 FIFA World Cup. *British Journal of Sports Medicine*, *46*(5), 374–376.

Dvorak, J. (2009). Give Hippocrates a jersey: promoting health through football/sport. *British Journal of Sports Medicine*, *43*(5), 317–322.

Dvorak, J., Grimm, K., Schmied, C. and Junge, A. (2009). Development and implementation of a standardized precompetition medical assessment of international elite football players – 2006 FIFA World Cup Germany. *Clinical Journal of Sport Medicine*, *19*(4), 316–321.

Dvorak, J., Kramer, E. B., Schmied, C. M., Drezner, J. A., Zideman, D., Patricios, J., Correia, L., Pedrinelli, A. and Mandelbaum, B. (2013). The FIFA medical emergency bag and FIFA 11 steps to prevent sudden cardiac death: setting a global standard and promoting consistent football field emergency care. *British Journal of Sports Medicine*, *47*(18), 1199–1202.

Ekstrand, J., Gillquist, J. and Liljedahl, S. O. (1983). Prevention of soccer injuries. Supervision by doctor and physiotherapist. *American Journal of Sports Medicine*, *11*(3), 116–120.

Impellizzeri, F. M., Bizzini, M., Dvorak, J., Pellegrini, B., Schena, F. and Junge, A. (2013). Physiological and performance responses to the FIFA 11+ (part 2): a randomised controlled trial on the training effects. *Journal of Sports Sciences*, *31*(13), 1491–1502.

Junge, A. and Dvorak, J. (2004). Soccer injuries: a review on incidence and prevention. *Sports Medicine*, *34*(13), 929–938.

Junge, A. and Dvorak, J. (2015). Football injuries during the 2014 FIFA World Cup. *British Journal of Sports Medicine*, *49*(9), 599–602.

Junge, A., Lamprecht, M., Stamm, H., Hasler, H., Bizzini, M., Tschopp, M., Reuter, H., Wyss, H., Chilvers, C. and Dvorak, J. (2011). Countrywide campaign to prevent soccer injuries in Swiss amateur players. *American Journal of Sports Medicine*, *39*(1), 57–63.

Junge, A., Rosch, D., Peterson, L., Graf-Baumann, T. and Dvorak, J. (2002). Prevention of soccer injuries: a prospective intervention study in youth amateur players. *American Journal of Sports Medicine*, *30*(5), 652–659.

Kramer, E. B., Dvorak, J., Schmied, C. and Meyer, T. (2015). F-MARC: promoting the prevention and management of sudden cardiac arrest in football. *British Journal of Sports Medicine*, *49*(9), 597–598.

Scharhag, J., Bohm, P., Dvorak, J. and Meyer, T. (2015). F-MARC: the FIFA Sudden Death Registry (FIFA-SDR). *British Journal of Sports Medicine*, *49*(9), 563–565.

Silvers-Granelli, H., Mandelbaum, B., Adeniji, O., Insler, S., Bizzini, M., Pohlig, R., Junge, A., Snyder-Mackler, L. and Dvorak, J. (2015). Efficacy of the FIFA 11+ Injury Prevention Program in the Collegiate Male Soccer Player. *American Journal of Sports Medicine*, *43*(11), 2628–2637.

Soligard, T., Myklebust, G., Steffen, K., Holme, I., Silvers, H., Bizzini, M., Junge, A., Dvorak, J., Bahr, R. and Andersen, T. E. (2008). Comprehensive warm-up programme to prevent injuries in young female footballers: cluster randomised controlled trial. *BMJ*, *337*, a2469.

Soligard, T., Nilstad, A., Steffen, K., Myklebust, G., Holme, I., Dvorak, J., Roald B. and Andersen, T. E. (2010). Compliance with a comprehensive warm-up programme to prevent injuries in youth football. *British Journal of Sports Medicine*, *44*(11), 787–793.

Steffen, K., Meeuwisse, W. H., Romiti, M., Kang, J., McKay, C., Bizzini, M., Dvorak, J., Finch, C., Myklebust, G. and Emery, C. A. (2013). Evaluation of how different implementation strategies of an injury prevention programme (FIFA 11+) impact team adherence and injury risk in Canadian female youth football players: a cluster-randomised trial. *British Journal of Sports Medicine*, *47*(8), 480–487.

13 Eccentric training as treatment of muscle–tendon injury

Per Aagaard and Jesper Løvind Andersen

Introduction

Tendon and muscle overuse injury is frequently observed in sports and exercise, including elite soccer (Askling et al., 2003; Croisier et al., 2008; Fredberg et al., 2008; Petersen et al., 2011). Despite a high injury incidence, the optimal treatment modalities for tendinopathy are not fully identified (Langberg and Kongsgaard, 2008; Malliaras et al., 2013; Rees et al., 2009).

In recent years, however, the use of eccentric (ECC) exercise for the muscle–tendon complex has been found to produce moderate-to-good clinical results for the rehabilitation of Achilles and patellar tendinopathy, while promising results also have been reported for shoulder rotator cuff tendinopathy and tennis elbow problems. In addition, ECC training seems to be useful for the rehabilitation and prevention of recurrent muscle strain injury.

The detailed physiological mechanisms responsible for these adaptations remain to be fully understood. Also, it should be recognized that only sparse clinical or mechanistic evidence exists for using eccentric-only muscle actions during the rehabilitation of tendon overuse injury, which underlines that coupled eccentric–concentric loading regimes should be considered alongside or instead of eccentric loading for the treatment of Achilles and patellar tendinopathy (Malliaras et al., 2013).

Rehabilitation of tendon overuse injury by use of eccentric training

ECC muscle–tendon loading regimes have demonstrated promising results in terms of tendon injury rehabilitation (for recent reviews, see Langberg and Kongsgaard, 2008; Rees et al., 2009). Thus, clinically effective treatment results have been reported in response to ECC training regimes during conditions of persistent ('chronic') tendon overuse injury such as Achilles tendinopathy (Alfredson et al., 1998; Jonsson et al., 2008; Langberg et al., 2007; Roos et al., 2004), patellar tendinopathy (jumper's knee) (Frohm et al., 2007; Jonsson and Alfredson, 2005; Purdam et al., 2004; Young et al., 2005), anterior patella–femoral pain (Werner and Eriksson, 1993), rotator cuff tendinopathy (Camargo et al., 2014), tibialis posterior tendinopathy (Kulig et al., 2009) and lateral elbow tendinopathy (Croisier et al., 2007; Peterson et al., 2014).

In terms of potential adaptation mechanisms, using microdialysis techniques we have previously observed that ECC training led to elevated type I collagen synthesis in the Achilles tendon of elite soccer players suffering from overload tendinopathy (Langberg et al., 2007). Further, based on ultrasonography evaluation ECC training appears to result in reduced tendon swelling, loss of focal hypo echoic areas, a more regular tendon fiber structure and decreased hyper vascularization in Achilles tendinopathy patients (Kongsgaard et al., 2009; Öhberg et al., 2004). High-frequency tendon oscillations during ECC training may be involved in the adaptive recovery (Henriksen et al., 2009; Rees et al., 2008), which seems to rely more on the magnitude of strain than the force stimulus imposed on the tendon tissue (Allison and Purdam 2009; Kjaer et al., 2009).

Reduced or removed symptoms of anterior patella pain and jumper's knee also were observed after ECC decline squat training (Jonsson and Alfredson, 2005; Purdam et al., 2004). Recent data suggest that the superior rehabilitation achieved with ECC decline vs. horizontal squats likely occurs as a result of greater tendon strain with this type of training (Kongsgaard et al., 2006). Interestingly, patella tendon stiffness appears to increase in response to of heavy-resistance strength training (HRST) in healthy, non-injured adults (Kongsgaard et al., 2007; Reeves et al., 2003; Seynnes et al., 2009), resulting in a reduced magnitude of tendon strain for a given level of muscle force production (Kongsgaard et al., 2007). In turn, this reduction in tendon strain contributes to a reduced risk of micro-ruptures in loaded tendon collagen fibrils (Haraldsson et al., 2005), hence potentially reducing the risk of tendon overuse injury.

Illustrating the adaptive plasticity in tendon morphology, patellar tendon cross-sectional area (CSA) increased 5–7 percent following nine to 12 weeks of HRST in young healthy adults (Kongsgaard et al., 2007; Seynnes et al., 2009) with comparable results observed in the Achilles tendon (Arampatzis et al., 2007), resulting in reduced levels of tensile tendon stress ($\downarrow$ tendon Force/CSA) that potentially provide increased protection against tendon overuse injury. In addition, slow-type HRST performed in tendinopatic patellar tendons led to a normalization in tendon microstructure reflected by an increased distribution of small-sized vs. large-sized collagen fibrils, along with removed hyper vascularization, reduced collagen cross-linking, elevated collagen concentration and a trend for increased type I collagen synthesis (Kongsgaard et al., 2010).

Notably, the use of HRST leg press and squat exercise (three times/week) using slow contraction cycles (6 s) and involving coupled concentric–eccentric muscle contractions appeared to be more effective than ECC training or corticosteroid injection in the long-term rehabilitation of patellar tendinopathy (Kongsgaard et al., 2009).

Rehabilitation and prevention of muscle strain disorders by use of eccentric training

Hamstring muscle strains represent a frequent injury type in both elite and sub-elite soccer players as well as in track and field sprinters, martial arts fighters, water-skiing athletes and ballet dancers (Croisier, 2004). Hamstring muscle strain injury arises from multifactorial problems. Thus, several 'intrinsic' factors appear to dispose for hamstring strain injury and reinjury: hamstring strength deficits, particularly eccentric strength deficits, reduced flexibility at hip joint, knee joint, muscle–tendon modifications from previous strain injury/reinjury, and inadequate rehabilitation from previous strain injury/reinjury (Croisier, 2004). In many cases muscle strain injury (affecting hamstrings, calf muscles and hip flexors) may become chronic, as manifested by recurrent incidents of strain injury located at the initial site of injury. Thus, soccer players with a previous history of hamstring strain injury demonstrate a five to seven times higher risk of sustaining another strain injury compared to previously uninjured players (Arnason et al., 2004; Petersen et al., 2011).

Hamstring muscle strain disorders appear to be highly effectively rehabilitated (Croisier et al., 2002, 2008) or prevented by use of ECC muscle training (Arnason et al., 2008; Askling et al., 2003; Croisier et al., 2002, 2008; Petersen et al., 2011) or high inherent levels of ECC hamstring muscle strength (Croisier et al., 2008). Somewhat surprisingly, given the persistent nature of recurrent muscle injury, athletes with a history of multiple recurrent hamstring muscle strain injuries may also show complete rehabilitation (Croisier et al., 2002). In addition to the substantial reduction (almost complete removal) in muscle strain incidence with ECC training, indications of performance enhancements may also be observed. Thus, 30-m maximal running speed was improved 2.4 percent in soccer players following ten weeks (16 sessions) of ECC hamstring muscle exercise using the Yo-Yo flywheel device, whereas sprint capacity remained unchanged in players not allocated to this training modality (Askling et al., 2003).

Although the involved adaptive mechanisms for the reduction in muscle strain injury with ECC resistance exercise largely remain unknown, several candidate mechanisms may be proposed. For instance, ECC strength training in rats resulted in increased collagen turnover and neoformation of vinculin and talin (Frenette and Côté, 2000). These cytoskeletal proteins are involved in the transduction of force between the interior of the muscle fiber and the outer cell membrane, including its surrounding collagen tissue (extracellular matrix: ECM). Increasing these force-bearing cytoskeletal proteins by means of ECC training is likely to reduce the risk of micro-injuries in the interface between myofibers and the surrounding ECM, hence potentially reducing the risk of muscle strain injury. In addition, the involved adaptive mechanisms may include an enhanced remodeling capacity of the muscle fiber-ECM structures due to the increase in local (muscular) IGF-1 production reported with maximal ECC muscle contractions (Bamman et al., 2001; Heinemeier et al. 2007). Furthermore, longitudinal (serial) sarcomere addition in active myofibers as a result of prolonged ECC muscle training has been observed in animal experiments (Butterfield and Herzog, 2006; Lynn and Morgan, 1994). Such serial sarcomere addition inevitably results in slightly longer muscle fibers, in turn reducing the magnitude of strain imposed on the single sarcomeres during maximal ECC muscle actions performed in a given range of motion, thereby reducing the risk of muscle strain injury during such high-risk movements. ECC muscle training in humans have been reported to result in elongated muscle fascicle lengths (Baroni et al., 2013 Blazevich et al., 2007; Duclay et al., 2009; Potier et al., 2007; Seynnes et al., 2007), indicating that serial sarcomere addition (i.e. increased myofiber lengths) may be achieved in human individuals in response to ECC training.

Conclusions

Growing evidence demonstrate that resistance training can be used to effectively prevent and rehabilitate overuse injury in human muscle and tendon tissue. In particular, exercise with emphasis on eccentric (ECC) muscle contractions seems to prove useful for the rehabilitation and prevention of chronic muscle strain disorders and various types of tendinopathy conditions. Recent findings suggest that slow-type heavy-resistance strength training (HRST) may have similar beneficial effects, at least in conditions of tendon overuse injury (tendinopathy).

However, as recently suggested by Malliaras and coworkers (2013), it should be recognized that only limited (Achilles) and conflicting (patellar) evidence exist to suggest that the clinical outcome related to tendinopathy problems are superior with ECC loading compared with other loading regimes. Thus, clinicians should consider coupled concentric–eccentric loading activities alongside or instead of eccentric exercise in the treatment of Achilles and patellar tendinopathy (Malliaras et al., 2013).

References

Alfredson, H., Pietilä, T., Jonsson, P. and Lorentzon, R. (1998). Heavy-load eccentric calf muscle training for the treatment of chronic Achilles tendinosis. *American Journal of Sports Medicine, 26*, 360–366.

Allison, G. T. and Purdam, C. (2009). Eccentric loading for Achilles tendinopathy – strengthening or stretching? *British Journal of Sports Medicine, 43*, 276–279.

Arampatzis, A., Karamanidis, K. and Albracht, K. (2007). Adaptational responses of the human Achilles tendon by modulation of the applied cyclic strain magnitude. *Journal of Experimental Biology, 210*, 2743–2753.

Arnason, A., Andersen, T. E., Holme, I., Engebretsen, L. and Bahr, R. (2008). Prevention of hamstring strains in elite soccer: an intervention study. *Scandinavian Journal of Medicine and Science in Sports, 18*, 40–48.

Arnason, A., Sigurdsson, S. B., Gudmundsson, A., Holme, I., Engebretsen, L. and Bahr, R. (2004). Risk factors for injuries in football. *American Journal of Sports Medicine, 32*(suppl. 1), 5S-16S.

Askling, C., Karlsson, J. and Thorstensson, A. (2003). Hamstring injury occurrence in elite soccer players after preseason strength training with eccentric overload. *Scandinavian Journal of Medicine and Science in Sports, 13*, 244–250.

Bamman, M. M., Shipp, J. R., Jiang, J., Gower, B. A., Hunter, G. R., Goodman, A., McLafferty, C. L. Jr. and Urban, R. J. (2001). Mechanical load increases muscle IGF-I and androgen receptor mRNA concentrations in humans. *American Journal of Physiology: Endocrinology and Metabolism, 280*, E383–390.

Baroni, B. M., Geremia, J. M., Rodrigues, R., De Azevedo Franke, R., Karamanidis, K. and Vaz, M. A. (2013). Muscle architecture adaptations to knee extensor eccentric training: rectus femoris vs. vastus lateralis. *Muscle Nerve, 48*, 498–506.

Blazevich, A. J., Cannavan, D., Coleman, D. R. and Horne, S. (2007). Influence of concentric and eccentric resistance training on architectural adaptation in human quadriceps muscles. *Journal of Applied Physiology (1985), 103*, 1565–1575.

Butterfield, T. A. and Herzog, W. (2006). The magnitude of muscle strain does not influence serial sarcomere number adaptations following eccentric exercise. *Pflugers Archiv, 451*, 688–700.

Camargo, P. R., Alburquerque-Sendín, F. and Salvini, T. F. (2014). Eccentric training as a new approach for rotator cuff tendinopathy: Review and perspectives. *World Journal of Orthopaedics, 5*, 634–644.

Croisier, J. L. (2004). Factors Associated with Recurrent Hamstring Injuries. *Sports Medicine, 34*, 681–695.

Croisier, J. L., Forthomme, B., Namurois, M. H., Vanderthommen, M. and Crielaard, J. M. (2002). Hamstring muscle strain recurrence and strength performance disorders. *American Journal of Sports Medicine, 30*, 199–203.

Croisier, J. L., Foidart-Dessalle, M., Tinant, F., Crielaard, J. M. and Forthomme, B. (2007). An isokinetic eccentric programme for the management of chronic lateral epicondylar tendinopathy. *British Journal of Sports Medicine, 41*, 269–275.

Croisier, J. L., Ganteaume, S., Binet, J., Genty, M. and Ferret, J. M. (2008). Strength imbalances and prevention of hamstring injury in professional soccer players: a prospective study. *American Journal of Sports Medicine, 36*, 1469–1475.

Duclay, J., Martin, A., Duclay, A., Cometti, G. and Pousson, M. (2009). Behavior of fascicles and the myotendinous junction of human medial gastrocnemius following eccentric strength training. *Muscle Nerve, 39*, 819–827.

Fredberg, U., Bolvig, L. and Andersen, N. T. (2008). Prophylactic training in asymptomatic soccer players with ultrasonographic abnormalities in Achilles and patellar tendons: the Danish Super League Study. *American Journal of Sports Medicine, 36*, 451–460.

Frenette, J. and Côté, C. H. (2000). Modulation of structural protein content of the myotendinous junction following eccentric contractions. *International Journal of Sports Medicine, 21*, 313–320.

Frohm, A., Saartok, T., Halvorsen, K. and Renström, P. (2007). Eccentric treatment for patellar tendinopathy: a prospective randomised short-term pilot study of two rehabilitation protocols. *British Journal of Sports Medicine, 41*, e1–e6.

Haraldsson, B. T., Aagaard, P., Krogsgaard, M., Alkjaer, T., Kjaer, M. and Magnusson, S. P. (2005). Region-specific mechanical properties of the human patella tendon. *Journal of Applied Physiology, 98*, 1006–1012.

Henriksen, M., Aaboe, J., Bliddal, H. and Langberg, H. (2009). Biomechanical characteristics of the eccentric Achilles tendon. exercise. *Journal of Biomechanics, 42*, 2702–2707.

Heinemeier, K. M., Olesen, J. L., Schjerling, P., Haddad, F., Langberg, H., Baldwin, K. M. and Kjaer, M. (2007). Short-term strength training and the expression of myostatin and IGF-I isoforms in rat muscle and tendon: differential effects of specific contraction types. *Journal of Applied Physiology (1985), 102*, 573–581.

Jonsson, P. and Alfredson, H. (2005). Superior results with eccentric compared to concentric quadriceps training in patients with jumper's knee: a prospective randomised study. *British Journal of Sports Medicine, 39*, 847–850.

Jonsson, P., Alfredson, H., Sunding, K., Fahlström, M. and Cook, J. (2008). New regimen for eccentric calf-muscle training in patients with chronic insertional Achilles tendinopathy: results of a pilot study. *British Journal of Sports Medicine, 42*, 746–749.

Kjaer, M., Langberg, H., Heinemeier, K., Bayer, M. L., Hansen, M., Holm, L., Doessing, S., Kongsgaard, M., Krogsgaard, M. R. and Magnusson, S. P. (2009). From mechanical loading to collagen synthesis, structural changes and function in human tendon. *Scandinavian Journal of Medicine and Science in Sports, 19*, 500–510.

Kongsgaard, M., Aagaard, P., Roikjaer, S., Olsen, D., Jensen, M., Langberg, H. and Magnusson, S.P. (2006). Decline eccentric squats increases patellar tendon loading compared to standard eccentric squats. *Clinical Biomechanics, 21*, 748–754.

Kongsgaard, M., Reitelseder, S., Pedersen, T.G., Holm, L., Aagaard, P., Kjaer, M. and Magnusson, S.P. (2007). Region specific patellar tendon hypertrophy in humans following resistance training. *Acta Physiologica, 191*, 111–121.

Kongsgaard, M., Vuokko, K., Aagaard, P., Doessing, S., Hansen, P., Laursen, A. H., Kaldau, N. C., Kjaer, M. and Magnusson, S. P. (2009). Corticosteroid injections, eccentric decline squat training and heavy slow resistance training in patella tendinopathy. *Scandinavian Journal of Medicine and Science in Sports, 19*, 790–802.

Kongsgaard, M., Qvortrup, K., Larsen, J., Aagaard, P., Doessing, S., Hansen, P. ... Magnusson, S.P. (2010). Fibril Morphology and Tendon Mechanical Properties in Patellar Tendinopathy : Effects of Heavy Slow Resistance Training. *American Journal of Sports Medicine, 38*, 749–756.

Kulig, K., Lederhaus, E. S., Reischl, S., Arya, S. and Bashford, G. (2009). Effect of eccentric exercise program for early tibialis posterior tendinopathy. *Foot Ankle International, 30*, 877–885.

Langberg, H., Ellingsgaard, H., Madsen, T., Jansson, J., Magnusson, S.P., Aagaard, P. and Kjaer, M. (2007). Eccentric rehabilitation exercise increases peritendinous type I collagen synthesis in humans with Achilles tendinosis. *Scandinavian Journal of Medicine and Science in Sports, 17*, 61–66.

Langberg, H. and Kongsgaard, M. (2008). Eccentric training in tendinopathy – More questions than answers. *Scandinavian Journal of Medicine and Science in Sports, 18*, 541–542.

Lynn, R. and Morgan, D.L. (1994). Decline running produces more sarcomeres in rat vastus intermedius muscle fibers than does incline running. *Journal of Applied Physiology, 77*, 1439–1444.

Malliaras, P., Barton, C.J., Reeves, N.D. and Langberg, H. (2013). Achilles and patellar tendinopathy loading programmes: a systematic review comparing clinical outcomes and identifying potential mechanisms for effectiveness. *Sports Medicine, 43*, 267–286.

Öhberg, L., Lorentzon, R. and Alfredson, H. (2004). Eccentric training in patients with chronic Achilles tendinosis: normalised tendon structure and decreased thickness at follow up. *British Journal of Sports Medicine, 38*, 8–11.

Petersen, J., Thorborg, K., Nielsen, M. B., Budtz-Jørgensen, E. and Hölmich, P. (2011). Preventive effect of eccentric training on acute hamstring injuries in men's soccer: a cluster-randomized controlled trial. *American Journal of Sports Medicine, 39*, 2296–2303.

Peterson, M., Butler, S., Eriksson, M. and Svärdsudd, K. (2014). A randomized controlled trial of eccentric vs. concentric graded exercise in chronic tennis elbow (lateral elbow tendinopathy). *Clinical Rehabilitation, 28*, 862–872.

Potier, T.G., Alexander, C.M. and Seynnes, O.R. (2009). Effects of eccentric strength training on biceps femoris muscle architecture and knee joint range of movement. *European Journal of Applied Physiology 105*, 939–944.

Purdam, C.R., Jonsson, P., Alfredson, H., Lorentzon, R., Cook, J.L. and Khan, K.M. (2004). A pilot study of the eccentric decline squat in the management of painful chronic patellar tendinopathy. *British Journal of Sports Medicine, 38*, 395–397.

Rees, J.D., Lichtwark, G.A., Wolman, R.L. and Wilson, A.M. (2008). The mechanism for efficacy of eccentric loading in Achilles tendon injury; an in vivo study in humans. *Rheumatology, 47*, 1493–1497.

Rees, J. D., Wolman, R. L. and Wilson, A. (2009). Eccentric exercises; why do they work, what are the problems and how can we improve them? *British Journal of Sports Medicine*, *43*, 242–246.

Reeves, N. D., Maganaris, C. N. and Narici, M. V. (2003). Effect of strength training on human patella tendon mechanical properties of older individuals. *Journal of Physiology*, *548* (Pt 3), 971–981.

Roos, E. M., Engström, M., Lagerquist, A. and Söderberg, B. (2004). Clinical improvement after 6 weeks of eccentric exercise in patients with mid-portion Achilles tendinopathy – A randomized trial with 1-year follow-up. *Scandinavian Journal of Medicine and Science in Sports*, *14*, 286–295.

Seynnes, O. R., Erskine, R. M., Maganaris, C. N., Longo, S., Simoneau, E. M., Grosset, J. F. and Narici, M. V. (2009). Training-induced changes in structural and mechanical properties of the patellar tendon are related to muscle hypertrophy but not to strength gains. *Journal of Applied Physiology*, *107*, 523–530.

Seynnes, O. R., de Boer, M. and Narici, M. V. (2007). Early skeletal muscle hypertrophy and architectural changes in response to high-intensity resistance training. *Journal of Applied Physiology (1985)* 102, 368–373.

Werner, S. and Eriksson, E. (1993). Isokinetic quadriceps training in patients with patellofemoral pain syndrome. *Knee Surgery, Sports Traumatology, Arthroscopy, 1*, 162–168.

Young, M. A., Cook, J. L., Purdam, C. R., Kiss, Z. S. and Alfredson, H. (2005). Eccentric decline squat protocol offers superior results at 12 months compared with traditional eccentric protocol for patellar tendinopathy in volleyball players. *British Journal of Sports Medicine*, *39*, 102–105.

Part II

Humanities and social sciences

Social sciences

14 Women's soccer

Historical development and current situation in Europe

Gertrud Pfister

Introduction: soccer, a men's game – the origins

Ball games existed – and still exist – in numerous time periods and in many regions and cultures. They have been played throughout the ages, for example in South America, in Greece as well as in China, and in many European countries. Players were children and adults, men and women, rich and poor, who used games as training or entertainment, or as a means of worshipping the gods. Kicking a ball was popular in many cultures, for instance in ancient China as well as among the Australian aborigines.

The roots of modern football were the wild folk games of the early modern age which attracted large crowds of participants, most of them boys and men, who tried to get hold of a ball and to transport it to a distant goal (Walvin, 1994). These games were 'tamed' in the English public schools, where middle- and upper-class boys were trained to follow rules by playing sport, in particular by playing football. The codification of rules encouraged competitions between schools and universities, but soon also between clubs, which emerged in the 1840s (Walvin, 2000). With the gradual reduction of working hours since the end of the nineteenth century, football began to attract male members of the working classes, not least because the game 'embodied' their values and their ideals of masculinity. Whereas the 'gentlemen' players, striving for social distinction, emphasized the values of amateurism, proletarian soccer players regarded soccer as work and became 'professionals' (Walvin, 2000).

After the turn of the century, soccer spread to other European countries and overseas, in particular to regions where Englishmen – sailors, soldiers or entrepreneurs – played the game and served as 'role models'. In the course of the twentieth century, men's soccer became the most popular sport worldwide, and today millions play the game and billions of fans watch the matches. The Soccer World Cup even exceeds the Olympic Games in popularity; in 2006, the World Cup had a total cumulative television audience of 26.29 billion viewers. The final match attracted an audience of 715 million.[1]

But soccer is more than a sport: soccer teams seem to represent their club, their city or their country and produce 'sites of memory,' i.e. remembrances which mirror the aims and values of their communities. A good example of the representative function of soccer is the interpretation of the German team's victory in the 1954 World Cup as a sign of the end of the country's ostracism after World War II. In postwar years, soccer played its part in contributing to a return to normality and became a symbol of reconciliation. Thus, Germany's victory in 1954, dubbed by Germans the 'miracle of Bern,' could be viewed as the return of the country to the world community. The increasing professionalization of the players in the 1960s and the new opportunities of consuming soccer via radio and then TV not only changed consumption habits but also contributed to the increasing importance of the game in the everyday lives of consumers and fans.

The popularity, the heroic image and the representative function of soccer, however, were reserved for the men's game. Women who played the game were considered outsiders, members of the 'weaker sex' who were trying to intrude into this male domain. The notion of women as the 'second sex,' unable to cope with the physical challenges of the game, hindered or even precluded the social acceptance of women's soccer for many years (Fan and Mangan, 2004).

In this chapter I will present a short overview of the emergence of women's soccer in Europe, describe the current situation and discuss explanations for the gender hierarchy in this game. Besides informing about general trends on the continent, I will provide examples primarily using the situation in the countries with the largest number of players, Germany, and the largest percentage of female soccer players, Denmark.

Women's soccer – developments

First attempts of women to play soccer can be traced to England and Scotland in the 1880s. Women's soccer experienced a considerable upswing during World War I, when matches of female teams drew large crowds, for instance in the UK. That women played a men's game was accepted and even welcomed because they donated the gate money for wounded soldiers. Particularly female workers in factories, such as the 'Dick, Kerr's Ladies,' loved the game because it provided a diversion from their tiresome everyday life. This team not only included some of the best players; it also survived the decline of women's soccer caused by – among other issues – the decision of the soccer federation to prohibit men's soccer clubs from supporting women's teams. Clubs were no longer allowed to make their fields available for women's matches. Female soccer players tried to solve these problems, for instance by founding a federation, but could not stop the decline of the women's soccer movement in England (Maguee, 2007; Williams, 2007).

In France, too, women's sport, including soccer, flourished after the turn of the century, and several women's sports clubs had already been founded before World War I. One of the most famous clubs was Femina, whose president in 1915, Alice Milliat, was also the president of the International Women's Sport Federation, an organization which conducted the Women's World Games. Soccer, however, was not included in the program of these events. The fierce competition between several women's teams contributed to the rise of women's soccer in the country. In 1920, a French team even traveled to England and engaged in the first international women's soccer matches with the Dick, Kerr's Ladies FC and other teams. In the same year the Ladies came to France (Pfister et al., 2002). One of the best all-round athletes in France and also of the best soccer players worldwide was Violette Morris, a member of Femina Sport and later Olympique de Paris. However, in 1928 she was denied a license and excluded from participation in the discus throw at the Olympic Games in 1928 because she dressed and behaved like a man. Not only in France but also in other countries playing sport was tolerated as long as the women respected the written and unwritten laws of the prevailing gender order (Michallat, 2005).

Other countries also hosted women's soccer teams, such as Belgium, the Netherlands, and Austria. In Germany, however, resistance to women's soccer was particularly strong. The following comment printed in a women's magazine represented the general opinion in the country: "Women may be playing soccer in England and America, but it is to be hoped that this bad example is not followed in German sport" (Pfister, 2012, p. 20). This hope was fulfilled as the very few attempts of German women to play soccer were doomed to failure. An initiative of young girls in Frankfurt in 1930 failed, for example, because of the resistance of their parents (Pfister, 2012). In the increasingly conservative climate of the 1930s and 1940s traditional ideals of femininity and attitudes toward women's participation in sport prevailed not only in Germany but in many other European countries.

In the 1950s, clever businessmen organized women's soccer matches between teams from Germany and the Netherlands. They used the 'spectacle' of soccer played by women to attract crowds and to make money. Although the skill of the players and the quality of the game surprised the audiences, decreasing interest, resistance from the German soccer federation (DFB), and bad management contributed to the decline of the first women's soccer movement in the country (Pfister, 2012).

From the end of the 1960s onward women in several countries started to play soccer as a leisure activity or as a competitive sport. However, the organization of matches and tournaments called for a certain form of governance and an umbrella organization. In Denmark, female soccer players organized a league of their own and even founded a women's soccer federation as early as 1968, which later merged with the Danish Soccer Federation (DBU) (Brus and Trangbaek, 2004).

In Germany, women played soccer in the 1960s 'just for fun,' but soon they demanded access to sport facilities and asked to be admitted to the DFB. The members of the president's committee were strongly opposed to this request and used medical and psychological arguments to legitimate the rejection of this application. They believed that participation in such a strenuous sport would damage the women's health as well as their feminine appeal. However, the increasing number of female players in the country and the rise of women's soccer movements in Europe and worldwide left the German soccer authorities no choice: they eventually accepted female players, but discussed numerous extra rules for the 'weaker sex,' for example the prohibition of cleated shoes and protection for the breast (Pfister, 2012). However, none of these rules were put into practice. In other European countries, too, women began to play soccer, and neither the disapproval of soccer organizations nor the alleged consequences for their health, fertility, and femininity deterred the female players. Despite the many obstacles, women's soccer came to stay. The number of female players grew slowly but continuously, at first in northern and central Europe but soon also in other European countries and on all continents. At the same time, the first national leagues and international competitions were organized. In 1991, the first 'official' FIFA World Championship took place in China; other events followed and soon filled the women's soccer calendar (Williams, 2011).

Women's soccer today

General situation

Although soccer still seems to epitomize masculinity, FIFA president Blatter claimed a 'female future' for the game as early as 1995 in a speech during the Women's World Cup in Sweden (Degun, 2013). His prophecy has come true, at least with regard to the expansion of women's soccer. The game has become the most popular female team sport in Europe, although there are decisive gender differences, in particular concerning the salary of the players.

The numbers of female players published by UEFA (2014, 2015), as well as numerous reports dealing with the game's development in different countries,[2] provide an overview of the situation of women's soccer in Europe: currently, more than 1.2 million girls and women are registered soccer players in the UEFA countries; in the UK, the Netherlands, and Sweden their numbers exceed 100,000. Germany is the country with the largest number of female soccer players: 258,000 girls and women play in one of the 12,900 women's or girls' teams in the country (DFB, 2015; UEFA, 2015). However, if we put these numbers in relation to the total number of players, girls and women form a relatively small minority: 7 percent of registered players in Europe are female; in four countries – Denmark, the Faroe Islands, Iceland, and Sweden – the percentage of girls and women among the players exceeds 20 percent. In other countries such as Turkey, Ukraine, Rumania, and Poland, less than 3 percent of players are girls or women (UEFA, 2015). Here, it must also be taken into consideration that a relatively large number of female players are not 'registered' as they do not take part in 'official' competitions. The latest figures provided for Germany by the DFB reveal that 758,441 women and 336,464 girls under 16 years of age are members of voluntary soccer clubs, many more than the registered players mentioned above. In addition, numerous females play the game outside clubs and federations, e.g. in schools or during leisure time in parks. Thus, there may be many more female soccer players in Europe than indicated in the UEFA report (DFB, 2015).

In Europe, soccer competitions are organized by clubs and federations. Female players are mostly members of local mixed-gender soccer clubs. In some countries women's soccer clubs with teams playing in the top leagues have emerged. Other top teams are attached to men's clubs.[3] In the German women's 'Bundesliga' two women's soccer clubs, Turbine Potsdam and 1. FFC Frankfurt, have dominated the women's soccer scene for many years. However, in recent years they have lost ground to teams attached to and supported by clubs with professional men's teams. In Sweden, a women-only club in Malmö, LdB FC Malmö, fielded one of the best European teams. But this club, too, merged with a club of male and female members.

The information presented above indicates that women's soccer is still a marginal sport compared with the men's game. However, soccer is the most popular women's team sports in some European countries like Germany. In Germany, 140,000 young women (19–26 years of age) play soccer – more than in all other team sports together.[4] The development during the past decade shows remarkable progress not only with regard to the numbers of players but also with regard to performance and public acceptance, indicated by the emergence of competitions and tournaments at national, regional, and international levels: female players compete in a quadrennial World Cup and a soccer tournament at the Olympics (since 1996), as well in continental competitions, e.g. the Euro and the UEFA Women's Champion League. In most countries league systems for women teams have been established which provide the opportunity of promotion and relegation. The prevalence of women's soccer has been accompanied by a continuous increase in the players' capabilities and performances, which has also had a positive influence on the quality of the matches and – as a further consequence – on the interest of soccer supporters and fans.

In the past decade the women's top events at the international level have gained considerable media attention and were followed by large audiences. The 2013 UEFA women's championship in Sweden broke the record in ticket sales, and the last mega event, the women's WC in 2015 in Canada, was covered by the "biggest and most advanced broadcast production for a women's soccer tournament" ever (FIFA, 2015). The 52 matches had a total attendance of 1.3 million. In many countries the viewing records of women's games have been broken. The final attracted 25 million Americans and was the most watched soccer match of men and women in the USA of all time; 25.4 million Americans followed their team's triumph on TV (Pingue, 2015).

Current issues

Despite the increasing number of female soccer players, above all in northern and central European countries, several issues must be taken into consideration as they may influence the development of women's soccer, in particular at the elite level (e.g. Williams, 2011). An overview provided by UEFA gives information about the budgets for women's soccer in the member countries, which vary between fewer than €100,000 and €15 million. Thirty out of 50 federations invest less than €1 million, and only the federations in France, Sweden, Norway, England, and Germany spend between €4 and €15 million on women's soccer (UEFA, 2015, p. 29).

The large majority of European soccer players are amateurs, but this is particularly true of women. In 22 of the 54 European soccer associations not a single professional female player is registered, and only 2,625 women play soccer professionally. However, most of them earn only a minimal salary (UEFA, 2015, p. 16).

In 2013/2014, the European Club Association (ECA) investigated 22 women's soccer teams in Europe. Special focus was placed on the budget, the salary of the players, and the number and qualification of the employees. One of the main questions was whether the teams were sufficiently supported and whether they could rely on professional staff. The results of this survey revealed that the lack of financial resources was one of the main problems in women's soccer. Only three of the clubs had a yearly budget larger than €1 million, but there were also three clubs which could only spend €50,000 or less. The players earned between €40 and €18,000. However, it seems to have been the Brazilian player Marta, playing for the Swedish club Rosengård, who earned this 'exceptional' sum (maybe paid by sponsors). The average salary was €545 in the clubs with a budget under €250,000 and €1,515 in the 'richer' clubs. Of the clubs, 41 percent had fewer than five employees, 36 percent between five and ten employees (ECA, n.d.). These numbers mirror the status of women in soccer: they are, at best, semi-professionals while men may earn millions.[5]

The financial situation of women's soccer has numerous consequences for the game. Small budgets mean a small number of staff – or none at all – with the result that many teams rely on the support of volunteers for carrying out the various daily tasks. As this situation may hinder an upwards trend in women's soccer, some of the European federations, such as the DBU, have taken action. Denmark is the country with the highest percentage of registered players due to the positive attitude toward girls' and women's soccer in the country. In 2012, the DBU decided on a 'development plan' for women's elite soccer (Vision 2020) which regulates the material conditions (including human resources) which clubs must provide if they wish to host a team in the top league. 'Poor' clubs can ask the DBU for financial support (DBU, n.d.).

Public interest in and media coverage of women's soccer

Despite numerous positive developments in recent decades, the lack of resources in women's soccer (as described above) is a decisive barrier impeding the professionalization of the players, and, in general, the advancement of the game. Resources are generated by entrance fees to matches, and, in particular, by sponsors who use soccer teams and players as endorsements for their products. Not only a team's positive image but also – and in particular – the coverage of the media, the media consumers, and the audiences of live events (their size and their demographic characteristics) are decisive criteria for sponsors' investments. Women's soccer differs from the men's game not only in the numbers of supporters and fans but also – and in particular – in the interest the media takes in the weekly matches.

Current information on public interest in soccer is provided by the results of a representative population survey conducted in eight countries in the context of the

FREE project (Football Research in an Enlarged Europe) which explored the role of soccer in the lives of Europeans.[6] Of the female respondents, 34.6 percent and 64.9 percent of the males reported that they were interested or very interested in soccer in general. However, there were large differences in soccer interest among the various countries: only 20.7 percent of the women but 71.4 percent of the men in Austria and 46 percent of German women but 64.9 percent of German men reported being (very) interested in the game. The country with the highest percentage of soccer consumers was Denmark: 48.8 percent of Danish women and 68.6 percent of the men stated that they were (very) interested in soccer, but only 22.8 percent of all respondents affirmed an interest in women's soccer matches.

Women showed no more interest in women's soccer than men. On the contrary, only 4.2 percent of the female and 7.1 percent of the male respondents on average reported any great interest. Women's soccer is most popular in the UK, where 29.5 percent of the female and 42.1 percent of the male respondents reported that they were (very) interested. In Poland only 2.6 percent of the women and 7.8 percent of the men declared any interest. In Denmark 19.5 percent of the women and 26.7 percent of the men while in Germany 26 percent of the women and 26.7 percent of the men reported that they were interested or very interested in women's matches. These results reveal quite clearly that male players, teams, and clubs are much more attractive for sponsors or advertisers than female players.

Interest in women's soccer may just mean following the top events; it does not necessarily mean interest in league matches, and it may also not lead to active consumption or attending matches at the stadium. As several studies show, league matches in Europe often take place in – almost – empty stadiums. In UEFA countries, matches between top women's teams are attended on average by 350 spectators, the highest average attendance figures at national league matches are attained in Germany with 2,500 spectators. Games of top teams may even attract more than 10,000 soccer supporters and fans. However, in eight UEFA countries only around 50 individuals, mostly family members, attend women's league games (UEFA, 2015). In contrast, men's matches reach attendance figures of up to 80,000.[7] The small numbers of spectators have a decisive impact on the clubs' budgets as gate receipts are an important revenue source.

Journalists, too, show little interest in women's soccer and female players, who receive scarcely any media exposure and attract few advertisement contracts or sponsorships. There is a large body of literature based on research in various European countries which provides convincing evidence that media sport in general and media soccer in particular are men's affairs (Peeters and Elling, 2015) – played by men, presented by men, focusing on men, and consumed by men. Men's teams and male players are, for example, testimonials for Pepsi, Turkish Airlines, or Mercedes. They often display a form of 'exaggerated masculinity' by starring as warriors, Ninjas, fighters in a cage or conducting duels on the soccer field. Not only their salaries as players but also their roles as testimonials for various products generate a large income. Thus, it is not surprising that 13 soccer players appear on the Forbes List of the world's 100 best earning athletes. Number 3 is Cristiano Ronaldo (after two boxers) with an income of $150 million a year. It goes without saying that no female soccer player is on this list, which names only three women: tennis and golf players.[8]

When one explores the reasons behind the gendered media coverage of soccer, gender theories as well as the concepts of 'agenda setting' and 'framing' provide clues for interpretations.

Gender has to be understood as a social construction at societal, interactional, and individual levels. It is embedded in social institutions and identity. Gender is not something we have but something we perform and do. Gender stereotypes and the 'doing gender' of players and fans construct 'real' soccer as a men's game and women's soccer as something different (Connell, 2002).

Soccer gains its importance to a large extent via media coverage. Journalists justify their lack of interest in women's soccer by referring to the expectations of their readers/viewers. However, it must be emphasized that the media have the power of agenda setting and framing and thus influence the tastes and consumption patterns of their consumers. Journalists (have to) select their topics from numerous issues and events, condense them and transform them into narratives. They set topics such as men's soccer 'on the agenda, creating and supporting interests of their consumers' (Fenton, 2000, p. 298).

But the media do not simply describe events; they give them meaning by 'framing' them, i.e. presenting them in specific contexts conveying specific messages and influencing the ways in which their consumers interpret and explain the world around them. Men's soccer is often presented – also in advertisements – as a battle and male player as heroes fighting for the honor of their clubs or their countries. Soccer played by women is considered a different game. The 'difference paradigm' is created by comparisons with men's matches, in particular men's performances and men's ways of playing, which sets the gender difference on the agenda. However, female players are faced with an additional dilemma as playing soccer and staging traditional femininity do not fit together, which may prevent sponsors and advertisers from staging female soccer players. Among many other voices, the *Washington Post* complained that the Women's World Cup in 2015 attracted far fewer of the "marketing blitzes or mega-deals seen in men's tournaments, and far less of the cash or corporate support, a glaring loss for players and fans of the world's most popular sport" (Harwell, 2015). In contrast to many other companies, Nike produced a commercial, showcasing powerful female soccer players.

Concluding remarks

Soccer has developed from a men's game to a sport which increasingly attracts girls and women. In many European countries women's soccer is thriving, in particular with regard to the quality of the game and the numbers of players. However, women's teams have on average few resources, and female players are either amateurs or semi-professionals. The main problem of players and teams is the lack of interest shown by the media and the small number of fans, which prevents advertisers and sponsors from focusing on female players. Whereas male soccer stars enact masculinity on and off the field, traditional femininity and playing soccer are incompatible. However, the latest developments signal a change: outstanding female players such as Marta have become stars on and off the field. It has to be hoped that these developments continue.

Notes

1 FIFA, InfoPlus, n.d. https://web.archive.org/web/20070614094554/www.fifa.com/mm/document/fifafacts/ffprojects/ip-401_06e_tv_2658.pdf
2 See e.g. the numbers of female members of the Danish Football Federation (DBU) www.dbu.dk/oevrigt_indhold/Om_DBU/DBUs%20historie/medlemstal.aspx or the membership statistics of the German Football Federation www.dfb.de/index.php?id=1000489.
3 See the teams which participated in the ECA study (European Club Association, n.d.). www.blossoming.it/portfolio-item/eca-womens-club-football-analysis
4 UEFA 2014–2015, 36; see also the numbers of members of the various sport federations in Germany, www.dosb.de/fileadmin/sharepoint/Materialien%20%7B82A97D74-2687-4A29-9C16-4232BAC7DC73%7D/Bestandserhebung_2014.pdf
5 See the list of the best earning sport stars www.forbes.com/athletes/list/#tab:overall
6 FREE Project (Football Research in an Enlarged Europe) (2014): "Survey on Football in European Public Opinion." For information about the project, see: www.free-project.eu/Pages/Welcome.aspx
7 See www.dfb.de/bundesliga/statistik/zuschauerzahlen
8 See www.forbes.com/athletes/list/#tab:overall

References

Brus, A. and Trangbæk, E. (2004). Asserting the Right to Play – Women's Football in Denmark. In F. Hong and J.A. Mangan (Eds.): *Soccer, Women, Sexual Liberation. Kicking Off a New Era* (pp. 95–111). London and Portland: Cass.

Connell, R.W. (2002). *Gender.* Malden: Blackwell.

Dansk Boldspil-Union (DBU) (n.d.). *Vision 2020.* Retrieved from www.dbu.dk/~/media/Files/DBU_Broendby/uddannelse_-_spiller/Vision2020.pdf (last accessed April 15, 2015).

Degun, T. (2013, January 2). The future of football is feminine, says Blatter. *Inside the games.* Retrieved from www.insidethegames.biz/articles/1012271/the-future-of-football-will-be-feminine-says-blatter (last accessed April 15, 2015).

Deutscher Fussball-Bund (DFB) (2015). *Mitglieder-Statistik.* Retrieved from www.dfb.de/fileadmin/_dfbdam/66210-Mitglieder-Statistik_2015.pdf (last accessed April 15, 2015).

European Club Association (ECA) (n.d.). *ECA Women's Club Football Analysis.* Retrieved from www.blossoming.it/portfolio-item/eca-womens-club-football-analysis (last accessed January 24, 2015).

Fan, H. and Mangan, J.A. (2004). *Soccer, Women, Sexual Liberation: Kicking off a New Era.* London: F. Cass.

Fédération Internationale de Football Association (FIFA) (n.d.) FIFA World Cup. *Fifa.com.* Retrieved from www.fifa.com/aboutfifa/worldcup (last accessed January 24, 2015).

Fédération Internationale de Football Association (FIFA) (2015, April 17). Canada set for biggest ever TV production in women's football. *Fifa.com.* Retrieved from www.fifa.com/womensworldcup/news/y=2015/m=4/news=canada-set-for-biggest-ever-tv-production-in-women-s-football-2591629.html (last accessed January 24, 2015).

Fenton, N. (2000). Mass Media. In S. Taylor (ed.): *Sociology* (pp. 297–321). New York: Palgrave.

Harwell, D. (2015, July 6). Why hardly anyone sponsored the most-watched soccer match in US history. *The Washington Post*. Retrieved from www.washingtonpost.com/news/wonkblog/wp/2015/07/06/the-sad-gender-economics-of-the-womens-world-cup (last accessed January 24, 2015).

Magee, J. (2007). *Women, Football, and Europe: Histories, Equity, and Experiences*. Oxford: Meyer & Meyer Sport.

Michallat, W. (2005). Droit au but: Violette Morris. *French Studies Bulletin*, 97, 13–17.

Peeters, R. and Elling, A. (2015). The coming of age of women's football in the Dutch sports media, 1995–2013. *Soccer and Society*, *16*, 620–638.

Pfister, G. U. (2002). Wem gehört der Fussball?: Wie ein englisches Spiel die Welt eroberte. In M. Fanizadeh and R. Diketmüller, R. (eds): *Global Players: Kultur, Ökonomie und Politik des Fussballs* (pp. 37–56). Frankfurt a. M: Brandes und Apsel.

Pfister, G. (2012). Frauen-Fussball-Geschichten. In S. Sinning (ed.): *Auf den Spuren des Frauen- und Mädchenfußballs* (pp. 14–17). Weinheim: Juventa.

Pfister, G. U., Fasting, K., Scraton, S., and Vázquez, B. (2002). Women and football – a contradiction? The beginnings of women's football in four European countries. In S. Scraton, and A. Flintoff (eds.): *Gender and Sport: A Reader* (pp. 66–77). London: Routledge.

Pingue, F. (2015, July 7). Women's World Cup final draws record audience for football in America as US beat Japan to seal third title in Canada. *Daily mail*. Retrieved from www.dailymail.co.uk/sport/football/article-3152577/Women-s-World-Cup-final-draws-record-audience-football-America-beat-Japan-seal-title-Canada.html#ixzz3hgFYYJa2 (last accessed January 24, 2015).

Pyta, W. and Havemann, N. (2015). *European Football and Collective Memory*. New York: Palgrave Macmillan.

Sonntag, A. (2008). *Gefühlsausbrüche: Europas Fußball zwischen Tradition und Postmoderne*. Wiesbaden: VS Verlag für Sozialwissenschaften.

Union of European Football Associations (UEFA) (2014). Women's football across the nations 2013/14. Retrieved from www.uefa.com/MultimediaFiles/Download/Women/WFDP/02/03/17/67/2031767_DOWNLOAD.pdf (last accessed January 24, 2015).

Union of European Football Associations (UEFA) (2015). Women's football across the nations 2014/15. Retrieved from www.uefa.com/MultimediaFiles/Download/Women/General/02/03/27/84/2032784_DOWNLOAD.pdf (last accessed March 8, 2015).

Viney, N., and Grant, N. (1978). *An Illustrated History of Ball Games*. London: Heinemann.

Walvin, J. (1994). *The People's Game: The History of Football Revisited*. Edinburgh: Mainstream.

Walvin, J. (2000). *The People's Game: The History of Football Revisited*. London: Mainstream Publishing.

Williams, J. (2007). *A Beautiful Game: International Perspectives on Women's Football*. Oxford: Berg.

Williams, J. (2011). Women's Football, Europe and Professionalization 1971–2011. UEFA research report. Retrieved from www.dora.dmu.ac.uk/bitstream/handle/2086/5806/Woman's%20football,%20Europe%20%26%20professionalization%201971–2011.pdf?sequence= (last accessed March 8, 2015).

Williams, J. (2013). *Globalizing Women's Football: Europe, Migration and Professionalization*. Bern: Peter Lang.

15 Development and voluntarism in soccer clubs

Siegfried Nagel and Torsten Schlesinger

Introduction

Sport clubs, especially soccer clubs, have a long tradition in many European countries and still play an important role by providing sporting activities for the whole population. However, future development of soccer and sport clubs presents significant challenges because of changes in society and in modern sport (e.g. Breuer et al., 2015). One significant problem is attracting enough members to volunteer in the long term. Recruiting and retaining volunteers for formal posts is a problem for nearly half of the clubs in Switzerland (Lamprecht et al., 2012), especially for soccer clubs. For example, a specific analysis of Swiss soccer clubs reveals that 60 percent of all clubs have major problems recruiting and retaining referees, coaches 47 percent, and staff 47 percent for formal positions on their boards (Lamprecht et al., 2012). Similar problems can be observed in other countries in and outside Europe (e.g. Breuer and Feiler, 2013; Cuskelly, 2005; Nichols and Shepherd, 2006; Scheerder and Vos, 2009). However, in nearly all European countries, voluntarism plays a central role in the organization of sport club activities (Breuer et al., 2015). The majority of board members, coaches, and referees in grass-roots soccer are volunteers, although there are a few instances of professionalization. Personal problems affect the work of clubs, such as ensuring their sporting services, and can also lead to sanctions by the soccer association, such as fines for missing referees, exclusion from playing in matches or tournaments. Furthermore, problems with volunteering in clubs also have noticeable consequences for the soccer association, for example, the promotion of talent or ensuring that regular matches and tournaments can be held. Therefore, for club management, a detailed understanding of how to attract and retain volunteers is becoming a high priority. In the context of these issues our research has posed the following two questions: (1) which *individual* characteristics and *organizational* conditions influence volunteering of members in sport clubs?; (2) which decision-making processes are related to the implementation of effective strategies for recruiting volunteers?

This chapter will give an overview of the main results of a larger research project "Personnel resource in sport clubs" (Schlesinger et al., 2014).

Theoretical framework

To analyze the research questions, we conceptualize sport clubs as corporative actors where the common goals of the members play an important role (Coleman, 1974; Nagel, 2006). Sport clubs are based on self-organization and on members pooling their resources in order to achieve shared interests. For example: when people want to play soccer together, they search for other team members, a soccer field, a trainer, etc. Soccer clubs can therefore be described as voluntary associations of members with the aim of realizing shared interests, in particular, practicing soccer together. The specific structural conditions of a sport club are subject to change by the corresponding impulses of the members. Nonetheless, these specific structural conditions, not the people, predominantly characterize the sport club as a corporate actor (Nagel et al., 2015).

It is also useful to consider a multilevel framework derived from the concepts of Esser (1999). This framework integrates different levels and perspectives of the development of sport clubs (see for detail, Nagel, 2006, 2007; Nagel et al., 2015):

1   *Macro-level*: sport club development has to be understood in the context of the broader development in society and modern sport. When analyzing the question of volunteering, we can assume that developments in society, such as processes of individualization, have led to problems with volunteering in sport clubs. In addition, it is interesting to note the role sport clubs play in the national and regional sport context as well as in national sport policy (e.g. Sport for All).
2   *Meso-level*: however, not all sport clubs in certain countries reveal the same structures and changes. According to Esser (1999), it is necessary to have a closer look at the meso-level: to consider sport clubs with their specific structures that are relevant to the members' decision to volunteer or not. We can assume that the specific organizational context influences the actions and decisions of the club. For example, the number of members, the financial resources, the clubs' goals or the importance of traditions and cultures in different kinds of sport may play a crucial role in the specific activities of club members, especially when volunteering.
3   *Micro-level*: furthermore, it is useful to look at the actions and decisions of the members that depend on club structures and also on specific interests and values. These interests and values in the context of the club can be particularly relevant to regulating action and engagement within their club (Schlesinger and Nagel, 2013; Wicker and Hallmann, 2013). Through collective action the members constitute and change the social structure of their sport club (e.g. club goals, sport activities), in this context it is appropriate to look at mutual correlations between the members and the club.

Multilevel model of long-term volunteering in sport clubs

In this general framework, we will now focus on the members' individual decision to volunteer or not (see Figure 15.1; according to Schlesinger and Nagel,

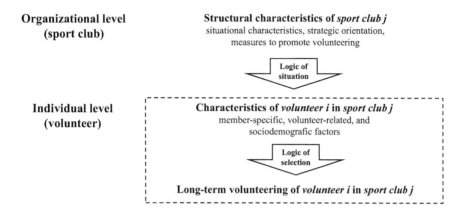

Figure 15.1 Multilevel model of volunteering in sports clubs

2013). The multilevel model assumes that both individual factors and the specific structural conditions of the club influence the members' willingness to volunteer within their club. Following the logic of the situation, the specific social structures of a club play a decisive role in the individual activities of club members (e.g. Coleman, 1990). Accordingly, club-specific structures such as particular material and non-material incentives are most likely to influence the individual decision for or against volunteering. Furthermore, the decision to volunteer or not could be dependent on the specific culture or structure of the club. The stronger the importance of volunteering is internalized in the club, the greater the individual utility of volunteering, and the higher the costs of non-volunteering. The status of volunteering can, for example, manifest in a strategic plan to promote and support volunteering in the club. There are numerous relevant factors at an individual level as to why club members actively volunteer in a sport club. For our research, the logic of selection is conceptualized in terms of an economic theory of behavior (Becker, 1976). The variety individual factors will be discussed in the results of our multilevel analysis.

Analyzing decision-making practices in sport clubs

The garbage can model is the framework used to analyze the decision-making process for effective strategies to recruit and retain volunteers (Cohen et al., 1972). This conceptual model focuses on actions (in form of decision-making processes) at a meso-level, which are dependent on the social structures and individual decisions of the members. The central idea of the garbage can model is that decision-making processes in organizations consist of four streams, namely:

1   *Problems*: problems are people's concerns in and outside the organization. Not every single problem is noted or dealt with in a decision-making process and not all problems confronted are solved.

2   *Choice opportunities*: these are situations and occasions where decisions are expected and made (e.g. board meetings of the sport club).
3   *Participants*: the outcome of the decision depends on the relevant problem and also on the individuals who deal with it and take the opportunity of decision making (e.g. club politically engaged members).
4   *Solutions*: these can be answers to the organization's problems. Very often they are also offers that search for demand and need. Aside from problem suitability, organization culture and negotiating practices also play an important role when searching for solutions.

These streams do not behave in factual and logical relation, but flow randomly together (Schlesinger et al., 2015).

Method

In order to analyze the different individual and structural determinants, members' surveys in selected Swiss sport clubs were carried out. The sampling procedure for the case studies was designed to encompass the full breadth of different types of structures in Swiss sport clubs in terms of number of members and types of sport as well as human resource management structures (Lamprecht et al., 2012). The first step of data collection obtained club-specific structural data from club managers (presidents, technical directors) through a paper-and-pencil questionnaire. The second step gathered individual-level data on factors of volunteering through an online survey to the members (for details of data collection, see Schlesinger et al., 2014). Forty-five clubs and 20 different sports (also soccer) were analyzed, and data was collected from 1,528 members, 441 of them volunteering regularly. The majority of respondents (62 percent) were male. This unequal gender distribution may be due to the fact that women are still underrepresented as members of sport clubs. According to the Swiss sport club report by Lamprecht et al. (2012), approximately 64 percent of sport club members are male and 36 percent female. A small percentage (5.6 percent) were aged less than 20 years, 49.5 percent were aged between 21 and 40 years, 36.2 percent were aged between 41 and 60 years, and 8.7 percent were aged over 60 years (for a detailed description of the sample, see Schlesinger et al., 2013). In a follow-up study "More volunteers in Soccer Clubs," data from 19 Swiss soccer clubs was collected and 600 members were questioned (291 of these were volunteers).

The analysis of contextual influences is linked to hierarchical data structures. Hierarchical data structures exist when the units of analysis are mostly individuals at a lower level (members) who are nested within contextual units at a higher level (sport club). The appropriate method for simultaneously assessing hierarchical data of both individual characteristics and structural factors is a multilevel analysis. This analysis highlights the effects between variables at several levels and identifies relationships that would remain undetected in conventional regression analyses (Hox, 2002). In addition, multilevel analyses require large sample sizes, but there is no consensus in the literature regarding the number of cases required at the second level. The usual recommendation is to take at least 25 cases at the highest level (the club level) and at least 20 observations within each lower level (the individual level; e.g. Hox, 2002). Accordingly, all sport clubs where fewer than 20 observations were available were excluded from the analysis.

To analyze decision-making processes in relation to recruiting volunteers, nine clubs were selected (from the whole sample of 45 sport clubs) for an in-depth analysis. These clubs all showed different aspects of decision-making processes and measures for recruiting new volunteers over the previous 12 months (e.g. reorganizing recruitment practices by making structural adjustments, developing new search strategies, or building up internal or external cooperation). Individual and/or group interviews were carried out with selected position holders and decision makers who were at that time (or previously) directly involved in current (or past) decision-making processes. Data was collected through problem-centered and thematically structured interviews designed to assess, as precisely as possible, the central process components of decisions (Schlesinger et al., 2015).

Results: individual and structural factors for volunteering

Several determinants are relevant when comparing, through a multilevel analysis, members who regularly volunteer with those who do not engage voluntarily (see Table 15.1). There is a significant effect of six variables at an individual

Table 15.1 Multilevel model analyzing volunteering in sport clubs, dichotomous yes = 1 (according to Schlesinger and Nagel, 2013)

		Random intercept (full) model
Fixed effects		.397*
Individual level	Age	.003
	Gender	−.021
	Working time	−.060*
	Income	.050*
	Human capital	.008
	Children	.003
	Children belonging to club	.066*
	Competition experiences	.104*
	Commitment to the club	.087***
	Length of club membership	.006**
Club level	Number of divisions	.012
	Settlement structure of the sports club	−.052*
	Goal: supporting competitive sports	.049
	Goal: supporting growth	−.068*
Variance components	Individual level (Var r_{ij})	.163
(Random part)	Structural level (Var u_{0j})	.008
	ICC (r)	.048
	Deviance (−2 log likelihood)	908.4

Note: *p ≤ .05; **p ≤ .01;***p ≤ .001

level. Looking at membership-related variables, it can be seen that *commitment to the club, length of membership, competition experiences*, and *children belonging to the sport club* increase the willingness to volunteer. In addition, the variable *income* promotes voluntary commitment. The negative of the significant coefficient *working time* indicates that longer working hours restrain volunteering. Gender, age, children, and education were not significant to the 5 percent level. Thus, female members are integrated into voluntary work in relation to the rate of membership. However, it should be noted that women are underrepresented in important board positions. Furthermore, results show that two structural variables were significant, and these could explain club-related differences in willingness to volunteer. Rural sport clubs revealed a higher willingness to volunteer independent from individual characteristics. In contrast, growth-oriented goals in a club have a negative effect. Therefore, any broadening of the sport for new member groups (e.g. soccer fitness) can reduce the willingness to volunteer.

What are the relevant individual and structural factors in the commitment of members to long-term volunteering? It must be noted that only respondents who hold a formal position (e.g. as coach, treasurer) within their club were considered as long-term volunteers. Due to data restriction (reduced sample size), multilevel models could not be developed for this research question. Only the findings at the individual level will be provided. Table 15.2 gives an overview of individual factors that play a role in long-term volunteering (for details of the analysis see Schlesinger et al., 2013, 2014).

Table 15.2 Determinants for long-term volunteering in sport clubs (estimated linear regression function, stepwise method)

Variable	Dependent variable: risk of terminating voluntary work				
	Non-standardized coefficients		Standardized coefficients		
	Regression coefficient B	SE	β	t	p
(Constant)	3.910	.583		6.710	.001
Orientation toward collective solidarity	−.190	.038	−.264	−4.984	.001
Volunteer job satisfaction	−.055	.017	−.177	−3.530	.001
Child belonging to sports club (dummy: yes = 0)	−.592	.155	−.175	−3.268	.001
Length of volunteering	.015	.006	.130	2.444	.015
Excluded variables:	age, gender, education, income, workload, length of membership, average time volunteered, job function (dummies)				
Explained variance	$R^2 = .25$ corr. $R^2 = .23$				

Results showed that the identification with the club as well as the orientation toward collective solidarity and volunteer job satisfaction positively correlate with long-term commitment of volunteers. The effect of the former was stronger than that of the latter. Volunteers with a higher orientation toward collective solidarity are unlikely to terminate their voluntary engagement in their club. The following conditions of volunteering are relevant to the volunteer satisfaction: *interesting workspace, support from other members, information on club affairs, recognition,* and *material incentives*. Incentives for volunteering seem to have a positive influence on commitment. Furthermore, having children in the club promotes long-term volunteering. Finally, it is interesting that there is a negative correlation between the period of volunteering and the commitment. After engagement of more than (approximately) ten years, most volunteers prefer to terminate. The specific data on soccer clubs in the follow up study reveal similar results. When considering structural aspects, long-term volunteering is more probable in rural sport clubs and clubs that set value on conviviality. However, surprisingly the results show that specific measures to promote volunteering have no significant effect on long-term volunteering.

Typology of decision-making practices

The analyses within the nine case studies show the following main characteristics of decision-making processes in sport clubs (in detail Schlesinger et al., 2015): decisions are often a response to acute recruiting problems rather than a pursuit of strategic goals, decisions take relatively long time, and the decision-making process is determined by key actors. In most cases, process control is initiated and shaped by a few dominant actors possessing a strong interest in club policy. When searching for suitable solutions to their specific problem situation, clubs frequently orient their response toward (proved) routines, and, finally, both formal meetings and informal opportunities are relevant.

Furthermore, we also plotted a typology of the analyzed decision-making practices (see Figure 15.2). The clubs were classified according to their specific decision-making practices in a four-part grid with the dimensions *process control* (top-down vs. bottom-up) on the horizontal axis and *problem processing* (situational vs. systematic) on the vertical axis. Clubs characterized by a systematic-strategic approach to decision making are in the two right-hand quadrants. Their decision-making process is characterized by a concrete planning and formalized organization of the actors involved, the decision-making opportunities to be used, and the courses of the decision (e.g. by initiating routines). Such action should avoid disorder and irrationality as far as possible, and go towards reducing the complexity of decision-making processes. The upper-right quadrant contains those clubs that not only take a systematic approach but also demonstrate a clear decision-making hierarchy in club policy. In these clubs, a small number of actors in the upper hierarchy (executive board) control the decision-making process in a more top-down way. The two left-hand quadrants are characterized by a situation-oriented processing of personnel problems. This keeps the

Top-down

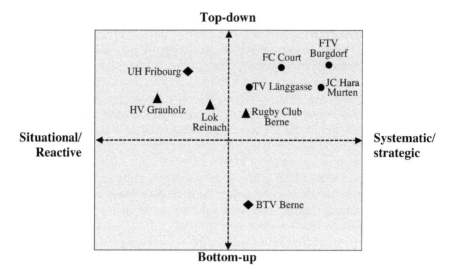

Bottom-up

Figure 15.2 Typology of decision-making practices

Note: = no effectiveness, = moderate effectiveness, and = effectiveness).

decision-making process more open and flexible. Both the inclusion of actors and the decision-making opportunities mostly emerge reactively and may be diffuse. As a result, the course of decision-making is more subject to random influence.

We further examined the extent to which particular decision-making practices succeed in solving the problem (of recruiting volunteers). Based on the reports from the clubs' actors, the consequences were categorized as: *no effectiveness* (no solution to the relevant recruitment problem), *moderate effectiveness* (a short-term/partial solution), and *effective* (a sustainable solution). Systematically designed decision-making processes with a clear regulation of responsibilities appear to solve personnel problems more purposefully and more quickly. Hence, top-down-controlled and systematically strategic decision-making practices are more appropriate. Obviously, sport clubs more likely succeed in solving problems concerning volunteering when they use more top-down and systematic decision-making processes.

Conclusion

To analyze individual and structural factors of long-term volunteering as well as decision-making processes questions, a multilevel framework was developed based on the structural–individualistic social theory. Individual and context factors for volunteering are estimated in different multilevel models based on a sample of n=1,434 sport club members from 36 sport clubs in Switzerland. Results indicate that volunteering is not just an outcome of individual characteristics such as lower workloads, higher income, children belonging to the sport club, longer club membership, or a strong commitment to the club. It is also influenced by club-specific structural conditions. An in-depth analysis of recruitment practices for volunteers was conducted in selected clubs (case study design) to look more closely at decision-making processes. The results show that systematically designed decision-making processes with a clear regulation of responsibilities appear to solve personnel problems more purposefully and more quickly.

What consequences can be drawn for volunteer management in sport clubs?

The analysis of decision-making processes implies that sport and soccer clubs should adopt a more systematic and strategic approach to volunteer management. The key to success lies in the commitment and competence of the central actors responsible for club policy. However, recruitment concepts in sport clubs cannot be completely oriented toward comparable practices in companies; in fact, their specific characteristics have to be considered.

The findings also indicate that an orientation toward collective solidarity is essential for the long-term commitment of volunteers. The promotion of a cooperative club atmosphere and the emotional and social attachment of club members need to be central elements for effectively managing volunteers and retaining them in sport clubs. It is necessary to provide high volunteer job satisfaction in order to ensure stability among volunteers. For long-term volunteers, recognition was particularly important. The need for recognition of their volunteering can be particularly well achieved through measures such as awarding honors for many years of volunteering or organizing specific volunteer events. Material incentives were particularly important for young volunteers and those in the sport domain. Finally, if a sport club wants to retain its volunteers, the individual expectations and needs of its club members, appropriate volunteering conditions, and incentive schemes that meet expectations (such as support, information) need to be considered.

References

Becker, G. S. (1976). *The economic approach to human behavior.* Chicago, IL: University of Chicago Press.

Breuer, C. and Feiler, S. (eds.). (2013). *Sportvereine in Deutschland. Sportentwicklungsbericht 2011/2012. Analyse zur Situation der Sportvereine in Deutschland* [Sport clubs in Germany. Sport development report 2011/2012. Analysis of the situation of sport clubs in Germany]. Köln: Deutsche Sporthochschule Köln.

Breuer, C., Hoekmann, R., Nagel, S., and van der Weerf, H. (Eds.) (2015). *Sport Clubs in Europe. A Cross-national Comparative Perspective.* New York, Heidelberg, London: Springer.

Cohen, M. D., March, J. G., and Olsen, J. P. (1972). A garbage can model of organizational choice. *Administrative Science Quarterly, 17,* 1–25.

Coleman, J. S. (1974). *Power and the Structure of Society.* New York: Norton.

Coleman, J. S. (1990). *Foundations of Social Theory.* Cambridge, MA: Belknap.

Cuskelly, G. (2005). Volunteer participation trends in Australian sport. In G. Nichols and M. Collins (eds.), *Volunteers in Sports Clubs* (pp. 87–104). Eastbourne, UK: Antony Rowe.

Esser, H. (1999). *Soziologie. Spezielle Grundlagen. Band 1: Situationslogik und Handeln* [Sociology. Special basics. Vol. 1: Situational logic and action]. Frankfurt a.M.: Campus.

Hox, J. J. (2002). *Multilevel Analysis: Techniques and Applications.* Mahwah, NJ: Erlbaum.

Lamprecht, M., Fischer, A., and Stamm, H.-P. (2012). *Die Schweizer Fussballvereine* [Swiss soccer clubs]. Zürich: SFA.

Nagel, S. (2006). *Sportvereine im Wandel. Akteurtheoretische Analysen zur Entwicklung von Sportvereinen* [Changing sport clubs: Actor theory analyses of trends in sport clubs]. Schorndorf: Hofmann.

Nagel, S. (2007). Akteurtheoretische Analyse der Sportvereinsentwicklung – Ein theoretisch-methodischer Bezugsrahmen [Actor theory analyses of sport club development – A theoretical and methodological framework]. *Sportwissenschaft, 37,* 186–201.

Nagel, S., Schlesinger, T., Wicker, P., Lucassen, J., Hoekmann, R., van der Weerf, H., and Breuer, C. (2015). Theoretical framework. In C. Breuer, R. Hoekman, S. Nagel, and H. van der Werff (eds.), *Sport Clubs in Europe. A Cross-national Comparative Perspective* (pp. 14–36). New York, Heidelberg, London: Springer.

Nichols, G. and Shepherd, M. (2006). Volunteering in sport: The use of ratio analysis to analyse volunteering and participation. *Managing Leisure, 11,* 205–216.

Scheerder, J. and Vos, S. (2009). *Panel van Sportclubs in Vlaanderen anno 2008. Eerste resultaten* [The Flemish sport club panel 2008: First results]. Leuven: K. U. Leuven, Research Unit of Social Kinesiology and Sport Management.

Schlesinger, T., Egli, B., and Nagel, S. (2013). 'Continue or terminate?' Determinants of long-term volunteering in sports clubs. *European Sport Management Quarterly, 13,* 32–53.

Schlesinger, T., Klenk, C., and Nagel, S. (2014). *Freiwillige Mitarbeit im Sportverein. Analyse individueller Faktoren und organisationaler Entscheidungen* [Voluntary collaboration in sport clubs. Analysis of individual factors and organizational decisions]. Zürich: Seismo.

Schlesinger, T., Klenk, C., and Nagel, S. (2015). How do sport clubs recruit volunteers? Analyzing and developing a typology of decision-making processes on recruiting volunteers in sport clubs. *Sport Management Review, 18,* 193–206.

Schlesinger, T. and Nagel, S. (2013). Who will volunteer? Analysing individual and structural factors of volunteering in Swiss sports clubs. *European Journal of Sport Science, 13,* 707–715.

Wicker, P. and Hallmann, K. (2013). A multi-level framework for investigating the engagement of sport volunteers. *European Sport Management Quarterly, 13,* 110–139.

16 The emergence of the Danish Soccer Fitness concept

Laila Susanne Ottesen, Søren Bennike and Lone Friis Thing

Taking a social science perspective, the aim of this chapter is to describe and analyze the Soccer Fitness concept and reveal the extent to which this design is innovative and viable. The chapter is structured in three parts. It starts with a short
introduction to the changing landscape of sport, which provides a framework for
understanding the link between football (i.e. soccer) and health, followed by the
results of an analysis of the changing landscape of soccer describing the thoughts
and ideas behind the design of the Soccer Fitness concept, and finishes with a
discussion and conclusion as to whether Soccer Fitness is sustainable as a health-
promoting concept.

Introduction: the changing landscape of sport

As Barrie Houlihan and others have described it, the landscape of sport is in
a period of change, both in terms of participation and sports policy at both
the government (municipal) level and in the sporting non-governmental bodies
(NGBs) (Bergsgard et al., 2007; Houlihan, 2012; Houlihan et al., 2009). Participation in sports in Denmark is generally high, particularly among children but
also among adults. Participation takes place in various settings; about one-third
of the population are active either on their own (self-organized, e.g. running
groups) or in commercial fitness centers, just over one-third are members of
a voluntary sports club, while the rest of the population is physically inactive
(Laub, 2013). However, the sports clubs and NGBs related to sport in Denmark
are being influenced by these changes in the patterns of sports participation,
and the funding of voluntary sport is being questioned in a recent report on
the economics and structure of the sports system in Denmark (Kulturministeriet, 2014), despite the fact that policymakers are increasingly recognizing
the value of advocating sport as a means of enhancing the overall health of the
population (Thing and Ottesen, 2010). In connection with the above-mentioned
changes, studies published in 2010 highlighting recreational small-sided soccer
as highly beneficial for enhancing overall fitness (Krustrup et al., 2010; Krustrup, Dvorak et al., 2010) and social capital (Ottesen et al., 2010) carried out at
the Department of Nutrition, Exercise and Sports (NEXS) at the University of

Copenhagen have led to the development of Soccer Fitness (Football Fitness), a soccer-based health-related activity launched in 2011 by the Danish Football Association (DFA).

Methods: a qualitative approach

The data analyzed in order to explore the Soccer Fitness concept are based on qualitative methods: document analysis (Hammersley and Atkinson, 2007), individual interviews (Kvale and Brinkmann, 2009), and focus group interviews (Morgan, 1997). The textual documents for analysis are papers and manuals describing Soccer Fitness before and during the process of implementation. The interviews include individual interviews with three key persons in the Soccer Fitness steering committee – three of the six members. The interviewees were selected because of their influence and different responsibilities in relation to the design of Soccer Fitness and their different tasks in the DFA. Seven focus group interviews were conducted, including one group of regional Soccer Fitness administrators and two groups of football development officers (FDOs) (all this done by Søren Bennike as a part of his PhD). Data were collected and analyzed concurrently from March to June 2013, which also meant that the data collection was continuously affected by the ongoing interpretation (Creswell, 2007). The data were collected in connection with a large-scale evaluation for the DFA concerning the implementation process of Soccer Fitness (Bennike et al., 2014a).

Analysis

The emergence of the Soccer Fitness concept

This section will examine the ideas behind the Soccer Fitness concept and the name itself. Apart from the empirical background mentioned in the section on methods, the analysis also builds on two articles (Bennike et al., 2014b; Ottesen et al., 2010), and two studies (Krustrup et al., 2011; Krustrup and Ottesen, 2014). According to the DFA (DBU, 2010), Soccer Fitness is organized in a:

> completely new way in both sporting and organizational terms, which breaks with the traditional organization, administration, and membership structure and combines Denmark's most popular ball-game with the flexibility offered by fitness centers.
>
> (DBU, 2010)

The design of the Soccer Fitness concept

As mentioned in the introduction, the board of the DFA was greatly inspired by the scientific work at NEXS, which showed that soccer could improve fitness and social capital. The DFA also carried out some soccer-related market analyses which showed that soccer is an extremely popular game among children and ado-lescents, but that this popularity tails off in men and women over the age of 25. This leaves a large unexploited potential market for new members among adults. An internal DFA proposal (DBU, 2010) states that:

> If it [Soccer Fitness] succeeds, we can also expect very great gains in mem-bership, with the associated membership fee income for the soccer clubs. On the other hand, if we do not succeed in this, we can expect to see much greater competition from other providers of soccer as exercise on the Danish market in the future.

The Soccer Fitness design is clearly inspired by the changing landscape of sport and the new focus on sport as a means to health promotion and includes a desire to reach out to new target groups. However, it is important to stress that, under the auspices of the DFA, Soccer Fitness is not treated as a short-term intervention but as a sustainable offer that the voluntary clubs are free to choose or reject. In an online proposal (DBU, 2010), it is stated that the primary aims of Soccer Fit-ness are to:

- Recruit more adult soccer players into the organized clubs
- Position soccer as a health-promoting activity
- Position the DIF, DFA and the local unions as the mass organizations for soccer
- Generate even greater interest in the use of soccer for training and exercise
- Assist the clubs in creating more flexibility in their offers to adult exercise soccer players
- Get even more people to use the facilities in the clubs at 'slack' times of the day
- Make contact with new clubs, e.g. based around housing associations etc.

The DFA board was also inspired by a trip to the UK where they took a closer look at the flexible and commercial five-a-side 'Pay and play soccer.' A representative from the steering group explained:

> We had been over in England and seen this five-a-side, which is growing fast. Very commercial in England, with companies building pitches like Fodbold-fabrikken [the Soccer Factory] at Vesterbro. They simply set up a facility like this, and just like a squash center in Denmark, they rent out the pitches and run tournaments for small teams. …We took a look at this and said, wasn't this something … to look into, maybe the soccer clubs could come up with an alternative offer … for busy fathers who might like to play a bit of soccer but don't have time for fixed training sessions and matches on Saturdays with 11 players and all that. But provide a flexible offer … We discussed it and out of that came … Soccer Fitness.

The flexibility that is stressed here is also picked up in the name Soccer Fitness, as it refers to the flexibility of fitness centers (DBU, 2014a). The DFA's Soccer Fitness project manager says:

> The name came about because we were inspired by the idea that soccer should be more flexible, and this flexibility basically comes from the fitness culture. At the same time, one of the things we wanted to provide was this online booking ... There was funding agreed for the purely technical work of producing this online booking system like they have in the fitness centers. So it looked a bit like we were trying to do the same thing as they were doing in the fitness centers. Online booking was easy to access and it was flexible.

The name Soccer Fitness was also inspired by the physiological data provided by researchers, which revealed the large improvement of fitness when playing soccer. These two sources of inspiration resulted in the name. The Soccer Fitness project manager further explains:

> Here in the organization we had a lot of discussions about what to call it. Exercise soccer was too boring. Flex soccer, which we thought was really exciting, was already taken by the DGI. That left Soccer Fitness. We were still afraid this might confuse people. Anyway, we called it Soccer Fitness because it is fun, healthy and social, and we set those targets beneath it which we hoped people would understand.

The above-mentioned concept of online booking was not part of the final design, as it proved impossible to apply in the voluntary soccer clubs. Given the DFA's desire to create something different organizationally, this was a cornerstone and top priority in the introductory phase. The actual online booking system was developed, but never took hold. The project manager explains:

> It [online booking] was also a pressure on the project and on those of us working on it. Well aware that we could see right away ... that it was completely unrealistic. Because soccer is a team sport, where the basic assumption is that you are together with others ... And often you are also there because they are people you get along with. That means that this way of thinking cannot be compared with fitness, which is individual. ... So this online booking turned out to be much too complex for the clubs. It actually stopped a lot of clubs from joining in. So the next year we told the clubs it was an option, and in the third year we actually played it down.

Instead, the clubs used Facebook and other online communication systems as a means of registration and for communication between the participants and, in addition, as a tool for the trainers or managers to prepare the training in the best possible way, or to cancel it if not enough participants sign up.

The changing landscape of soccer: three types of soccer in Denmark

Inspired by a discussion in Rowe et al. (2013), which places cycling in three categories labeled *competition, leisure,* and *transport,* we aim to show how Soccer Fitness differs with regard to its sporting principles and its organization from other forms of soccer run by the DFA, namely recreational and professional soccer (this does not include the DFA's organization of futsal). Before we can make use of this distinction, it is necessary to define recreational soccer and professional soccer. The analysis, which compares the three forms of football, is summarized in Figure 16.1. The concept of recreational soccer is linked to the Danish club tradition, which can be traced back to the Danish Constitution of 1849, which guaranteed the right to freedom of association. Since KB ('Kjøbenhavns Boldklub') organized soccer in 1879, recreational soccer has been organized within the Danish sports clubs and has played a key role in Danish sport practices. The fact that recreational soccer is organized in clubs means that it is non-profit, receives public funding, and has a democratic structure, i.e. the participants in recreational soccer pay a membership fee and have a say at the general meeting of the club.

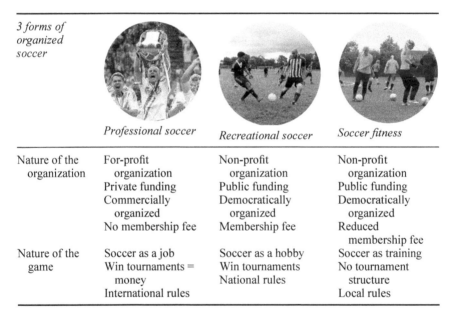

	Professional soccer	Recreational soccer	Soccer fitness
3 forms of organized soccer			
Nature of the organization	For-profit organization Private funding Commercially organized No membership fee	Non-profit organization Public funding Democratically organized Membership fee	Non-profit organization Public funding Democratically organized Reduced membership fee
Nature of the game	Soccer as a job Win tournaments = money International rules	Soccer as a hobby Win tournaments National rules	Soccer as training No tournament structure Local rules

Figure 16.1 In the changing landscape of soccer, Soccer Fitness is shown as a third form of soccer. Recreational soccer is placed in the middle because the two other forms of organized soccer are built on the foundations of recreational soccer and have similarities with it. The DFA wants Soccer Fitness to differentiate itself from recreational soccer. The way in which this is to be realized is explained in the figure, which illustrates that there are now three forms of organized adult soccer

Sources: pictures with permission of photographers Anders Kjærbye/fodboldbilleder.dk and Mia Kjærgaard, Danish Football Association.

The teams participate in a tournament structure with a national and sometimes regional set of rules. These rules are closely linked to, but not necessarily the same as, the international rules of the game. The success of recreational soccer and the advantageous conditions for setting up clubs in Denmark, together with strong amateur ideals in the sports system and the late arrival of professionalism in soccer, has helped recreational soccer establish a particularly strong position in the field of sport participation.

It was not until 1978, close to 100 years after recreational soccer was first organized, that the DFA modified its amateur ideals and introduced professional soccer, where the players received a salary (Grønkjær and Olsen, 2007). The DFA was reacting to both national and international pressure to organize soccer in a way where the Danish teams could compete internationally. The clubs whose teams competed at the highest level gradually changed their organization, and many clubs formed professional superstructures in the form of limited companies. Today, all these professional clubs are profit-driven and privatized, with a hierarchical bureaucratic structure. The players are employed on contracts; they do not pay membership fees and have no say in the management of the clubs. The matches follow internationally defined rules. The game is basically the same as in recreational soccer, while the organizational structure of the club is strikingly different. These differences in the characteristics of the organization and of the game are summarized in Figure 16.1.

How does Soccer Fitness differ from the DFA's other forms of soccer?

Four aspects of Soccer Fitness should be highlighted as characteristic of the concept compared to recreational and professional soccer. First, Soccer Fitness has a pronounced *health perspective*. Second, Soccer Fitness does not include a *tournament structure* (so team selection does not take place). Third, participants in Soccer Fitness pay a *reduced membership fee* compared to recreational soccer. And, fourth, the concept has been designed by the management of the DFA for a *specific target group*, i.e. players 25 years and older (with no requirement of previous soccer experience or skills).

The health perspective

As mentioned, the DFA developed Soccer Fitness with the intention to "position soccer as a health-promoting activity" and "generate even greater interest in the use of soccer for training and exercise" (DBU, 2010). Soccer is thus seen as a means to improve the health of the participants (DBU, 2012). The DFA has produced training booklets for both men and women with both soccer drills and fitness exercises (DBU, 2014b, 2014c, 2014d, 2014e). These booklets, which serve as inspiration for clubs that organize Soccer Fitness, emphasize that the DFA wants the clubs to practice soccer fitness differently than recreational soccer. As emphasized in these booklets, the aim of Soccer Fitness is that the participants are physically active and have fun rather than acquiring soccer skills and winning matches. The latter is further reinforced by the fact the teams do not participate in tournaments.

No tournament structure

The fact that there is no tournament structure is particularly important, because this makes it possible to modify the rules to the local setting. This means that every club can organize Soccer Fitness in a way that suits them and their participants.

In the first phase of the Soccer Fitness design, the DFA aimed to organize Soccer Fitness in a flexible way, much like in a fitness center, so the participants would be able to train when they wanted. However, this form of flexibility could not be realized in Soccer Fitness. This may have been the intention of the DFA in the beginning, but it was not possible to include flexible training times in a concept like Soccer Fitness, as the soccer clubs often face challenges when it comes to pitch bookings. Another challenge is the number of participants, because Soccer Fitness requires at least enough players to make two teams. But the participants do experience Soccer Fitness as flexible, and this can be partly attributed to the fact that they do not have to participate in tournaments. One administrator explains:

> It is soccer when people have time for it. … It is not compulsory in the same way as traditional soccer, it's not about training twice a week with a match at the weekend, it's more flexible in that way.

There is nobody relying on your presence for the team to function, so it's not a problem if you miss a week, and this makes Soccer Fitness flexible compared to professional and recreational soccer. This also means that the players do not compete with each other for places on a team to play on the weekend.

Reduced membership fee

The fact that there is no tournament structure also means that Soccer Fitness can be provided for a reduced membership fee compared to recreational soccer, as there are no fees – neither for referees nor for tournament administration.

Specific target group

Soccer Fitness targets a specific group of the population as indicated by a press release from the DFA:

> The DFA and the Sports Confederation of Denmark (DIF) are collaborating on a three-year project which aims to develop and offer soccer as fitness with a completely new sporting and organizational approach for both men and

women over 25. This should lay the foundation for attracting a completely new group of people.

(DFA, 2010)

This approach meant that the clubs were free to organize Soccer Fitness according to their wishes and needs, with a large degree of freedom in their choice of target groups and activities. It is highlighted as a benefit and 'sales argument' in a mini-manual for the clubs (DBU, 2014c) that clubs can administer Soccer Fitness as it best suits them and the group(s) they want to focus on. In order to make Soccer Fitness accessible to new target groups, the training in the concept is designed so no previous soccer experience or skills are required.

Soccer Fitness – a path-breaking concept

As it was the case with the DFA's decision to introduce professional soccer in 1978, there is also a tide of change behind the decision to implement Soccer Fitness. The shift to professional soccer brought a change in the organizational structure of both the DFA and some clubs, whereas the shift to Soccer Fitness has more impact on the nature of the game. The concept is designed to fit into the organizational structure that already exists in the clubs. In both cases, there were and are some groups pressing for a change, although the momentum for change may be generated in different ways. When professional soccer was introduced, the change was a bottom-up process (Jansen, 2004), with several forces slowly pushing the DFA into a shift that the organization finally could not avoid. In contrast, with the introduction of Soccer Fitness the change is based on a top-down process (Jansen, 2004) where an executive committee and the board of the DFA have decided to launch Soccer Fitness. The DFA is trying to prepare for the future patterns of sports participation, as shown by the internal proposal (DBU, 2010), and is intentionally breaking with the path that exists within recreational soccer. This proposal presents a scenario in which the DFA will face major challenges if it is not able to rethink its product and adapt to the changing landscape of sport. These challenges are also outlined in the report "Soccer in Denmark" (Kirkegaard et al., 2014), which came out a few years after the introduction of Soccer Fitness, and backs the new health-oriented strategy.

Within the DFA, the advocates of Soccer Fitness have been able to mobilize sufficient momentum for change to realize the concept. The implementation of Soccer Fitness has not been an easy process because of the resistance against change in the DFA, in local unions, and in soccer clubs. At first, the Soccer Fitness project in the DFA was only meant to be a three-year project, but although the management of the DFA sometimes felt the implementation could have gone faster, Soccer Fitness was a success in the clubs that introduced the concept. There were particularly large numbers of women who saw an opportunity to start playing soccer although they were complete beginners, and for whom Soccer Fitness was an activity they could fit into their daily routine. That is why the Soccer Fitness project was extended, and the DFA continued to set aside resources for the project.

Discussion and conclusion: is Soccer Fitness sustainable as a health-promoting concept?

Several studies highlight that organized sport is an ideal setting to promote community-wide participation in physical activity due to its societal position and reach into the local community (Casey et al., 2009; Crisp and Swerissen, 2003; Dobbinson et al., 2006; Eime et al., 2008). Soccer Fitness is a good example of this. Soccer Fitness uses the popular game soccer as an instrument of health policy with the specific aim of increasing the number of adult members in the soccer clubs and, in addition, of engaging more adults in physical activity. Considering the strong position of the organized sport, Priest et al. (2008) highlight the importance of identifying the most effective programs that sporting organizations can use to increase people's participation in physical activity. In addition, the authors state that the organized sport setting as a means of health promotion is a topic, which needs more attention from scholars and of practitioners. Casey et al. (2009) and Ooms et al. (2015) suggest that further research should focus on exploring factors influencing the long-term sustainability of health enhancing physical activity programs in the organized sports setting. If Soccer Fitness proves to be viable, this may be because Soccer Fitness has taken on a design, which is based on certain possibilities that soccer and team sports offer, which differ from the possibilities in the commercial centers, the opportunities of self-organized exercise, and the existing offers of the sports clubs. Even though challenges concerning the implementation have been detected (Bennike and Ottesen, manus), the Soccer Fitness concept is still growing and has even expanded to other countries as a model for engaging more people in physical activity within the context of sports clubs. One of the main questions is, whether Soccer Fitness is sustainable in the long term. It is central to both research and health promotion activities to identify enabling and constraining factors that influence the process of introduction and establishment of Soccer Fitness, and also to determine what makes soccer (as a team sport) effective as a health-promoting initiative.

A discussion of these questions can draw on Elias and Dunning's (1966) considerations on soccer. They emphasize that sport games like soccer are "largely ends in themselves. Their purpose, if they have a purpose, is to give people pleasure" (1996, p. 400). Although Soccer Fitness is primarily marketed as a health or fitness initiative, the DFA also emphasizes that this is not the only purpose of Soccer Fitness – other benefits include pleasure and friendship, which the DFA accentuates in the marketing with the subheading "Fun, Fitness, and Friendship." According to Elias and Dunning, sport is a creative playground where the participants are liberated from the daily humdrum and a place where emotions can be loosened. Sport is a 'mimetic event,' which allows people to slacken their self-restraints, and enjoy the pleasure of play and the 'leisure-gemeinschaften,' which reinforces our commitment (Elias and Dunning, 1986, p. 123). And this is exactly what the Soccer Fitness concept embodies.

Another important element in soccer is also stressed by Elias and Dunning (1966): soccer (and other team games) involves upholding a complex 'tension-balance,' which is only maintained by constantly producing a balance between a complex of interdependent polarities (p. 398). The first polarity is concerned with the group dynamic between the two subgroups represented by the teams. In order for the game to maintain a tension-balance, the teams should ideally be equally strong; if one team is much stronger, the game loses its dynamic, and the pleasure in playing vanishes (p. 397). The second polarity is the balance between cooperation and tension between the two teams. The third polarity is the balance between cooperation and tension between the players within each team. Tension control and conflicts are an inevitable part of the dynamic of the game of soccer, just as there is also a high degree of cooperation and harmony on a variety of levels (pp. 391, 399). The battle between the teams and the tension with regard to the outcome might be mechanisms that produce fitness or the medical health aspect of Soccer Fitness, as studies have shown that the players push themselves hard physically without it feeling exhausting, because the game provides enough diversion and gives them pleasure (Elbe et al., 2010).

In conclusion, we can say that Soccer Fitness manages to maintain a tension-balance and most of the other mechanisms that Elias and Dunning consider crucial to the success of the game. The DFA and the clubs have managed to organize and administer Soccer Fitness in new ways by the use of reduced membership fees (while retaining democratic influence) and the communication concerning the training happening via social media. In terms of flexibility, they have not been able to create the same flexibility with regard to attendance as there is in fitness centers, but the organization with teams formed of those players who turn up for training means that the participants experience attendance as being flexible.

To sum up, the development of Soccer Fitness is an example of sport used as a health-enhancing concept by way of a de-sportification process that so far has turned out successfully.

References

All links last accessed August 15, 2015, unless otherwise indicated.

Bennike, S., and Ottesen, L. (2016). How does interorganisational implementation behaviour challenge the success of Football Fitness? *European Journal for Sport and Society,* *13*(1), 19–37.

Bennike, S., Wikman, J.M., and Ottesen, L. (2014a). *Fodbold Fitness – Implementeringsstudie. 2013* [Football Fitness – Implementation study. 2013]. Copenhagen: Copenhagen Center for Team Sport and Health. Department of Nutrition, Exercise and Sports. University of Copenhagen.

Bennike, S., Wikman, J.M., and Ottesen, L. (2014b). Football Fitness – A new version of football? A concept for adult players in Danish football clubs. *Scandinavian Journal of Medicine and Science in Sports, 24* (S1), 138–146.

Bergsgard, N.A., Houlihan, B., Mangset, P., Nodland, S.I., and Rommetveldt, H. (2007). *Sport Policy: A Comparative Analysis of Stability and Change.* London: Elsevier.

Casey M.M., Payne W.R., Brown S.J., and Eime, R.M. (2009). Engaging community sport and recreation organisations in population health interventions: Factors affecting the formation, implementation, and institutionalization of partnerships efforts. *Annals of Leisure Research, 12*(2), 129–147.

Casey M. M., Payne W. R., Eime R. M., and Brown, S. J. (2009). Sustaining health promotion programs within sport and recreation organisations. *Journal of Science and Medicine in Sport*, *12*(1), 113–118.

Creswell, J. W. (2007). *Qualitative Inquiry and Research: Choosing among Five Approaches.* Thousand Oaks: SAGE.

Crisp, B. R., and Swerissen, H. (2003). Critical processes for creating health-promoting sporting environments in Australia. *Health Promotion International*, *18*(2), 145–152.

DBU (2010). *Fodbold Fitness (motionsfodbold)* [Football fitness (exercise football)] [booklet]. Brøndby: DBU.

DBU (2012). *Brug bolden – Forebyg livsstilssygdomme og aktiver udsatte borgere* [Use the ball – Prevent lifestyle diseases and activate at risk citizens] [booklet]. Retrieved from www.dbu.dk/~/media/Files/DBU_Broendby/Fodbold_Fitness/Materiale_til_klubber/ Materiale%202012/FF_Kommunemanual_dec2012.pdf

DBU (2014a). *Fodbold Fitness – Din sunde og fleksible mulighed* [Football Fitness – Your healthy and flexible option] [booklet]. Retrieved from www.dbu.dk/~/media/ Files/DBU_Broendby/Fodbold_Fitness/Materiale_til_klubber/Materiale_marts_2014/ Fodboldogsundhed_FF_2014.pdf

DBU (2014b). *Fodbold Fitness for kvinder – Øvelseskort med 12 ugers fitnesstræning* [Football Fitness for women – 12 weeks of fitness exercises] [booklet]. Retrieved from www.dbu.dk/~/media/Files/DBU_Broendby/Fodbold_Fitness/Materiale_til_klubber/ Materiale_marts_2014/FFQ_fitnessoevelser_2014.pdf

DBU (2014c). *Fodbold Fitness for kvinder – Øvelseskort med 12 ugers fodboldtræning* [Football Fitness for women – 12 weeks of football exercises] [booklet]. Retrieved from www.dbu.dk/~/media/Files/DBU_Broendby/Fodbold_Fitness/Materiale_til_klubber/ Materiale_marts_2014/FFQ_fodboldoevelser_2014.pdf

DBU (2014d). *Fodbold Fitness – Spiløvelser for mænd* [Football Fitness – Drills for men] [booklet]. Retrieved from www.dbu.dk/~/media/Files/DBU_Broendby/Fod bold_Fitness/Materiale_til_klubber/Materiale_marts_2014/FFM_fodboldoevelser_ 2014.pdf

DBU (2014e). *Fodbold Fitness – Styrkeøvelser for mænd* [Football Fitness – Strength exercises for men] [booklet]. Retrieved from www.dbu.dk/~/media/Files/DBU_Broendby/ Fodbold_Fitness/Materiale_til_klubber/Materiale_marts_2014/FFM_styrkeoevelser_ 2014.pdf

Dobbinson, J. S., Hayman, J. A., and Livingston, P. M. (2006). Prevalence of health promotion policies in sports clubs in Victoria, Australia. *Health Promotion International*, *21*(2), 121–129.

Eime, R. M., Payne, W. R., and Harvey, J. T. (2008). Making sporting clubs healthy and welcoming environments: A strategy to increase participation. *Journal of Science and Medicine in Sport*, *11*(2), 146–154.

Elbe, A. M., Strahler, K., Krustrup, P., Wikman, J., and Stelter, R. (2010). Experiencing flow in different types of physical activity intervention programs: Three randomized studies. *Scandinavian Journal of Medicine and Science in Sports*, *20*(S1), 111–117.

Elias, N., and Dunning, E. (1966). Dynamics of group sports with special reference to football. *British Journal of Sociology*, *17*(4), 388–402.

Elias, N., and Dunning, E. (1986). *Quest for Excitement: Sport and Leisure in the Civilizing Process.* Oxford: Blackwell.

Grønkjær, A., and Olsen, D. H. (2007). *Fodbold, fair play og forretning – Dansk klubfodbolds historie* [Football, fair play, and business – The history of Danish club football]. Århus: Turbine Forlaget.

Hammersly, M., and Atkinson, P. (2007). *Ethnography – Principles in practice* (3rd ed.). London: Routledge.

Houlihan, B. M. J. (2012). Sport policy convergence: A framework for analysis. *European Sport Management Quarterly*, *12*(2), 111–135.

Houlihan, B. M. J., Bloyce, D., and Smith, A. (2009). Developing the research agenda in sport policy. *International Journal of Sport Policy*, *1*(1), 1–12.

Jansen, K. J. (2004). From persistence to pursuit: A longitudinal examination of momentum during the early stages of strategic change. *Organization Science*, *15*(3), 276–294.

Kirkegaard, K. L., Fester, M., and Gottlieb, P. (2014). *Fodbold i Danmark – Kulturer, status og udvikling* [Football in Denmark – Cultures, status, and development]. Brøndby: Danmarks Idrætsforbund, Team Analyse.

Krustrup, B. R., Nielsen, S. F., and Ottesen, L. S. (2011). *Åbne fodboldbaner i dagtimerne. Igangsættelse af motionstiltag for inaktive grupper – en Hvidbog om sundhedsfremme i kommunalt regi* [Open football fields in the daylight houes. The start-up of exercise initiatives for inactive groups – A white paper on health promotion in the context of the municipalities]. Copenhagen: Department of Exercise and Sport Science. University of Copenhagen.

Krustrup, B. R., and Ottesen, L. (2014). *Fodbold Fitness – Pilotstudie. 2011* [Football Fitness – Pilot study. 2011]. Copenhagen: Copenhagen Center for Team Sport and Health. Department of Nutrition, Exercise and Sports. University of Copenhagen.

Krustrup, P., Aagaard, P., Nybo, L., Petersen, J., Mohr, M., and Bangsbo, J. (2010). Recreational football as a health promoting activity: A topical review. *Scandinavian Journal of Medicine and Science in Sports*, *20*(S1), 1–13.

Krustrup, P., Dvorak, J., Junge, A., and Bangsbo, J. (2010). Executive summary: The health and fitness benefits of regular participation in small-sided football games. *Scandinavian Journal of Medicine and Science in Sports*, *20*(S1), 132–135.

Kulturministeriet (2014). *Udredning af idrættens økonomi og struktur. Analyse* [Report on the economy and structure of sport in Denmark. Analysis]. Retrieved at http://kum.dk/fileadmin/KUM/Documents/Temaer/Midlertidig_mappe_juni_2014/Idraetsudredning_filer_juni_2014/Udredning_af_idraettens_oekonomi_og_struktur__Analyse_1.pdf

Kvale, S., and Brinkmann, S. (2009). *Inter View – Introduktion til et håndværk* (2. udg.). København: Hans Reitzels Forlag.

Laub, T. B. (2013). *Sports participation in Denmark 2011. National Survey – English Version*. Copenhagen: Danish Institute for Sports Studies.

Morgan, L. M. (1997). *Focus Groups as Qualitative Research* (2nd ed.). London: SAGE Publications.

Ooms, L., Veenhof, C., Veldhoven, N. S., and Bakker, D. H. (2015). Sporting programs for inactive population groups: Factors influencing implementation in the organized sports setting. *BMC Sports Science, Medicine, and Rehabilitation*, *7*(1), 12.

Ottesen, L., Jeppesen, R. S., and Krustrup, B. R. (2010). The development of social capital through football and running: Studying an intervention program for inactive women. *Scandinavian Journal of Medicine and Science in Sports*, *20*(S1), 118–131.

Priest, N., Armstrong, R., Doyle, J., and Waters, E. (2008). Interventions implemented through sporting organisations for increasing participation in sport. *Cochrane Database of Systematic Reviews*, *2008*(3), 1–15.

Rowe, K., Shilbury, D., Ferkins, L., and Hinckson, E. (2013). Sport development and physical activity promotion: An integrated model to enhance collaboration and understanding. *Sport Management Review*, *16*(3), 364–377.

Thing, L. F., and Ottesen, L. S. (2010). The autonomy of sports: Negotiating boundaries between sports governance and government policy in the Danish welfare state. *International Journal of Sport Policy and Politics*, *2*(2), 223–235.

17 Smart consumers and hopeless romantics

Albrecht Sonntag

A child of modernity in postmodern times

Contemporary soccer is a child of modernity. Born in England in 1863, it was raised in an environment of distinctly modern values and grew up under the influence of a strong political and cultural nationalism that held the entire continent in its firm grip.

In such a context, it is hardly surprising that from the beginning of the twentieth century, when the first international matches were played, soccer was, due to its intrinsic territorial layout and battlefield terminology ('attack,' 'defense,' 'wings,' 'shots,' 'captain,' etc.), understood everywhere as a mock confrontation of nations – "war minus the shooting," as George Orwell famously called it half a century and two world wars later (Orwell, 1945). At a moment where 'social Darwinism underwent considerable vulgarization' and where the principle of 'struggle – between animal species, social classes, capitalistic enterprises – started to be conceived as the main motor of life' (Ehrenberg, 1984), the organizers of international soccer fixtures very quickly saw the extraordinary identification potential that this sport held for crowds already prepared by massive nationalistic brainwash (Wahl, 1989; Hobsbawm, 1990).

A look at the chronological tables of the first international matches on the continent – putting aside the so-called 'international' matches between the British home nations, the first one of which was played as early as 1872 – is revealing: it is striking to see the speed with which encounters between national teams became a regular fixture in the soccer calendar during the first decade of the twentieth century. France played its first international match in 1904 in Belgium, but by the outbreak of the Great War only ten years later, it had already played 34 against a total of eight national teams! For Germany, the figures are comparable: its first match took place in 1908 in Switzerland; six years later 30 matches against nine different opponents had already been played (Sonntag, 2008, p. 101).

For more than a century, the modern values soccer thrived upon since its beginnings have underpinned its development, especially in the international arena. Over the last 25 years, however, there have been significant changes. Not in the rules of the game, whose remarkable stability over soccer's entire history accounts for a good deal of its worldwide success, but in the way it is organized, experienced, and narrated.

The present contribution is based on the assumption that these changes are nothing short of a paradigm shift that has brought international soccer to emancipate, albeit not entirely, from its 'upbringing' in modernity and embrace postmodern values. Soccer's new postmodern 'character traits' can be traced back to a series of events that took place in the 1990s, a decade which may be considered as the tipping point in the game's biography.

Paradigm shifts

Within a few years, soccer has undergone fundamental change. The following subsections will briefly discuss five events that occurred between 1991 and 1998 and whose long-term impact can today be assessed with the necessary distance.

1991 – the Premier League: introducing a new economic model

The agreement, signed on July 17, 1991, to create the English Premier League as a private limited company, clearly dissociated and independent from the associative structure that had organized top-flight soccer since the very beginning of professionalism, was nothing short of a revolution. Given financial and administrative autonomy, the Premier League has succeeded, in just a quarter of a century, to become an economic model of its own, envied and emulated by other major leagues in Europe.

In retrospect, the Premier League stands first and foremost for the unrestricted commodification of the game and a significant professionalization of its management. It turned club soccer into a 'premium product' of the entertainment business. The change in this product's distribution model was perfectly in line with the liberalization of the media landscape that had already started in the 1980s. The capitalization of the clubs brought in new types of investors, whose fundamental interest for the game itself may be open to speculation, but who fueled the new economic model to an extent that went beyond expectations.

As a result of the above (and also partly of other continent-wide changes discussed below), the Premier League has become the epitome of world club soccer, at least when it comes to the economic exploitation of soccer's potential. The exponential development of revenues from television has reached unprecedented heights for the broadcasting rights 2016–2019. Due to its deep and massive internationalization – on the pitch, in the stands, in the boardroom and in front of TV screens – it has truly become "The Global Soccer League," as Peter Millward put it (2011).

1992 – the Champions League: branding a new competition

On a European level the UEFA Champions League, which was introduced in 1992, was much more than just a new format for a long-established competition. Commissioned by UEFA in part as response to the menace of a secessionist 'super-league' made up of major European clubs, the Champions League was the application of contemporary branding techniques to a transnational event. The new brand was meant to be bigger than its participants and winners, similar to the Tour de France. Created by the Lucerne-based agency TEAM, the Champions League not only introduced perfect simultaneity of fixtures across the entire continent, but most of all was endowed with a particularly strong and all-encompassing audio-visual identity, leading to a genuine 'ritualization' of the event (King, 2003).

The Champions League opened new avenues for the commercialization of the top European club competition, contributing to the 'Europeanization' of the game (Niemann et al., 2011). Its most important innovation, however, was to give priority to market potential over sporting success in redistributing the enormous revenues it created. Almost 25 years later, it has become clear that this model has led to a concentration of financial, human and symbolic resources in the hands of a few clubs, which may eventually well be detrimental to the very idea of an open European club competition. It is not excluded that the development of the Champions League will inevitably lead to the de facto emergence of the closed private league that it was created to avoid in the first place.

This perspective notwithstanding, the Champions League is a model case study of how to 'update,' with the help of state-of-the-art marketing techniques, a relatively simple competition firmly rooted in the modern values soccer was nurtured upon, and turn it into an almost post-national, global brand.

1992 – Fever Pitch: changing the soccer narrative

At the same moment, with an amazing sense for the dusk of an epoch, the autobiographical first novel of an unknown author changed the manner in which soccer was written and talked about. Nick Hornby's reflexive account of his own soccer craziness introduced a new tone in narrating the individual and collective soccer experience. His self-mocking, often hilarious description of the eternal frustration and suffering of the ordinary supporter gave evidence to the fact that soccer fans were perfectly capable of adopting a critical distance to their own passion (Hornby, 1992).

Hornby's novel gave birth to an entire genre, in which new and different self-perceptions of soccer supporters were expressed with an irony that may be qualified as 'postmodern,' for want of a better term. It also echoed the phenomenon of popular appropriation and interiorization of knowledge generated by the social sciences that has been termed 'reflexivity' and defined as a characteristic feature of 'late modernity' by scholars like Anthony Giddens (1990) or Ulrich Beck (1994, 1997).

1995 – The Bosman ruling: imposing European labor law on soccer

The *Bosman* ruling of December 1995 has become probably the single most quoted ruling of the European Court of Justice, at least in the general media. It has also been the object of massive academic comment, especially in the field of legal studies. The decision to apply the principle of free movement of workers enshrined in the European treaties to the labor market of professional soccer players put an end to the quotas of 'foreign players' traditionally imposed by the leagues on their clubs. The ruling initially only concerned players from within the European Union, but several leagues and federations seized the opportunity to extend it to other countries of origin and virtually liberated professional clubs from any previously existing restrictions based on the nationality of players (Lanfranchi and Taylor, 2001). As a result, today the mobility of players is basically unrestricted, and professional squads have become multinational to the point that some of them often no longer count any home-born national player in their line-ups.

The long-term consequences of the *Bosman* ruling are controversial. Many commentators were (and still are) deeply nostalgic about the days when national teams had been a simple extension of club soccer, with players selected from the best clubs of each country. They feared that national teams would lose their 'identity,' together with their traditional playing style narrative (as imaginary as the latter may have been in reality). At the same time clubs were believed to inevitably lose their local support, with next to no player from their home region in their line-up.

Time and scholarly research (Sonntag, 2008; Ranc, 2011) have shown that both fears were perfectly unfounded. Still the *Bosman* ruling is a paradigm shift, not only for its massive impact on player mobility and team compositions, but also for the precedent it created in making European governance trump over the famous 'autonomy of sport' and its national regulations. It is not exaggerated to say that the *Bosman* ruling and the Champions League were made for each other and have mutually reinforced their effects on the development of contemporary European soccer.

1998 – France 98: serving the romantics

Only six years after the creation of the Champions League and three years after the *Bosman* ruling, the FIFA World Cup 1998 in France turned out to be a 'watershed' event (Sonntag, 2014).

First of all, it was a major logistical challenge. For the first time 32 teams (among which 15 from Europe) were qualified for a tournament that was organized in a country which is already in normal times the world's number one tourist destination. Moreover, the liberalization of European air traffic, Western Europe's highly developed high-speed rail grid and the excellent motorway infrastructure brought a number of potential spectators to France that the relatively small stadiums were perfectly incapable of absorbing.

Against the backdrop of disappointed fans, in many cases abused by ticket frauds, especially in Japan, the organizers had no choice but to provide alternative solutions. As a result, the huge asymmetry between demand and supply of available tickets both for the domestic and foreign public eventually had an unexpected side effect, which turned out to be a major asset of the French World Cup and has since changed the way the event is experienced and shared: the invention of large-scale 'public viewing.'

France 98 was the first World Cup that was shown on a significant number of giant screens on town squares and in sport arenas, in parks and on beaches. These screenings gained an immediate and lasting popularity and contributed massively to the atmosphere in the country and the appropriation of the World Cup by the French population.

The emergence of 'public viewing' – initially a pseudo-anglicism coined in Germany, now the official term used by FIFA and public authorities – cannot be overestimated in its lasting impact. Not only has it massively increased the number of spectators that can experience the games together in a stadium-like atmosphere, but it has put the crowd in the center of the show. What was observed with amused curiosity in 1998 (Augé, 1998) has today become an indispensable part of the event itself: the unfiltered emotional reactions of the crowd huddled together in front of the screens, its noisy and colorful self-celebration – complete with make-up, clothing, wigs, and hats, etc. – have become trademarks of soccer mega-events (Alpan et al., 2015).

Most of all, France 98 was a powerful demonstration for the unbroken appeal of national teams. The unprecedented public display of national identities actually revealed an entirely new, and strengthened, positioning of the national teams, which had occurred not *despite* but *because of* the combined effects of the Premier League, the Champions League, and the *Bosman* ruling.

At the end of the twentieth century soccer had undergone dramatic change, which became more and more visible in the years that followed. Today the game is organized, experienced and narrated in a different manner; it is played and watched in a substantially different environment of accelerated cultural globalization. In the twentieth century, characterized by contradictory phenomena of postmodern consumer trends and modern social needs, there is no longer one uniform game, but two different soccers, embodied in European club soccer and periodic international events contested by national teams.

The age of two soccers

Until the 1980s national teams had been very closely linked to the domestic leagues. When Bayern Munich won the European Cup in 1974, it fielded ten German players, seven of whom were from Bavaria! The World Cup final of the same year, between Germany and the Netherlands, came close to an opposition between Bayern and Ajax, enriched by a handful of players from other major clubs in the respective countries. In contrast, the victorious French team of 1998 only counted two players who still played for French clubs!

In other words: there has been a 'divorce' between club soccer and national teams, and it can be said to be a mutually beneficial one, since both types of soccer, epitomized, on the one hand, in the Premier League and the Champions League and, on the other hand, in the World Cup and the Euro, have not only stabilized but actually increased their appeal (given television's seemingly insatiable appetite for soccer, one may replace 'appeal' by 'revenues'). They have been able to do so because in the imagination of their public they are now perceived as 'antithetical' to one other.

This 'antithetical' configuration is based on two antagonistic sets of representation that have emerged and consolidated over the last 15 years. While the postmodern world of club soccer now reflects unlimited mobility and multiculturalism, national teams still stand for strong local roots and a kind of imaginary, untainted cultural 'purity' (note that this imagined 'purity' is no longer based on ethnic criteria in most Western European societies).

While leagues and clubs appear as giving priority to economic value and maximum commercialization, national teams represent cultural values and not-for-profit idealism. Needless to say this idealism is partly imaginary – after all, national teams are the revenue-generating cash cows of the federations – but it is also founded on the perfectly credible assumption that professional players are not motivated by money when they play for the national 'colors' (Sonntag, 2008).

This 'tale of two soccers' brings to mind the famous distinction between 'society' ('*Gesellschaft*') and 'community' ('*Gemeinschaft*') formulated by the German sociologist Ferdinand Tönnies in 1887 (Tönnies, 1957). Under globalization pressure this seminal dichotomy seems to have become even more relevant today than it was at the end of nineteenth century (Barber, 1995). Interestingly, in a contribution to a sociology handbook 40 years after his groundbreaking book, Tönnies emphasized that society and community are not mutually exclusive, but actually mutually reinforcing within the framework of what he referred to as '*Samtschaft*,' a neologism that should be understood as an umbrella term for what is usually called 'people' or 'nation' (Tönnies, 1959). The '*Samtschaft*' is thus a very ambiguous, even contradictory concept. Its members oscillate between the societal and communitarian logic, which they activate at different moments, depending on their contextual sociopsychological needs.

At the beginning of the twentieth century, what Tönnies described as 'society' could be referred to as the 'socio-economic marketplace,' subject to and shaped by the rules of free-market economy, supply and demand. It's a world in where individualism reigns, where the customer is king, and which is based on the principle of hedonistic choice. Socioeconomic bonds, such as loyalties between employer and employees, are increasingly flexible, less and less stable.

There is, however, another world that still remains deeply attractive to human beings, where free-market economy does not make the rules, where choice is almost inexistent, where loyalties are forever. It is the community of destiny, firmly anchored in modernity, a community one cannot escape and which provides reliable, emotional bonds between the individuals that compose it. In stark opposition to the profane marketplace of 'society,' the community of destiny triggers deep collective feelings of belonging, that are attributed to the realm of the 'sacred' (Eliade, 1965).

Soccer is compatible with both worlds, with postmodern hedonism and modern belonging, with the profane and the sacred. It serves at the same time the smart, individualist lifestyle consumers of the twenty-first century, and the helpless community romantics whose social needs of 'togetherness' makes them prisoners of the legacy of the nineteenth-century's 'nationalization of the masses' (Mosse, 1975).

As interviews with major actors of the European soccer scene have shown, the process of 'divorce' that has led to the present configuration has by no means been an intentional one (Sonntag, 2008), neither from the side of the leagues or 'big clubs,' nor from the side of the national associations, which are in charge of the national teams. This is perhaps the reason why both sides are winners.

Some lessons from the FREE project

The FREE Project (Football Research in an Enlarged Europe), which was carried out between 2012 and 2015 has, in some of its research streams, tried to study the oscillation of soccer fans' behavior between modern and postmodern values and attitudes. While the space of this contribution does of course not allow an in-depth discussion of the findings, some points may be summarized in a succinct manner.

In the large quantitative survey, for instance, carried out in 2014, a series of questions were linked to attitudes with regard to the dichotomy between patriotic–traditionalist values and more critical–postnational values (FREE, 2014). Among many other questions, respondents were asked whether they agreed or disagreed (on a four-point scale) with the following statements:

- The victories of our national soccer team are a source of pride for me.
- When my national team loses an important match, I am sad or upset.
- National teams should have a coach from the same country.
- Players with migrant background should play for the country of their family.
- It is an honor for a soccer player to play for the national team.
- The national team is nothing sacred; I can easily make fun of it.
- It is fun to joke around with national stereotypes when two teams meet.

To no surprise, both patriotic–traditionalist and critical–postnational values are significantly present among soccer fans. The degree to which an individual fan tends toward critical-postnational (or 'cosmopolitan') attitudes is directly affected by the migrant status of the respondents themselves and by the country of residence. Soccer patriotism is for instance particularly strong in the UK, Spain, or Turkey, while respondents from Germany, Austria, or Denmark tend to show more relaxed arrangements with their national identity (at least when it comes to soccer). Interestingly, across all variables, players with migrant origins in the national team were clearly perceived as positive integration models.

The findings from the survey are corroborated by the extensive qualitative research carried out by the FREE project consortium across nine European target countries. European soccer fans accept increasingly fluid loyalties and transnational standardization, while appreciating punctual nostalgic reassurance of national singularity (Alpan et al., 2015). They are clearly both 'smart consumers,' shopping for hedonistic pleasure, and 'hopeless romantics' who long for authentic emotions.

The next 25 years

The heritage of the paradigm shifts from the 1990s is no doubt a rather sustainable one. There will be no 'remarriage' between the two soccers. The divorce has been too beneficial to all parties to be put into question again. The enormous financial benefits that reside in the ever clearer cut between club soccer and national teams are however likely to be too tempting for all stakeholders involved to keep them from overblowing the bubble.

There will be, in the coming years, a further 'Disneyization' of European top-flight soccer. The focus in the soccer entertainment industry will be on market share, risk management and planning security rather than on the traditional principles of modern sport. The redistribution of revenues is likely to result in a further concentration of financial and sportive power in the hands of a small élite. And the logical end of this evolution will necessarily be a kind of closed league on the European level, no matter how loudly the main actors currently protest against this idea.

At the same time there will be a further, intensified exploitation of the enormous emotional potential of the national teams. The imagined 'purity' and 'authenticity' of this symbolic embodiment of the modern community of destiny will continue to be perceived as a necessary counter-weight to the anxiety produced by a rootless and borderless postmodern society. In addition to the World Cup and European Championship, which are already reliable producers of emotional outbursts every second year, a new competition named 'Nations League' will be launched by UEFA as of 2018.

Will the soccer bubble burst at one point? Given the context of accelerated globalization, a sudden burst is not very likely. What the FREE research has shown, however, is that the continuous flow of money into the game is perceived by many as too destabilizing. As a result, there are increasing calls for more regulation. In their postmodern business euphoria, the next generation of soccer leaders would be well advised to keep in mind that the smart consumers, whose purchase power they target, are also hopeless romantics in search of more than just entertainment.

References

Alpan, B., Schwell, A., and Sonntag, A. (eds.) (2015). *The European Championship: Mega-Event and Vanity Fair*. Basingstoke: Palgrave Macmillan.

Augé, M. (1998). 'Un ethnologue au Mondial.' In: *Le Monde diplomatique*, August 1998.

Barber, B. (1995). *Jihad vs. McWorld: How Globalism and Tribalism Are Reshaping the World*. New York: Crown.

Beck, U. (1997). *Was ist Globalisierung?* Frankfurt: Suhrkamp.

Beck, U., Giddens, A., and Lash, S. (1994). *Reflexive Modernization: Politics, Tradition and Aesthetics in the Modern Social Order*. Redwood, CA: Stanford University Press.

Eliade, M. (1965). *Le sacré et le profane*, Paris: Gallimard.

Ehrenberg, A. (1984). 'Le football et ses imaginaires,' *Les Temps Modernes*, *460*, November 1984, 841–884.

FREE (Football Research in an Enlarged Europe) (2014). European Football Fans Survey (Unpublished data).

Giddens, A. (1990). *The Consequences of Modernity*. Redwood, CA: Stanford University Press.

Hobsbawm, E. (1990). *Nations and Nationalism since 1780*. Cambridge: Cambridge University Press.

Hornby, N. (1992). *Fever Pitch*. London: Victor Gollancz.

King, A. (2003). *The European Ritual*. Aldershot: Ashgate.

Lanfranchi, P. and Taylor, M. (2001). *Moving with the Ball*. Oxford: Berg.

Millward, P. (2011). *The Global Football League. Transnational Networks, Social Movements and Sport in the New Media Age*. Basingstoke: Palgrave Macmillan, 2011.

Mosse, G. (1975). *The Nationalization of the Masses*. New York: Howard Fertig.

Niemann, A., Garcia, B., and Grant, W. (2011). *The Transformation of European Football. Towards the Europeanisation of the national game*. Manchester: Manchester University Press.

Orwell, G. (1945). 'The sporting spirit,' *Tribune*, 14 December 1945.

Ranc, D. (2011). *Foreign Players and Football Supporters: The Old Firm, Arsenal, Paris Saint-Germain*. Manchester: Manchester University Press.

Sonntag, A. (2008). *Les identités du football européen*. Grenoble: Presses Universitaires de Grenoble.

Sonntag, A. (2014). 'France 98 – A Watershed World Cup.' In S. Rinke and K. Schiller (eds.): *The FIFA World Cup 1930–2010 – Politics, Commerce, Spectacle and Identities*. Göttingen: Wallstein, 318–336.

Tönnies, F. (1959). 'Gemeinschaft und Gesellschaft.' In A. Vierkandt (ed.): *Handwörterbuch der Soziologie*, [1931]. Stuttgart: Ferdinand Enke, 180–191.

Tönnies, F. (1957). *Community and Association (Gemeinschaft und Gesellschaft)*. London: Routledge & Kegan Paul.

Wahl, A. (1989). *Les archives du football. Sport et société en France (1880–1980)*. Paris: Gallimard.

18 American football

Ideology and national identity

Gerald R. Gems

Introduction

This study presents an interdisciplinary approach to deconstruct the American national game of football to determine its characteristics, values, and meanings and the role it plays in the American culture. The history of the game, an anthropological assessment of its martial qualities, and a linguistic analysis of its terminology will provide greater understanding of the roots of American ideology and its ramifications for political decision making.

Americans gained their independence from Great Britain after their Revolutionary War in the late eighteenth century; but it took another century for them to fashion the game that would define American culture. In the aftermath of the Revolutionary War, Americans struggled to agree upon the nature of democracy, the relationship between the disparate states, human rights, and the economy. The British practice of impressment of American sailors resulted in a second war with the monarchy in 1812. In its aftermath Americans began to distance themselves from British culture by creating their own national literature replete with American heroes, emblematic of their frontier experience, eventually leading to a belief in American exceptionalism. In the wake of the American Civil War the first intercollegiate football contest was played in 1869, spawning the game that would surpass baseball to become the national sport, and the one that defines American character (Blum et al., 1981; Gems, 2000).

Evolution of the game

Versions of football had been played by American students on college campuses for decades, usually as a means for older students to pummel younger ones in an initiation rite. In 1868 the Princeton College club adopted the London Football Association Rules, and traveled to nearby Rutgers College a year later to undertake the first contest between academic institutions, won by Rutgers, 6–4. The two teams competed again a week later in a game won by Princeton, 8–0. Both teams used 25 players per side. In 1872 Harvard University adopted rugby rules, necessitating deliberations between teams over the nature of any future contests between schools (Gems, 2000). Such contests were organized by student clubs that identified themselves with the colleges although they had no formal affiliation with it.

Rules committees composed of members of the eastern college teams gradually adopted rugby football rules throughout the remainder of the decade. By 1876 Yale claimed a 'national championship' when it defeated Princeton, a rival school. The designation of 'national champion' earned greater social capital. By that time the interscholastic matches had already become commercialized spectacles with thousands of paying spectators and the game soon spread to the Midwest region of the country. The game further evolved under Walter Camp, captain of the Yale team and head of the rules committee, which he chaired until his death in 1925, earning him the sobriquet of 'the father of American football.' Camp's innovations included a line of scrimmage, similar to rugby, which started each play. Further departures from European soccer and rugby ensued with the introduction of a rule requiring teams to gain 5 yards within three tries to retain possession of the ball (later changed to 10 yards in four tries). The innovation required greater attention to offensive strategy and brute force as teams plowed forward, not unlike in actual warfare, in an attempt to advance through the opponents' territory and reach the ultimate goal line to score points. The mass plays and attacks directed at weak points in the opponents' line resembled actual warfare and engendered numerous casualties and a mounting number of actual deaths as the game spread throughout the nation. Like the ancient Romans who congregated in the Colosseum, fans flocked to the games to witness the violent carnage (Gems, 2000).

Militarism

Journalists drew comparisons to actual warfare where "two armies are managed on military principles ... where players worked with 'clock-work precision'" (Johnston, 1887, pp. 891–893). In the modern world, football thus served as a training ground for the aggressive, competitive industrialized capitalist system as the Americans prepared to challenge the British for global supremacy and coaches extolled the leadership qualities inherent in the game that would transfer to the business world.

As early as 1890 *The Nation*, a prominent publication asserted that:

> The spirit of American youth, as of the man, is to win, to 'get there,' by fair means or foul; and the lack of moral scruple which pervades the struggle of the business world meets with temptations equally irresistible in the miniature contests of the football field.
>
> (*Nation*, 1890, p. 895)

By 1898 the American economy surpassed British production and Americans rationalized such expansion as 'the survival of the fittest' in a Social Darwinian battle for markets (Brands, 1995).

The rivalries fostered by the interscholastic competitions caused a further departure from the British ideals of sportsmanship. For many Americans, winning surpassed sportsmanship as a means to social capital and national distinction among universities. Walter Camp proclaimed that "our players have strayed away from the original Rugby [*sic*] rules, but in so doing they have built up a game and rules of their own more suited to American needs" (1888, pp. 858–859). Another writer explained that "football … embodies so many factors that are typically American … virile, intensive, aggressive energy that makes for progress is the root which upholds and feeds American supremacy and American football" (Blanchard, 1923, pp. 389–390).

Senator Henry Cabot Lodge rationalized that

> such injuries incurred on the playing field are part of the price which the English-speaking race has paid for being world conquerors … victories … are the manifestation and evidence of a spirit which is all important … this great democracy is moving onward to its great destiny. Woe to the men or nations that bar its imperial march.
>
> (*Harvard Graduates Magazine*, 1896, pp. 66–68)

The United States soon embraced its belief in manifest destiny by embarking on the Spanish–American War in 1898.

Violence and deaths continued to mount on the football fields as well, with 18 fatalities and 159 serious injuries in the 1905 season and another 33 deaths in 1909. College presidents and clergy clamored for a ban on the game; but political leaders extolled it as a necessity to build the martial qualities required for warfare and imperial ventures to match the Europeans' global colonies. Despite the death of one of his own players at the University of Virginia in 1909, the school president, Edwin Alderman, refused to ban the sport, claiming that "in dealing with this game you are dealing with our national characteristics" (Watterson, 1993, p. 159).

President Theodore Roosevelt proved an ardent supporter of the game for similar reasons. As women assumed a greater role in society and eroded male dominance in political, educational, and economic domains Roosevelt claimed that the "football field is the only place where masculine supremacy is incontestable" (Hult, 1994, p. 84). By the turn of the twentieth century, football had spread throughout the secondary schools as youth teams traveled across the country to claim their own national championships. Urban athletic clubs, small towns, and industrial teams also formed to challenge their rivals with large wagers at stake. Such intense gambling necessitated a quest for the best players regardless of pedigree or social status, allowing working class participation and a growing professionalization within the sport. The incorporation of the lower classes, ethnic immigrant youth, and African Americans also promoted the perception of a meritocracy within the American society. The physical prowess required and celebrated by the game held special appeal for the habitus of the lower classes. In that sense, the game had become "a weekly anthropological play that celebrated American might and vitality, as it signaled the transition in power relations, both internally and abroad" (Gems, 2000, p. 24).

The National Collegiate Athletic Association was formed as a governing body in 1906 to address the mounting casualty rate, and the following year the rules committee introduced a new statute that allowed the ball to be thrown forward as a means to advance the offense and by 1912 the game had assumed the characteristics by which it is played today. With the advent of World War I the military formally adopted the game as part of its training. The Rose Bowl game, the most prominent football spectacle of the era, featured military teams rather than university squads in both 1918 and 1919 (Hibner, 1993). In the wake of the war football stadiums were built throughout the nation to commemorate the deaths of the military veterans. One of them, the aptly named Soldier Field in Chicago, hosted the annual city championship game between the winners of the Public High School League and the Catholic schools. Such contests served to integrate the largely outcast and suspect Catholics into the mainstream Protestant culture. The 1937 contest drew 120,000 spectators to the stadium, a measure of the importance attached to a game between two teams composed of teenagers (Gems, 1996). With the outbreak of World War II, American football assumed greater prominence in sustaining the morale of its military forces. Military bases formed their own baseball and football teams and engaged in international competitions to be recognized as champions. Amid the rubble caused by the nuclear bombs that ended the war, the Americans even staged the scornfully named Atom Bowl football game in Nagasaki, Japan. By 1950, 80 admirals in the American navy and 98 generals had played the game, seemingly a necessity for leadership in the military (Higgs, 1982; Siegfried and Katz, 2011).

By the 1960s, professional football surpassed baseball as the national game and the National Football League (NFL) increasingly tied itself to the military in the staging of its weekly spectacles and its national championship known as the Super Bowl. The current contest serves as a two week long national festival promoting such American values as nationalism, civic pride, capitalist excess, and consumption, with particular attention to militaristic displays of power (Oates and Furness, 2014). Football games are often accompanied by thunderous flyovers by military jets. Steve Sabol, president of NFL Films, stated that "perhaps the most impressive moment of the NFL pregame pageantry is the shock and awe of the flyover" (Butterworth, 2014, p. 205). Military personnel are then often involved in ceremonial functions, such as the coin toss to determine which team will get the ball first, the presentation of the American flag, the singing of the national anthem, and tributes or medal presentations to personnel wounded in wars, none of which have anything to do with the actual playing of the game other than the symbolic portrayal of nationalism and the warrior ethic (Butterworth, 2014).

The personal costs of football

Upon the field, high priced gladiators charge each other in individual and group combat, sacrificing their bodies for temporary wealth and celebrity. Their average career lasts fewer than four years and most players end up in financial straits. With no guaranteed health insurance and broken bodies, their life expectancy is about 20 years less than that of the average American male. Many players suffer from brain damage due to repeated concussions, consequent depression, and a high rate of suicide (Lazar, 2013). Still the media extols the violence inherent in the game and the NFL glories in its militaristic associations. The American people largely dismiss their warlike tendencies and seemingly take pride in the fact that every American generation has fought in a war. Children are socialized to accept such values at an early age (Oates and Furness, 2014).

Football terminology

The language of football represents the close association with war and violence. Among the terminology of the sport, by no means complete are: bomb, blitz, in the trenches, coffin corner, gunner, sack, suicide squad, aerial attack, run and shoot, shotgun, sudden death, and field general. Such terminology portrays the American affinity with violence. The United States was forged in war and its entire national history is littered with violence. When it was not engaged in war with other nations it sanctioned violence against its own populace. Frontier pioneers, cowboys, and soldiers assumed iconic and heroic roles in the conquest of the American West by killing its native inhabitants. Lynchings, or informal group killings, took the lives of many thousands of non-whites, mostly African Americans; but also Hispanics, Native American Indians, Asians, and Italians over the nineteenth and twentieth centuries (Pfeifer, 2014). Gun violence remains a prodigious cause of death throughout the United States, accounting for more than 33,000 mortalities in 2013 (Statistics USA, 2013). During the football season, sanctioned violence is publicly exhibited and praised daily by both broadcast and social media platforms.

Heroization

The NFL tried to manipulate the merger of football, war, and violence in the construction of a national hero in 2004. In the aftermath of the 9/11 attacks in 2001, Pat Tillman, a professional football player, eschewed his $3.6 million dollar contract to join the US Army in 2002. Two years later he was killed in a firefight with the Taliban in Afghanistan. The Army awarded him a Silver Star medal, one of the highest honors for valor presented to American heroes. He was extolled by the White House, lauded by celebrities and politicians, and praised as a role model by the NFL. Three thousand people showed up at his memorial service, which was televised by two television networks. Senator John McCain, a former prisoner of war in Vietnam, and Maria Shriver, a member of the Kennedy family and wife of then California governor Arnold Schwarzenegger, delivered speeches in Tillman's honor. Arizona, the state in which he played football at the university and professional levels, flew its flags at half-mast in recognition of his sacrifice. The professional team for which he played permanently retired his jersey, a distinct honor as no one else will ever be allowed to wear it, erected a statue of him outside the stadium and named the adjoining plaza after him as a lasting memorial. Fans travel to the site not unlike a religious pilgrimage to bask in the graces of a holy martyr.

Sports Illustrated, a popular magazine, stated that:

> In a country where no civilians have been asked to sacrifice anything and where even the cost of the war is being forwarded to their children and their children's children, a man had sacrificed the biggest dream of all. The NFL.
>
> (King, 2014, p. 198)

Despite the fact that an investigation revealed that Tillman was actually killed by friendly fire, i.e. mistakenly by his own troops, his "story being relentlessly told and retold to this end, a ceremony to honor his death became a vehicle through which sport and war were once again rendered equivalent" (King, 2014, pp. 198–199). Even though his family revealed that Tillman had become disenchanted with and actually opposed the war, the NFL continued with the charade.

The NFL had already marked its close relationship with the military after 9/11 by sending players to visit wounded veterans of the Iraq war in hospitals, sending football equipment to military teams, and partnering with the federal government to sponsor a program known as Operation Tribute to Freedom to promote patriotism, nationalism, and support for the war being conducted in the Mideast. To open the 2003 football season the government gave the NFL, a private entity, permission to commandeer the public space on the National Mall in Washington, DC for an entire week to deliver its $10,000,000 theatrical production featuring a series of popular musical stars in a festive atmosphere, which was attended by 300,000 fans, including 25,000 military veterans and their families. The joint venture honored the military, offered support for the so-called 'war on terrorism,' and linked the effort to the NFL, which culminated the event with the inaugural game beamed to American military bases around the world (King, 2014). The production provided a justification for American retaliation and equated the military warriors with the warrior ethic that had been trained on the football fields for more than a century.

At the 2004 NFL draft, a public ceremony in which the professional teams select the best players from the college ranks as potential warriors, the commissioner of the league stated that:

> "Pat Tillman personified the best values of America and of the National Football League.... Like other men and women protecting our freedom around the globe, he made the ultimate sacrifice and gave his life for his country"..
> After a moment of silence, the assembled crowd of fans erupted in the 'USA, USA' chant, continuing to link nationalism, patriotism, and football with the perception of heroic martyrdom.
>
> (King, 2014, p. 198)

Conclusion

Such manifestations of heroic militarism are evident throughout the football season, which starts in August and continues into February, in which high school, intercollegiate, and professional games are televised almost daily, thus reinforcing such cultural values. Another American scholar has determined that "Football is a kind of work, organized in accordance with military images, that requires the body to be used as an instrument of sanctioned aggression and violence" (Butterworth, 2014, p. 210).

Football serves Americans as a form of a secular religion, reinforcing its norms, values, and standards. It is a highly competitive and commercialized enterprise reflecting the countries' capitalist economy, played out in a game that requires a public demonstration of aggressive masculinity, cloaked in the trappings of patriotism. The game is exemplary of American national identity historically forged by the violent acquisition of territory. Its heroes are enshrined in halls of fame where believers travel to worship in the glory of their deeds that tie the past to the present and reinforce the ethnocentric belief in American exceptionalism (Gems and Pfister, 2009).

References

Blanchard, J.A. (ed.) (1923). *The H Book of Harvard Athletics, 1852–1922*. Harvard Varsity Club.

Blum, J.M., Morgan, E.S., Rose, W.L., Schlesinger, Jr., A.M., Stampp, K.M., and Woodward., C.V. (1981). *The National Experience: A History of the United States*. New York: Harcourt, Brace, Jovanovich.

Brands, H.W. (1995). *The Reckless Decade: America in the 1890s*. New York: St. Martin's Press.

Butterworth, M.L. (2014). NFL Films and the Militarization of Professional Football. In Oates, T.P. and Furness, Z. (eds.) (2014): *The NFL: Critical and Cultural Perspectives*, 205–225. Philadelphia: Temple University Press.

Camp, W. (1888). The American Game of Football. *Harper's Weekly*, November 10.

Garaty, J.A. (1983). *The American Nation: A History of the United States*. New York: Harper and Row.

Gems, G.R. (1996). The Prep Bowl: Sport, Religion, and Americanization in Chicago. *Journal of Sport History*, (Fall), 284–302.

Gems, G.R. (2000). *For Pride, Profit and Patriarchy: Football and the Incorporation of American Cultural Values*. Lanham, MD: Scarecrow Press.

Gems, G.R. and Pfister, G. (2009). *Understanding American Sport*. New York: Routledge.

Harvard Graduates Magazine (1896). 5:17 (September).

Hibner, J.C. (1993). *The Rose Bowl, 1902–1929*. Jefferson, NC: McFarland and Co.

Higgs, R.J. (1982). *Sports: A Reference Guide*. Westport, CT: Greenwood Press.

Hult, J.S. (1994). The Story of Women's Athletics: Manipulating a Dream, 1890–1985. In Costa, D.M. and Guthrie, S.A. (Eds.): *Women and Sport*, 83–106. Champaign, IL: Human Kinetics.

Johnston, A. (1887). The American Game of Football, *Century, 12*, 891–893.

King, S. (2014). Offensive Lines: Sport-State Synergy in an Era of Perpetual War. In Oates, T.P. and Furness, Z. (eds.) (2014): *The NFL: Critical and Cultural* Perspectives, 191–204. Philadelphia: Temple University Press.

Lazar, K. (2013). NFL players union and Harvard team up on landmark study of football injuries and illness. *Boston Globe*, January 29. Retrieved February 25, 2015 from www.

boston.com/lifestyle/health/2013/01/29/nfl-players-union-and-harvard-team-landmark-study-football-injuries-and-illness/aCGnf96h7ptWX2Lnp5MIiP/story.html

Oates, T. P. and Furness, Z. (eds.) (2014). *The NFL: Critical and Cultural Perspectives.* Philadelphia: Temple University Press.

Pfeifer, M. J. (2014). At the Hands of Parties Unknown? The State of the Field of Lynching Scholarship. *Journal of American History*, *101*(3), 832–846.

Siegfried, C. S. and M. Katz (2011). The Creation of Domestic and International Bowl Games from 1942 to 1964: The United States Military and Football as Conjoined Twins. *Sport History Review*, *42*(2), 153–175.

Statistics USA (2013). *Mortality.* Retrieved February 28, 2015 from www.cdc.gov/nchs/fastats/injury.htm

Watterson, J. S. (1993). The Death of Archer Christian: College Presidents and the Reform of College Football. *Journal of Sport History*, *22*(2), 149–167.

19 Gaelic football in a sociological perspective

John Connolly and Paddy Dolan

Introduction

We have previously written from a sociological perspective on many aspects of Gaelic football, and Gaelic games more generally, including player and spectator violence (Connolly and Dolan, 2010; Dolan and Connolly, 2009, 2014), media relations (Connolly and Dolan, 2012), organizational tensions (Connolly, 2015; Connolly and Dolan, 2011, 2013a) and the tension between amateurism and professionalism (Connolly and Dolan, 2013b). It is to this latter aspect we return here. The sports of Gaelic football, handball and hurling (collectively referred to as 'Gaelic games') remain one of the few remaining amateur sports in the world today. This is somewhat remarkable given the gradual erosion of the amateur ethos across a whole range of sporting domains that has occurred over the course of the last 130 years, including sports such as rugby union which held a strong amateur ethos until relatively recently. Moreover, the Gaelic Athletic Association (GAA), the entity with responsibility for the organization of games, is one of the largest sports bodies in Ireland. It has 500,000[1] members worldwide and significant financial revenues generated directly and indirectly from spectators – through gate-taking and broadcast rights. Indeed, over €29m was generated from gate-taking in 2013.[2] We emphasize this last point because financial dependence on spectators has been connected to professionalizing pressures (Dunning and Sheard, 1979).

In recent years professionalizing tensions within the GAA have escalated. Moreover, given the emotional charge, the issue generates debates and disputes between different groups and individuals comprising the GAA have tended to mask a more sociologically informed picture of the amateur–professional structure of Gaelic games and the GAA. Previously we explained how amateurism came to be framed and institutionalized, while we also outlined how and why discourses associated with both amateurism and professionalism were increasingly amplified since the 1960s (Connolly and Dolan, 2013b). However, these changes were not merely discursive. Over the last 40 years, in particular, professionalization has advanced – particularly at the elite level, though also at lower tiers but in a more uneven and limited way. This contention – that professionalization has advanced[3] in the GAA – is somewhat controversial and perhaps, stripped of its theoretical underpinning, misunderstood. We are not suggesting the Gaelic games are professional; they remain essentially amateur games and the GAA a primarily amateur sporting organization. Professionalism at a sporting level, i.e. the payment of wages for playing does not take place and is considered a contravention of the rules. However, over the course of the last 40 years many characteristics of professional sport have become a feature of Gaelic games and some players, particularly, at the elite level, do receive non-financial and indirect financial recompense for playing. It is in that sense we contend that professionalization has advanced; the balance between amateurism and professionalism changed in the direction of the latter.

Our aim in this chapter, based on the figurational–sociological approach of Norbert Elias (Elias, 2000; Elias and Dunning, 1986; Elias and Scotson, 1994) is to sketch an outline of the various interwoven social processes that have led to shifts in the balance between amateurism and professionalization. We also illustrate how the changing social structure in Ireland post the 1960s, involving a shift in the intergenerational power ratio, facilitated the development of an organized elite players' union which further increased professionalizing pressures. That said, it is important to emphasize that the advance of professionalism remains confined to relatively small, though influential and functionally important, groups of the GAA overall.

The amateur ethos

While the GAA was established as an amateur sorting organization the rules and ethos institutionalized never reflected a pristine form of amateurism. As we explained elsewhere this ambivalence was connected to the structure of ethnic and class relations that had emerged in Ireland in the 1880s (Connolly, 2015; Connolly and Dolan, 2013b). Though the social make-up of the GAA has never been thoroughly examined and accessed – and remains a point of contest – the available evidence would suggest that the GAA's membership was primarily lower middle-class with others drawn from sections of the urban working class or similar rural lower class groups (Garnham, 2004a; Hunt, 2008, 2009; McMullan, 1995). Consequently, the importance of work and the necessity to earn money was part of the values and interest of many GAA activists from the outset; their commitment to pristine amateurism was never absolute. They fully understood that both players and administrators could not generally be 'out of pocket' and needed to be reimbursed for losses incurred due to playing or organizational activities. Thus, from the very start the payment of expenses or compensation, where possible, was instigated with little or no opposition. Indeed, the sport was monetized very early through gate-taking (Garnham, 2004a).

The balance between amateurism and professionalism, which lay firmly in the former, began to shift somewhat in the direction of professionalization in the 1930s and 1940s. The sport, at the highest level, took on greater features of professional sport – greater emphasis on success striving in formal competitions and greater commitment in terms of time and seriousness of involvement in pre-match preparation. In turn, reimbursement of lost wages became an aspect of the sport in the 1930s and 1940s, while players were compensated for travel and related costs for playing (McAnallen, 2009).

However, despite this movement, the sport still remained strongly amateur. There were several reasons for this, yet a crucial facilitating condition was the structure of the competing sports of soccer (Association football) and rugby union in Ireland at that time. Although soccer in Ireland had become a 'professional' sport in 1894 (Garnham, 2004b) (rugby remained amateur), and GAA activists had used, and continued to use, this as an opportunity to denigrate and stigmatize it in an effort to discourage people from partaking in the sport rather than Gaelic games, soccer was primarily an amateur sport in Ireland. Consequently, the real competitive pressures and related threat to GAA administrators in the struggle to maintain and expand its playing and support base came from amateur sports – soccer and rugby. It was in that context that soccer become vilified within a wider narrative which sought to present the sport as "professional," "effeminate," "British," and "foreign," and which constituted a form of blame gossip (Elias and Scotson, 1994) for GAA activists. This vilification of professionalism took place against a backdrop in which amateurism, the very antonym of professionalism, rarely featured as an aspect of GAA "praise gossip" (Elias and Scotson, 1994) of its own games. While this deamplifying of amateurism remained up to and including the 1930s a praise-gossip regarding amateurism did emerge in the 1940s. Furthermore, the fact that the real threat to the GAA came from competing amateur sports meant professionalizing pressures were subdued greatly and tended to emanate from the 'internal' competitive sporting relations that GAA units exercised upon one another. Indeed, this became a key factor in the reamplifying of an 'amateur' praise gossip that would subsequently emerge.

The competitive pressures had reached new heights by the 1940s and early 1950s, with the emergence of 'whole time' training camps. Here entire teams of players trained collectively for periods of two to six weeks with players often accommodated in hotels for the period involved (McAnallen, 2009). Players also received financial allowances or broken-time payments on top of this. The fears this generated for various GAA administrators, and the different concerns and interests behind them, certainly led to the amplification of the amateur ideal in the 1950s and greater efforts to thwart aspects of the sport than were deemed close to, or a form of, 'professionalism.'

In spite of this, professionalizing pressures soon re-emerged by the 1960s. Over the next 50 years the balance between professionalism and amateurism shifted more significantly, and more rapidly, in the direction of professionalism. This was neither a mono-causal development nor a planned or intended development. It took its impetus from a constellation of social processes that occurred at different, yet interconnected, levels of social integration.

Inter-unit competitiveness, underpinned by strong local identifications, continued to exert professionalizing pressures as it led to an increase in the seriousness of involvement and achievement striving of players. There was a gradual, cumulative increase in the scale and intensity of training by players and relatedly in the activities of those concerned with preparing teams. Team preparation and the abilities of those responsible for this, took on greater functional importance. Of course, the practice of 'coaching,' and the function of 'coach' was no mere innovation of the 1960s, rather its functional importance to achieving or maintaining success simply increased. Furthermore, given the identity and meaning functions that the Gaelic games provided, and the social value connected with this for the wider community, a pressure was placed on those deemed responsible for achieving success – players and coaches but also administrators. This in turn led to a spiral of innovation and emulation concerning pre-match preparations and in the material and financial resources made available to facilitate this. Greater specialization and scientific knowledge were brought to bear upon on the games. Coaching, and specific forms and types of skill and knowledge transfer, were deemed crucial to attaining success. Consequently, administrators who were responsible for the appointment of 'specialists' deemed to hold such skills (various managers and trainers) became more dependent on these very specialists. A feature of this shift in interdependency was a more even power ratio between coaches and administrators. The effect of this was that coaches were capable of demanding greater concessions from administrators in terms of resources and organizational arrangements connected with team preparation. Combined, these develops meant players, coaches and other support personal were required to devote greater time and serious of involvement to the sport while the provision of material and financial resources to sustain this similarly increased.

The enhanced status of coaching was not only connected with intra-unit competitive relations. Interorganizational tensions also served to elevate its import. It was now seen as crucial in integrating 'youth' into the association – a primary concern for senior central GAA administrators post the 1960s (Connolly and Dolan, 2012). Nationalist rhetoric no longer appeared as effective at integrating young people into the GAA as in the past, generating both insecurities among GAA administrators and a compulsion to find alternatives. The parallel processes of advancing individualization and a widening of the scope of identification between people in Ireland more broadly (Dolan, 2009, 2014) meant younger people, in particular, were more discerning in their uptake of sports, being more reluctant to accept or acquiesce to the prevailing social norms and standards of older generations. It was in this social context that coaching, among other activities, was now elevated as one strategy in the contest to integrate youth in to the GAA rather than other sporting and leisure organizations. Appeals to the Irishness of Gaelic games (reflecting strong national we-feelings and we-identities) was now replaced by efforts to attract youth to Gaelic games through greater consideration of their felt needs and desires (I-feelings and I-identities). One manifestation of this was the move toward the greater use of communications to present Gaelic games as an attractive sport, and a concern with how young people experienced Gaelic games. Consequently, coaching became indirectly part of this new strategy to appeal and attract youth people into the GAA for it choreographed and shaped how the games were physically embodied and thus both experienced and visually perceived (see *Gaelic Sport*, 1974, August,

p. 3; *Gaelic Sport*, 1976, February, p. 17; *Gaelic World*, 1980, January, p. 37; *Gaelic World*, 1980, June, pp. 16–17).

Indeed, these interorganizational pressures also partly underpinned the increasing commercialization of the Gaelic games and the growth of the professional bureaucracy of the GAA charged with organizing and administering the sport. While a professional bureaucracy to administer the 'amateur' game had existed since the foundation of the association, expanding slighting in the proceeding decades, it was the 1960s and beyond which saw the period of greatest expansion (Connolly, 2015). However, the increasing professionalization of administrative functions occurred without generating anything like the concern or tension that would subsequently emerge over movements in the direction of professionalization at the playing level. Central to understanding this, and the advance in professionalism that did occur, was a strengthening of 'player power' at the elite level.

'Player power'

Although various groups of inter-county[4] players had at different stages sought greater concessions in terms of financial and non-financial resources as far back as the 1930s, it was the 1980s before any cross-county[5] effort emerged. In 1982 several inter-county players came together and formed the Gaelic Players Association – a union of sorts for Gaelic players. In a sense it reflected a widening of the emotional identification between players from across Ireland[6] (32 counties). Perhaps more significantly it was based more on a desire for greater social contact between players rather than as a means to promote and advocate the interests of players.[7] Indeed, it was open to all adult players at all levels across the GAA – not just inter-county players. While short lived, its later reincarnation, in 1999, also known as the Gaelic Players Association (GPA), but with membership confined to inter-county players only, was a more organized entity which extracted considerable financial and non-financial resources for inter-county players. It is in that sense too, that this development, among others, has led to a movement toward professionalism relative to amateurism.

That players were able to extract these concessions can be traced to a number of interconnected processes. The competitive tensions generated by the GAA inter-county competitions combined with the increasing social significance of sport referred to earlier continued and further escalated. This involved and propelled a further reciprocal spiral of innovations and emulations in relation to pre-match preparation, training, and what can be described as the 'intellectualization' (Dunning and Sheard, 1979) of the games as more time was given to thinking and planning around the games. One barometer of this has been the stratospheric rise in financial resources dedicated to inter-county teams by administrators.

As before, the increase in the functional importance of coaching and team preparation meant the power balance between coaches and administrators, which lay in favor of the latter, declined even further, as did that between players and administrators. One aspect of this was that administrators were now required to take into consideration, and accede to, many of the demands of coaches and players. The winning of the senior men's inter-county competition had become the pinnacle of achievement for players and those they were representative of – their wider 'county' communities. Indeed, inter-unit competition and the we-feelings connected with this impelled a pressure on players to compete more intensely. More broadly, it led to a spiral of increasing competitiveness which was pervasive across all levels. This exerted a considerable pressure on administrators, particularly for the preparation of inter-county teams, to increase the financial resources to facilitate this. The fact that county administrators also constituted an element of the intra-unit competitive figuration that exerted a strong social pressure for sporting success certainly contributed to this. But so too did change in the structure of interdependency between administrators and players (and coaches). The successful expansion of Gaelic games, and, interrelated with this, the social desire for success from within the wider communities of which administrators were representative, had increased administrator dependence on those functionaries who could attain this (through winning) – players and coaches. Furthermore, the same processes meant central administrators were now also more dependent on players for it was through their on-field performances and completion of inter-county competitions, which attracted spectators and generated directly and indirectly the vast bulk of the GAA's revenues. Players too were becoming more aware of this and of the physical, temporal and social commitments they gave which sustained this. Consequently, as the pressures on inter-county players continued to increase players sought greater recompense. Indeed, the 1970s, 1980s and 1990s saw an increasing number of contests of control between players and administrators over resources and functions.

However, this emergence of what the media increasingly labeled 'player power' in the 1990s was also connected to changes in the structure of social interdependencies more broadly in Irish society. From the 1960s, individualization processes in Ireland advanced significantly (Dolan, 2009). A feature of this was more equal intergenerational power relations. As the power ratio between the younger and older generations in Ireland became less unequal, it initially led to a heightening of tensions as younger groups sought to have more of their interests and values reflected across different strands of Irish social life and older generations sought to retain their position of authority, status and a way of life commensurate with their values and ideals. This struggle and the tensions connected with it were also manifest within the GAA. For instance, during a debate on removing the ban on 'foreign games'[8] at a meeting of the GAA's annual congress in 1962, one administrator, Micheal O' Ruairc, asserted:

> it had often been stated that the voice of the players was not heard, but he saw no reason why it should be. In schools, colleges' and universities the students had no say in the curriculum, because they were too immature to make decisions of major importance.
>
> (cited in *Irish Independent*, 1962 April 23, p. 17)

In a response penned by Eamonn Young in a GAA magazine of the day, *Gaelic Sport*, under the heading 'Why should the players pipe down?' he stated:

> At home we listen even to the voices of children and, indeed, parents who don't soon see the children go. Players are not children; yet Miceal O Ruairc I suspect, regards them as such by drawing a parallel with college students.
>
> (*Gaelic Sport*, 1962, March–May, p. 33)

This interaction illustrates both the sense of superiority, condescending tone, and the general authoritarian approach to players taken by some administrators at the time but also embers of the changes underway. Despite the pronouncements of some from the older generations, the views and interests of children, and young people more generally, were now being given greater consideration and with more benign understanding (Dolan, 2015). Moreover, it is clear that young people would not stand for the status quo without presenting some form of opposition or resistance.

By the late 1970s, the relationship between players and administrators had become even more equal and was felt to be so in comparison with times past. For instance, in 1979 one writer in the GAA themed magazine *Gaelic Word* (1979 November, p. 11) noted:

> [In the past] The climate abroad such times dictated that players, like children, should be seen, not heard. To speak out on such issues was to rock the boat and one ran the risk of sinking without a trace from the scene.
>
> Happily, a more informed light shines down on the G.A.A. today. It is recognised that players have a not inconsiderable influence on the Association . . . [*sic*] no longer are they regarded as a lower order.
>
> That the players have a powerful voice is a fact of life. Their silent vigil is part of history.
>
> (1979 November, p. 11)

Through the 1980s the felt pressures on players increased further. Many exasperated by the situation spoke out individually or as part of their inter-county teams. By the 1990s the 'we-identity' of inter-county players as a distinct group had hardened and manifested itself in efforts to form a national representative body to push their interests. The GPA was formed in 1999, which unlike its predecessor of the early 1980s, restricted membership to inter-county players. This group now sought to establish its legitimacy as the voice of 'elite' Gaelic players and push their interests and a struggle ensued with the central administrators of the GAA. For instance, shortly after the formation of the GPA the then president of the GAA, Joe MacDonagh, himself a former inter-county player in 1970s and 1980s, stated: "We take serious issue with any group which would negotiate a sponsorship at national level outside of our organization on behalf of our members as long as they remain members of our association" (cited in *Sunday Independent*, March 19, 2000, p. 30). Despite this declaration, and indicative of the strength of the players' position relative to the central administrators of the GAA, within a few years the GPA negotiated several sponsorship deals, while their efforts to obtain other concessions and benefits for inter-county players were also successful to varying degrees. These included individual financial grants,[9] a financial payment if attending third level education, clothing and sportswear, and sponsored cars. They also benefited from enhanced team holidays financed by the GAA, better training and playing facilities and social and material supports connected with this including physiotherapy, food, bio-medical advice and monitoring.

Over the course of the last decade, as the power deferential between players and central administrators became more even, and despite the initial enmity, mutual trust and identification re-emerged. The longstanding strength and scale of mutual dependencies and the emotional connections between elite players and central administrators certainly facilitated this. The GPA became more greatly integrated into the existing institutional structures of the GAA, legitimated and accepted. More of their interests have catered for and elite players have secured greater financial and non-financial rewards.

Recent decades have seen further efforts to commercialize the games and further monetization of the games has occurred. Commercial sponsorship were introduced in the 1980s and expanded while media agreements have become more varied generating enhanced revenue streams. The scale and scope of organizational and administrative tasks generated by expansion and interorganizational competitive pressures also led to the further professional bureaucratization of the central administrative units particularly post the early 1970s. Indeed, this process expanded, percolating down to lower-tier units and functions in recent years. Another feature of this since the 1960s has been the legitimization of professional administrative functions. These developments, paradoxically as Dunning and Sheard (1979, p. 242) suggested in the case of rugby in England in the late 1970s, serve

> only to undermine amateurism even further since, to the extent that the paid administrators bring rationality and efficiency to the performance of their task, the game's expansion is facilitated and the trend towards bureaucracy and professionalism, of which their own existence is an expression, is reinforced.

It is unsurprising, then, that an ambivalence toward professionalism remains among some players and administrators. A small number of players continue to go to the USA to play Gaelic games during the summer months where they receive cash payments or some form of benefit in kind – though these games are governed by the GAA. Equally, rumors have persisted for several decades now around under-the-counter payments to inter-county and club coaches. Combined, these developments have served to erode further the amateur aspects of Gaelic games and replace them with characteristics associated with professional sport.

Conclusion

Despite the advance of professionalization, the amateur and voluntary conception, and organization, of sport within the GAA remains strong. Notwithstanding, it would be remiss not to suggest that both amateurism and voluntarism have been eroded somewhat over the decades. In seeking to understand these movements and developments it is crucial to move beyond static conceptions of amateurism and professionalism and instead view this dynamic in a more processual and relational way. Furthermore, although particular individuals and groups have at times sought, and had different motivations for seeking, to 'professionalize' aspects of Gaelic games and their organization, the shift in the balance between amateurism and professionalism that has occurred has been largely unintended and unplanned.

Notes

1 www.gaa.ie/clubzone/club-info/membership (last accessed April 10, 2015).
2 Annual Report of the GAA, 2013.
3 Of course it is difficult to be certain of the absolute extent and scale of professionalization across the association given that certain practices are deemed in contravention of the association's rules on amateurism and therefore remain hidden.
4 An inter-county player refers to a GAA player who is selected to play for the county he lives in or was born. The GAA is structured along similar lines to the geopolitical administrative structures of Ireland (both the republic and Ireland and Northern Ireland). All GAA members are members of clubs which are organized around parishes. The inter-county team is selected from a combination of what are deemed the best players from all the clubs within a county. The male senior inter-county competitions are considered the elite and the pinnacle for those playing Gaelic games.
5 The coming together of inter-county players from different counties across Ireland.
6 The GAA is an All-Ireland 32 county organization. Ireland was partitioned in 1921 following the War of Independence with Britain. The 26 counties that became independent later became known as the Republic of Ireland, while the six counties within the jurisdiction of Britain were referred to as Northern Ireland.
7 Constitution of the Gaelic Players Association, 1981.
8 The ban on foreign games referred to a GAA rule which prohibited GAA members from not only playing 'foreign sports' (pseudo for British sports) – soccer, rugby, cricket and hockey – but actually attending as spectators at these games. The ban was only removed in 1971.
9 These grants were paid by Irish state authorities as a part of an agreement with the Irish Sports Council rather than the GAA.

References

Connolly, J. (2015). Elias and habitus: Explaining bureaucratisation processes in the Gaelic Athletic Association. *Culture and Organization* [online first].
Connolly, J. and Dolan, P. (2010).The civilizing and sportization of Gaelic football in Ireland: 1884–2009. *Journal of Historical Sociology*, *23*(4), 570–598.
Connolly, J. and Dolan, P. (2011). Organizational centralization as figurational dynamics: Movements and counter-movements in the Gaelic Athletic Association. *Management and Organizational History*, *6*(1), 37–58.
Connolly, J. and Dolan, P. (2012). Sport, media and the Gaelic Athletic Association: the quest for the 'youth' of Ireland. *Media, Culture and Society*, *34*(4), 407–423.
Connolly, J. and Dolan, P. (2013a). Re-theorizing the 'structure–agency' relationship: Figurational theory, organizational change and the Gaelic Athletic Association. *Organization*, *20*(4), 491–511.

Connolly, J. and Dolan, P. (2013b). The amplification and de-amplification of amateurism and professionalism in the Gaelic Athletic Association. *International Journal of the History of Sport*, *30*(8), 826–853.

Dolan, P. (2009). Developing consumer subjectivity in Ireland: 1900–80. *Journal of Consumer Culture*, *9*(1), 117–141.

Dolan, P. (2014). Cultural cosmopolitanization and the politics of television in 1960s Ireland, *Media, Culture and Society*, *36*(7): 952–965.

Dolan, P. (2015). Balances between civilising processes and offensives: Adult–child relations in Irish primary schools from the mid-nineteenth century. *Human Figurations*, *4*(1).

Dolan, P. and Connolly, J. (2009). The civilizing of hurling in Ireland. *Sport in Society*, *12*(2), 196–211.

Dolan, P. and Connolly, J. (2014). Emotions, violence and social belonging: An Eliasian analysis of sports spectatorship. *Sociology*, *28*(2), 279–294.

Dunning, E. and Sheard, K. (1979). *Barbarians, Gentlemen and Players: A Sociological Study of the Development of Rugby Football*. Canberra: Australian National University Press.

Elias, N. (2000). *The Civilizing Process: Sociogenetic and Psychogenetic Investigations* (rev. ed.). Oxford: Blackwell.

Elias, N. and Dunning, E. (1986). *Quest for Excitement: Sport and Leisure in the Civilizing Process*. New York: Basil Blackwell.

Elias, N. and Scotson, J.L. (1994). *The Established and the Outsiders* (2nd ed.). London: Sage.

Garnham, N. (2004a). Accounting for the early success of the Gaelic Athletic Association. *Irish Historical Studies*, *34*(133), 65–78.

Garnham, N. (2004b). *Association football and society in pre-partition Ireland*. Belfast: Ulster Historical Foundation.

Hunt, T. (2008). *Sport and Society in Victorian Ireland. The Case of Westmeath*. Cork: Cork University Press.

Hunt, T. (2009). The GAA: social structure and associated clubs. In M. Cronin, W. Murphy and P. Rouse (eds.), *The Gaelic Athletic Association 1884–2009*. Dublin: Irish Academic Press.

McAnallen, D. (2009). The Greatest Amateur Association in the World? The GAA and Amateurism. In M. Cronin, W. Murphy and P. Rouse (eds.), *The Gaelic Athletic Association 1884–2009*. Dublin: Irish Academic Press.

McMullan, M. (1995). Opposition, social closure, and sport: The Gaelic Athletic Association in the 19th century. *Sociology of Sport Journal*, *12*, 268–289.

20 Sports teams as complex social entities

Tensions and potentials

Lars Tore Ronglan

Introduction

Much of the literature on team dynamics of sport teams is based on the notion that there exist unifying as well as fractious forces in such groups. Often the former is seen as positive and the latter as negative. For example, cohesion and unity is regarded positive for collective performance, whereas tensions and conflicts are supposed to threaten team functioning and productivity (Carron et al., 2007). Consequently, tensions and conflicts should be worked upon in order to be solved. Such a conception supposes that the 'ideal state' of a sports team is to appear as a harmonious social group focusing its effort toward agreed common goals. Although the literature acknowledge that such a state may not be easy to reach, an underlying assumption is that it is a desirable goal to strive for.

In this chapter the aim is to argue that this is a simplistic conception of a sports team, and to suggest a more context sensitive approach in observing and understanding social interaction in this kind of groups. The argument is developed along two lines. The starting point is a description of some unique characteristics of a sports team in competitive sports. Basic to sport researchers is to pay attention to such distinct features and thereby strive to develop knowledge that is contextually grounded. Second, based on this description I argue that complexity theory may be a promising framework for investigating sport teams. Such a 'context driven' reasoning (from context to theory) leads to a shift from viewing a sports team as a unity to viewing the team as complexity, with important consequences to sports team researchers.

The chapter is structured as follows. First, I briefly describe some features characterizing sport and sport teams that contribute to distinguish sport teams from teams in general. This gives a glimpse into the difference, pluralism, and ambiguities marking a sports team. Second, I sketch out some sensitizing concepts of complexity theory and link this way of thinking to the team sport context. In specific, emergence, causality, and paradox are focused upon. Third, paradox in a sports team is illustrated by giving a brief empirical example of the handling of competition immanent in a collaborating team. In conclusion, the chapter summarizes some consequences for researchers if complexity thinking is applied as a framework for empirical studies of sport teams.

Immanent features of sport teams

What characterizes the context in which athletes and coaches as team members operate? Below I will highlight six aspects: (a) competition; (b) collaboration and complementarity; (c) goals and interests; (d) social relationships; and (e) the contexts on and off the court. Far from giving any complete picture, these points give examples of the uniqueness, tensions, and diversity marking sport teams.

Competition

One thing impossible to ignore, is the competitive aspect. Competition is not unique for sport; there is competition also in school, in organizations, and in research communities. However, competition is a more constitutive feature of the sporting context. Athletes practice to learn, develop, and improve, and in recurring contests performances are demonstrated and measured. Players compete against opponents, try to do their best and overcome resistance. The genuine openness of the contest means that the game is far from stable; in contrast, it is genuinely unstable and unpredictable. "The sweet tension of uncertainty of outcome" (Kretchmar, 1975) applies at both a social and individual level, and in competition as well as practice. Here, the point is not to advocate specific coaching or coping strategies, but to underline that this feature of sport has to be taken into consideration and managed by the participants.

In addition to external competition; that is, competition against opponents, research has begun to explore how sport teams are marked by a duality of internal collaboration and internal competition (Agergaard and Ronglan, 2014; Taylor and Bruner, 2012). Teammates cooperate to develop as a strong collective unit, but at the same time, they compete to be picked on the team and gain playing time on court. Particularly in high-performance sport, such internal competition will add to the tensions and instability marking the context in which the collaboration takes place.

Collaboration and complementarity

When looking more closely into how sport teams try to improve their internal collaboration, *relational* and *complementary* skills stands out as main aims. Teammates practice to develop relational skills; that is, skills or competencies that some players possess together. For example, passing as a relational skill, supposing individual techniques in kicking and receiving the ball, but also a dynamic interaction (MacPhail et al., 2008). Relational skills are expressed as precisely timed and coordinated interaction between teammates. It supposes mutual understanding of play sequences and each other's movements, and sport teams work to develop this kind of collaboration on a daily basis.

At the same time, team collaboration supposes players that complement each other. A team is in a need of so many role-specific and situation-specific competencies that players have to be different to contribute to a balanced and powerful team performance. Even 11 Lionel Messis would not make up the best soccer team in the world. Both disciplined, hard-working guys keeping strict to the game plan and creative players thinking out of the box are needed. Any team strives for an appropriate composition of different competencies. Hence, sport teams do not suppose players that are identical concerning personalities and skills, on the contrary, difference and complementarity is needed and valued (Ruigrok et al., 2011).

Goals and interests

Sport teams strive to establish common goals; team goals that the members are more or less committed to. However, although the team goals may be widely shared, it is naive to suppose that personal goals and individual interests will disappear. A more realistic view would be that collective goals and individual goals and interests coexist and may either pull in the same direction, or collide, depending on the situation at hand. As pointed out by Jones and Wallace, short-time and long-time goals present in a team are "diverse, some are highly diffuse, others are inherently incompatible" (2005, p. 125), leading to compromises or dilemmas. Although players identify with the team and the team objectives, they indeed keep their own wishes and desires. For example, most players want to be on the pitch and not on the bench. Common goals are accompanied by individual interests, and the amount of different goals and interests in a team contribute to complexity and tensions.

Number of relationships

In studying pedagogical strategies in school, Axley and McMahon stated that "it is undeniable that a classroom of people qualifies as a complex adaptive system in itself" (2006, p. 303). To illustrate that this also applies to sport teams, a single element as the number of participants can provide a glimpse of the diversity. With increasing number of members on a team the number of relationships rapidly increases. Whereas a team of five participants constitute ten relationships (in terms of dyads) a team of 20 participants make up 190 relationships (formula: (n x n−1): 2). In addition, there are numerous constellations of players; three to four individuals composing different kinds of performance units within the team, e.g. based on interrelated playing positions. In sum, if we consider social relationships as basic units of a team, the complexity explodes with increasing team size.

The contexts on and off the court

A final point that contributes to increase team diversity is the on-court–off-court distinction. Rather than looking at the team as one group moving between different arenas, on court–off court can be seen as distinct contexts shaping, structuring an enabling different interaction patterns and communication forms to evolve. Such an approach would again, related to the paragraphs above, further increase the number and types of relationships and values emerging from team interaction as a whole.

In previous work (Ronglan, 2000, 2010), I have explored how elite players themselves make a clear distinction between the two spheres. Different logics seem to shape interaction and meaning making processes. On court, improving performance constitute the implicit code for action and interaction. Interaction and identity are linked to the continuous work related to develop collaboration and handle competition, and players have to demonstrate willingness to work hard for the benefit of the team to appear as a legitimate and valued member. Off court, a social community, or several communities within the group, develops at another pace and based on other criteria. Interaction and identity are formed on a different basis, expressed through storytelling, humor, jargon, etc. Teammates have to demonstrate social adaptability and to prove themselves as human beings that deserve to be trusted in social relationships. Observations of a team on court and observations of the same team in the locker room, or at a McDonald's on the way home after a match, may give an impression of two quite different groups in terms of roles, communication, and social relationships.

The team as difference

Taken together, what I have suggested so far points toward approaching a sports team in terms of difference and complexity rather in terms of a stable unity. What is present and constitutive in the social life of a team is likely to be a diversity of values, interests, goals, perceptions, and relationships, that come to expression and is made significant in specific social situations or team contexts. This does not mean that there are no cohesive and unifying forces at play, indeed, there are, and a team is at one level continuously working to strengthen such forces and appear as a collective unit. Nevertheless, a closer look may probably give a glimpse into a complexity that invites us to consider the team as pluralism. This pluralism does only on very rare occasions lead to a breakdown of the team. Moreover, I would argue that pluralism and heterogeneity, rather than being perceived as 'dangerous,' should be seen as a logical (and more or less wanted) consequence of the sporting context and the characteristics of a sports team.

Now, where does this bring us? Our prior expectations as researchers sensitize us in specific ways; they guide what we see and how we interpret it when observing team interaction. If we imagine two extremes: (a) the team is marked by harmony, balance, and stability; or (b) the team contains ambiguity, tensions and ongoing change, I would suggest that researchers should be open to expect findings that tend toward (b) rather than seeing the opposite as the expected condition. The term 'sensitizing concepts' originated with the American sociologist Blumer, as "a general sense of reference and guidance in approaching empirical instances" (1954, p. 7). Sensitizing concepts are background ideas that inform the overall research problem and they offer ways of seeing, organizing and understanding experience (Charmaz, 2003). Based on the previous description of sports team characteristics, I propose ideas from complexity thinking as promising sensitizing concepts in investigating sport teams.

Complexity theory

"Complexity theory" does not refer to a specific body of literature (Haggis, 2008). In an overview article, Richardson and Cilliers (2001) define three themes in the literature: "hard complexity science" (the principles of complex systems), "soft complexity science" (complexity as a metaphorical tool to understand organizations) and "complexity thinking" (assuming "the ubiquity of complexity"). The latter assumes that individual human beings (here: players and coaches), associations of individuals (teams, games), and human endeavor (such as sports coaching) are multidimensional, non-linear, interconnected, far from equilibrium and unpredictable. This implies that not everything that is complicated manifests features of complexity. Cilliers (1998) distinguishes between "complicated" (having many parts, but each part can be explained – e.g. a mechanical engine) and "complex" (having many parts, but not all of which can be named, and not all processes involved can be tracked or described). Thus, complex problems can encompass complicated ones but not be reduced to such, because they carry with them significant elements of ambiguity and uncertainty (Mason, 2008).

A mistaken interpretation of complexity theory is that it somehow can "account for" or model the totality of things (Cilliers, 1998). That is not the case. The approach invites us to focus on relationships and interactions rather than static categories. Further, the interactions are multiple, and multiply connected, and it is the multiplicity of interactions *through time* that produce effects (Haggis, 2008). With its emphasis on non-linear and dynamic interactions between multiple variables, complexity thinking supports the case for connectionist and holistic analyses. The focus thus shifts from a concern with decontextualized and universalized essence to contextualized and contingent complex wholes. Complexity theory "suggests the need for case study methodology, qualitative research and participatory, multi-perspectival and collaborative forms of research" (Mason, 2008, p. 6).

Applying a complexity framework will sensitize scientific investigations of sport teams in certain directions. The world of a sports team can be viewed as a thumbnail of society. In line with the classic sociologist Georg Simmel's relational turning point, supposing that society *is* (not 'has') relations, complexity theory supposes that a team basically consists of relationships. From this perspective relations, rather than the individuals, form the 'building blocks' of the team. Hence, a complexity point of departure reaches far beyond merely stating that interaction is relevant to understand the team. Viewing the team as multiple and interconnected relations means a shift of attention: from action to *interaction*, from cause–effect to *reciprocity*, and from 'one plus one is two' to *emergent* effects.

Emergence

A simple understanding of emergent phenomena is that a whole is something more than the sum of its parts. More specifically, the notion of emergence implies that new properties and behaviors emerge that are not contained in the essence of the constituent elements, or able to be predicted from a knowledge of initial conditions (Mason, 2008). In other words, collectives and relations possess emergent properties that cannot be reduced to individual properties (Sawyer, 2001). To illustrate, we can take the social relation 'friendship,' which does not belong to either of the friends but is shared and valued by both. Relational goods reside in the relationships that link or bond the members concerned. In the same way, "no-one can take away part of the orchestra of soccer game as their personal property; they can only take themselves away from the orchestra or the team" (Donati, 2010, p. xi). Thus, the social order is a relational entity and emergent in kind.

A soccer game is relational and thus emergent as the game displays flow and dynamics that is collectively produced but not able to predict from initial knowledge of the participating players. Nor is it possible to reduce rhythmic interplay between two teammates to the 'sum' of their individual actions, because 'collective rhythm' on the pitch emerges *between* interacting players and remains invisible when observing the actions separately. To players, then, the ability to mutual bodily adjustment to the other stands out as a basic competence. To coaches, orchestrating relations become vital; which supposes the ability to notice carefully what is going on between players (*inter*action). To sports team researchers, the challenge is to observe and understand emergent phenomena on and off court, and try to trace how emergent effects are shaped by multiple, mutual interconnections across the team (players, coaches, and context) over time.

From 'causes' to 'effects'

Complexity thinking directs the attention toward relationships and interactions, and thus puts reciprocity and circularity to the foreground instead of linearity and simple cause–effect correlations. This does not mean that that there are no (systemic) effects of the interactions. However, as the interactions are seen as multiple, and multiply connected, the conception of causality has to be redefined (Haggis, 2008). Causality in such a situation cannot be reduced to a single or limited number of factors, as the factors are crucially implicated in relation to each other. Byrne (2005) suggests a shift from the habitual preoccupation with *causes* to a focus on *effects* due to the impossibility of tracking these multiple interaction processes. Such a shift echoes the metaphor of coach orchestration (Jones and Wallace, 2005), which also directs the attention toward the outcome of processes. Conceptualizing causation as multidimensional and decentered (Haggis, 2008) is parallel to the logic of orchestration: what is needed of the coach in contributing to achieve a team goal can vary considerably depending on the web of interrelated interactions influencing the process.

Shifting focus from causes to effects acknowledges the interdependency that contribute to shape a sports team. Thus, interaction effects are seen as systemic. Reciprocity exists between for example athletes and coaches, meaning that a certain conduct from party A may stimulate or provoke certain responses from party

B, again strengthening the typical conduct from party A, and so forth. Such kind of circularities may create stable interaction patterns, leading to more or less unintended consequences (Ronglan, 2011). Rather than searching for single 'causes' leading to specific effects, a shift of focus may lead to breaking the circularity or to expanding the gaze for potential alternatives.

Dealing with paradox

A substantial amount of empirical research based on complexity thinking and theories are occupied with the contextual handling of diversity, ambiguity, insecurity, nonlinearity, and not the least: paradox (Axley and McMahon, 2006; Haggis, 2008; Lewis and Dehler, 2000). Acknowledging complexity means acknowledging paradox, and working with it in a continuous process. This implies working with "contradictory, mutually exclusive elements that exist simultaneously and for which no synthesis or choice is possible nor necessarily desirable" (Lewis and Dehler, 2000, p. 708). Paradox may appear as mixed messages (praising teamwork while rewarding individual performance), opposing perspectives (short term and long term, people and productivity), or conflicting demands (creativity and efficiency, cooperation and competition). In team sport processes, as in any complex system, paradox is immanent. It should be handled rather than hidden away, and accommodates a potential for learning and development. Axley and McMahon (2006) suggest that a leader's role in working with paradox is to maintain and hold it at to preserve the creative tension and uncertainty that it provides, and Lewis and Dehler (2000) advocate learning through paradox as a pedagogical strategy for exploring contradictions and complexity.

This may be a promising approach also to coaches and athletes in their efforts to deal with team processes, adapt to constantly changing condition, and become comfortable with ambiguity and paradox. To researchers, an interesting question is how and to what extent sport teams and team members recognize and deal with paradox in the tension between hiding it away and embracing it.

An empirical example: collaboration and competition

To illustrate paradox in a sports team I will give a brief example of the handling of competition immanent in a collaborating team. Internal competition is inherent in elite teams due to the selection from the squad (e.g. 20 players) to the team-in-match (11 players) going on prior to every match during a season. Thus, internal competition is a result of the structuring of the practice (a surplus of participants), meaning that selections have to be made. This creates 'internal competition' as an inherent feature of the group, independent of the individuals' motivation or attitude. The recurring selection process will influence team dynamics, communication, collaboration, and emotions in different ways depending on the handling of the paradox. (Note that such a recurring selection process is primarily faced by sport teams and not teams in general; strengthening the argument to be context specific when investigating sports teams.)

A few quotes from elite team players illustrate some dimensions of this paradox. First, internal competition is by these informants regarded positive in terms of team performance:

> There has never before been such a fight for the starting positions. Now it is tough. It doesn't matter how you compose the teams in training sessions – they are equally strong anyway. We have never had a better possibility to win the championship.
>
> (female handball player)

> That's how it is, it has to be competition. That's then we are getting better, when there is real competition to qualify to the team.
>
> (male soccer player)

Second, it is not always easy to handle the personal stress created by the internal competition:

> I don't necessarily like it [the competition], but maybe I work a bit harder. It is keeping me on the toes. I just have to handle the discomfort.
>
> (male ice hockey player)

Third, the handling is also a joint effort:

> When I am picked for a match then I know who is not going to play. I know how they feel and that they have to work it out. When included in the team for a match, we don't cheer in front of the others, you know, I cheer inside. And the other way around; if I am dropped I support those who are going to play. I go somewhere else to blow out my frustration alone. I have been into this for a while and learned a lesson; it's not everything you say or show in public.
>
> (female handball player)

In sum, these participants seem to acknowledge that the duality collaboration–competition is immanent in the team context; competition is unavoidable and from a team performance perspective, it is wanted. On the other side, from a personal point of view it is not pleasant and not always easy to handle. Competition within collaboration has to be handled carefully both as an individually and socially experienced paradox.

Concluding thoughts

In this chapter the main argument has been to advocate complexity thinking and sensitizing concepts from this framework as a means to develop contextually grounded knowledge of sport teams. The point of departure was a description of some characteristics of teams in the sporting context, leading to the argument that complexity thinking seems relevant to grasp diversity and ambiguity.

A challenge when trying to understand interaction and dynamics in sport teams is that the inner diversity makes it difficult to portray the team as one, unambiguous, stable group. Inspired by a complexity approach some possible alternatives can be suggested as points of departure:

(a) One option is to deconstruct the understanding of 'a team,' understood as a 'fixed' totality. Rather than looking at the team as consisting of individual members, it is possible to observe the social phenomenon as *webs of relationships* or as constituted of recurring situations embedded in specific contexts.
(b) Then it becomes important to paying attention to (recurring) *social situations* – and ask what logics are at play, what kinds of intra-team approaches come to expression and how these shape relationships and interaction patterns.
(c) Further, it is possible to distinguish between *different contexts* (e.g. on/off court) and look for their particularities and interconnections. Although the contexts may appear as distinct spheres, they are defined in relation to each other and there are obviously interconnections linking them together.
(d) By extension, it is relevant to trace social *processes* within and across contexts. Looking at the team as 'a process' rather than as 'a group' may make it easier to observe ongoing change and apparently contradicting tendencies.

Replacing action with 'interaction' and individuals with 'relationships' as core concepts in research on sport teams might be a fruitful point of departure in exploring sport teams as complex social entities.

References

Agergaard, S. and Ronglan, L. T. (2015). Player migration and talent development in elite sports teams. A comparative analysis of inbound and outbound career trajectories in Danish and Norwegian women's handball. *Scandinavian Sport Study Forum*, 6, 1–26.

Axley, S. R. and McMahon, T. R. (2006). Complexity: a frontier for management education. *Journal of Management Education*, 30(2), 295–315.

Blumer, H. (1954). What is wrong with social theory? *American Sociological Review*, 18, 3–10.

Byrne, D. (2005). Complexity, configurations and cases. *Theory, Culture and Society*, 22(5), 95–111.

Carron, A. V., Eys, M. A., and Burke, S. M. (2007). Team cohesion: nature, correlates and development. In S. Jowett and D. Lavallee (Eds.): *Social psychology in sport* (pp. 91–101). Champaign: Human Kinetics.

Charmaz, K. (2003). Grounded theory: Objectivist and constructivist methods. In N. K. Denzin and Y. S. Lincoln (eds.): *Strategies for qualitative inquiry* (2nd ed., pp. 249–291). Thousand Oaks, CA: Sage.

Cilliers, P. (1998). *Complexity and postmodernism*. London: Routledge.

Donati, P. (2010). *Relational sociology. A new paradigm for the social sciences*. London: Routledge.

Haggis, T. (2008). "Knowledge must be contextual": Some possible implications of complexity and dynamic systems theories for educational research. *Educational Philosophy and Theory*, 40(1), 158–176.

Jones, R. L. and Wallace, M. (2005). Another bad day at the training ground: Coping with ambiguity in the coaching context. *Sport, Education and Society*, *10*(1), 119–134.

Kretchmar, S. (1975). From test to contest. An analysis of two kinds of counterpoint in sport. *Journal of the Philosophy of Sport*, *2*(1), 23–30.

Lewis, M. W. and Dehler, G. E. (2000). Learning through paradox: a pedagogical strategy for exploring contradictions and complexity. *Journal of Management Education*, *24*(6), 708–725.

MacPhail, A., Kirk, D., and Griffin, L. (2008). Throwing and catching as relational skills in game play: situated learning in a modified game unit. *Journal of Teaching in Physical Education*, *27*(1), 100–115.

Mason, M. (2008). Complexity theory and the philosophy of education. *Educational Philosophy and Theory*, *40*(1), 4–18.

Richardson, K. and Cilliers, P. (2001) What is complexity science? A view from different directions. *Emergence*, *3*(1), 5–22.

Ronglan, L. T. (2000). *Gjennom sesongen. En sosiologisk studie av det norske kvinnelandslaget i håndball på og utenfor banen.* [During the season. A sociological analysis of the female Norwegian national handball team on and off the court] Oslo: PhD thesis, Norwegian School of Sport Sciences.

Ronglan, L. T. (2010). Grasping complexity in social interaction: Communication systems in an elite sport team. In U. Wagner, R. Storm, and J. Hoberman. (Eds): *Observing sport – modern system theoretical approaches* (pp. 197–216). Schorndorf: Hofmann Verlag.

Ronglan, L. T. (2011). Social interaction in coaching. In R. L. Jones, P. Portac, C. Cushion and L. T. Ronglan (Eds): *The sociology of sports coaching* (pp. 151–165). London: Routledge.

Ruigrok, W., Greve, P. and Engeler, M. (2011). International experiential diversity and performance at project organizations: The case of national soccer teams. *Sport, Business and Management: An International Journal*, *1*(3), 267–283.

Sawyer, R. K. (2001). Emergence in sociology: contemporary philosophy of mind and some implications for sociological theory. *American Journal of Sociology*, *107*(3), 551–585.

Taylor, I. M. and Bruner, M. W. (2012). The social environment and developmental experiences in elite youth soccer. *Psychology of Sport and Exercise*, *13*(4), 390–396.

Psychology

21 Flow experiences in soccer

The key to a successful physical activity intervention?

Anne-Marie Elbe

Flow is defined as a psychological state "in which the person feels simultaneously cognitively efficient, motivated, and happy" (Moneta and Csikszentmihalyi, 1996, p. 277). It is further described as a "subjective state that people report when they are completely involved in something to the point of forgetting time, fatigue, and everything else but the activity itself" (Czikszentmihalyi and Rathunde, 1992, p. 59). According to Csikszentmihalyi (1997), such a peak experience may emerge in any activity. It is a widely researched phenomenon that has been analyzed in many areas of human life (Jackson and Roberts, 1992). Researchers observed flow during the execution of a large number of different activities, including sports (e.g. Catley and Duda, 1997; Jackson and Csikszentmihalyi, 1999; Jackson and Marsh, 1996), music, art, and even paid work (Bakker, 2005, 2008; Demerouti, 2006). This positive experience of flow is seen as being so rewarding that individuals want to experience it again and again. Therefore flow can be viewed as being intrinsically motivating and a factor that influences future motivation to perform a certain activity.

In order to experience flow, people have to experience an optimal combination of personal skills and external challenges. Czikszentmihalyi and Czikszentmihalyi (1988) report that when individuals perceive the challenge and their available skills as both high and broadly in balance, they experience this highly intrinsically motivated state of flow. This means that the tasks individuals are currently performing have to fit their performance level optimally. The ability to appraise one's own skills in regard to the demands is therefore crucial for experiencing flow. If the task is perceived as too easy, individuals experience boredom; and if it is perceived as too difficult, they experience anxiety. Jackson (2007) points out several precursors of flow, such as optimal physical preparedness, good team interaction and motivation to perform. A factor that can impair the ability to experience flow is worrying thoughts; worry is therefore often assessed in connection with flow (Rheinberg et al., 2003).

There are many studies looking into the flow experiences of athletes especially in connection with peak performance (for a comprehensive review, see Swann et al., 2012). According to Czikszentmihalyi and Jackson (2000) athletes often experience flow during peak performances, but experiencing flow does not necessarily have to go along with peak performances and can be experienced by all athletes in all sports or forms of physical activity. In comparison to that of elite sports, research into the significance of flow in relation to physical activity intervention programs and other related areas like recreational sport and exercise is not as extensive. It has been suggested that elite athletes, who have higher athletic abilities, experience higher flow values (Engeser and Rheinberg, 2008), and that optimal experiences might not occur in non-elite contexts like physical activity or leisure sports (Jackson and Kimiecik, 2008). On the contrary, it has been proposed that non elite sport participants "may have an advantage over elite athletes in being more able to control their sporting environment in a way that optimizes the quality of their experience" (Swann et al., 2012, p. 808). Reinhardt et al. (2008) were able to show that flow could be induced in a running intervention for individuals suffering from depression by adjusting the treadmill to about 80–90 percent of the participants' maximum heart rate. Physical activity performed at this heart rate is perceived to be of above average difficulty but manageable. However, so far there has been little research into the significance of flow in relation to sports or physical activity intervention programs. Schüler and Brunner (2009) put forward that experiencing flow may contribute to the long-term adherence to physical activity because individuals, rewarded for their activity, are likely to seek this activity again. Experiencing flow has been connected to an increase in well-being (Haworth, 1993) and improved self-concept (Jackson et al., 2001) and therefore, could contribute to long-term beneficial health effects which are especially relevant for the physical activity context.

The role of gender differences in athletes experiencing flow so far has not been widely researched either. Several studies that did investigate gender differences in the experience of flow in sport found no significant differences between males and females in their general flow experience (Murcia et al., 2008; Russell, 2001).

Flow in sports has been analyzed in participants involved in mostly individual sports. The experience of flow in team sports is under-researched. However, there is evidence that flow is also experienced in teams (Bakker et al., 2011), and more so by team members that feel socially connected (Kowal and Fortier, 1999). Qualitative data has further indicated that a good interaction between teammates helps individuals to attain flow (Jackson, 1996, 2007). Bakker et al. (2011) demonstrated that young soccer talents' flow experiences were connected to performance feedback and support from the coach. Following on from Swann et al. (2012), more research is needed on whether team sports and individual sports make a difference in if and how flow occurs and how it is experienced.

It can be summarized that studies concerning flow and physical activity interventions are almost nonexistent, and that information about gender aspects and type of activity (e.g. team vs. individual sports) is lacking. Therefore, the following questions will be addressed in this chapter. It will be investigated whether participants in a soccer physical activity intervention can experience flow and, if so, if higher flow experiences are connected to higher physiological improvements during the intervention. Furthermore, gender differences with regard to the flow experiences of participants will be analyzed. And lastly, it will be assessed whether a soccer physical activity intervention elicits different flow experiences for participants in comparison to those involved in a physical activity intervention incorporating individual sports (e.g. jogging, Zumba).

Two studies aimed at answering the previously raised questions will be described in the following. Study 1 investigated whether inactive individuals attending a physical activity intervention program experience flow and if, so, if these flow experiences are connected to physiological improvements. Furthermore, gender differences will be investigated as well as the question of how soccer compares to the individual sport of jogging when it comes to eliciting flow experiences. Study 2 investigated the flow experiences of female healthcare workers involved in a workplace physical activity intervention including both soccer and Zumba. Again their flow experiences were assessed. Additionally, it was investigated whether soccer elicited higher flow values than Zumba and if flow was connected to physiological improvements achieved during and adherence to physical activity after the intervention.

Study 1

In study 1, 12- to 16-week exercise interventions which included continuous running and soccer were conducted with a total of four randomized intervention groups, two female and two male groups of previously inactive participants (Elbe et al., 2010). In addition, one female and one male control group were recruited for the study. All male participants completed a 12-week intervention phase with two to three weekly one-hour training sessions (Krustrup et al., 2009; Nybo et al., 2010). One group took part in a soccer intervention (n=10) with small-sided games performed outdoors; a second group completed a jogging intervention (n=12) with continuous outdoor running. All females completed a 16-week intervention period with two weekly one-hour training sessions. One group took part in a soccer intervention with small-sided games performed outdoors (n=21). The second group completed a jogging intervention with continuous outdoor running at the same average heart rate as the soccer players (n=20).

The physiological improvements of the participants in all groups were determined by the Yo-Yo Intermittent Endurance level 2 test (Yo-Yo IE2; see Bangsbo 1995; Bangsbo et al., 2006), and by a maximal oxygen uptake test on a rating scale from 0 (no improvement) to three (major improvement).

The participants' flow states were measured once midway into the intervention program. The midway measurement was chosen in order to enable the inactive participants to get used to the exercise intervention itself. To measure flow the Danish version of the 13 item Flow Kurz Skala (FKS: Rheinberg et al., 2003) which assesses the flow total score (10 items) on a 7-point Likert scale was applied. Values closer to seven indicate very high flow rates, whereas values closer to one indicate very low flow experiences. High flow values are described as being greater than five (Reinhardt et al., 2006; Reinhardt et al., 2008). The FKS also assesses the worry component with a total of three items, as worry can counteract the flow experience. The questionnaires were filled out by the participants right at the end of a training session. In addition to assessing flow, participants were requested to assess their rate of perceived exertion. The Rate of Perceived Exertion was used for this (Borg, 1982). After four to six weeks of training, the participants were asked after three different training sessions how hard they felt the training session had been in general.

The results indicate that both intervention groups experienced levels of flow that can be characterized as being high (Reinhardt et al., 2006, 2008). The highest levels of flow were experienced by the female runners and the lowest values by the male soccer players. In the female sample, runners experienced higher flow values than the soccer participants. In the male sample there were no significant differences in flow between the runners and soccer players. Concerning worry, there were very high values in the male runners, with low worry in the female and male soccer players as well as the female runners. In the male sample, soccer players experienced significantly lower worry than the runners whereas as there were no significant differences in the female sample. The male runners experienced the highest levels of perceived exertion and the male soccer player the lowest. The differences in perceived exertion were significant for the male sample whereas the female sample showed no significant differences with regard to perceived exertion between the two groups. The exact values are presented in Table 21.1.

In addition, all groups showed physiological improvement measured by the Yo-Yo Intermittent Endurance level 2 test (IE2) and a maximal oxygen uptake test. A connection between experiencing flow and physiological improvement measured by VO2 max and the Yo-Yo test could not be found.

This first study could identify that previously inactive male and female participants can experience high flow values in a soccer intervention and that gender differences with regard to how soccer and running are experienced, exist. For male participants, involvement in a soccer physical activity intervention can achieve higher physiological improvements and elicits lower feelings of worry and perceived exertion than participation in a running physical activity intervention. Low feelings of worry are important when attempting to create flow experiences because as previously mentioned, worry can impair the ability to experience flow (Rheinberg et al., 2003). The results, however, cannot be transferred to female participants. For female participants running can elicit higher flow values than soccer.

Table 21.1 Means and standard deviations regarding the scales flow total, worry, perceived exertion and physiological improvement

	Flow total	*Worry*	*Physiological improvement*	*Perceived exertion*
Sample 1 (male)				
Running	4.99± 0.60	4.05 ± 0.99 }*	1.50 ± 1.08 }*	6.0* ± 1.3 }*
Football	4.78 ±0.78	2.83 ± 1.06	2.45 ± 0.69	3.9 ± 1.8
Sample 2 (female)				
Running	6.01± 0.52 }**	2.81 ± 1.22	1.75 ± 0.79	5.5 ± 2.9
Football	5.0 ± 0.83	2.83 ± 1.25	2.05 ± 0.92	5.8 ± 1.8

Notes: * p ≤ .05; ** p ≤ .01

However, there are some limitations to this research that need to be addressed. The results apply only to experiencing flow midway into an intervention program, and in this study only one measurement for experiencing flow was collected. Flow was also only measured towards the end of the training session and not at the beginning or midway into the session, for example. Due to ongoing physiological measurements it was not possible to interrupt the participants during the exercise session and ask them to complete the flow questionnaire then. Furthermore, the small sample makes statistical analyses difficult. However, due to the extensive physiological testing, it was not possible to conduct the study with a larger sample. A final limitation to this study is that no follow-up data on the participants was available to answer the question of whether they continued their sport involvement after the end of the intervention. This, however, in addition to physiological improvement, is an important success factor of physical activity interventions. A second study tried to address some of the limitations of this first research by including larger samples, several flow measurements as well as a follow-up of participants.

Study 2

Study 2 explored healthcare workers' flow experiences during a workplace exercise intervention (Elbe et al., 2106). A difference to the first study was that this study included only female participants and that these participants were not necessarily inactive in their leisure time, which was a precondition for participation in the first study. Sixty-five female nurses who fulfilled the inclusion criteria (i.e. hospital employees, aged 25–65, female) were assigned to either a 12-week soccer (FG, n=41) or Zumba intervention (SG, n=38).

The soccer group performed sessions consisting of three-a-side/four-a-side soccer matches in a gym (10x20 m) owned by the hospital and/or five-a-side/six-a-side/ seven-a-side matches in a municipal sports hall (20x40 m) located three km from the hospital. Each training session was initiated by a 5-min low-intensity warm-up period and a 5-min rest after half-time. The soccer sessions were initially supervised by an instructor then gradually taken over by the participants themselves.

The Zumba group performed sessions of Zumba, supervised by a certified Zumba instructor in a fitness center three km from the hospital. The sessions consisted of continuous dance movements to Latin music with varying intensity levels throughout the sessions. Each session started with low-intensity movements for the first five minutes, followed by increasing intensity throughout the rest of the workout. At the end of the session, the intensity was gradually reduced.

After the end of the organized intervention, 12 of the soccer participants and 15 of the Zumba participants continued in self-organized regular physical activity. These participants were categorized as 'adherers'. The 'adherers' were still active 30 weeks after the start of the intervention and 18 weeks after the end of the intervention.

To measure flow the Norwegian version Flow Kurz Skala (FKS: Rheinberg et al., 2003) was applied. The flow questionnaire was administered at the beginning, four weeks into the intervention program and at the end (after 12 weeks) always directly at the end of each training session. To evaluate the physiological effects of the training intervention, pulmonary gas exchange (VMAX Spectra Series, SensorMedics Corporation, US) was conducted at baseline and after 12 weeks.

The results showed that both intervention groups experienced medium levels of flow (Reinhardt et al., 2006; Reinhardt et al., 2008) and an increase in flow values over time. At measurement 1 the soccer group experienced significantly higher flow values than the Zumba group. All values of the three measurement points are presented in Table 21.2.

A correlation was conducted to investigate the relationship between flow values and improvements in VO_2 max. No significant correlation was found between the increase in VO_2 max between T1 and T3 and experiencing flow at any of the three measurement points.

A significant positive correlation ($r = .28$; $p < .05$), however, could be found between higher flow value experienced at the second measurement and if participants continued with regular physical activity after the end of the intervention in week 12 and were still active 40 weeks after the beginning of the intervention.

Furthermore, repeated measures throughout the intervention period showed a significantly different development of flow values over time for the adherers and non-adherers. These results indicate that already at T1 adherers were characterized by significantly higher flow values.

In conclusion, the results of both studies show that soccer is an activity that can elicit high flow values in previously inactive participants and medium flow values in female participants of a workplace physical activity intervention. For inactive male participants, soccer creates less worrying thoughts and less perceived exertion as well as more physiological improvements than running. These differences cannot be seen in inactive female participants, and, overall, inactive females perceive higher flow in running than in soccer. A workplace intervention with female healthcare workers showed that soccer can elicit higher flow values than Zumba already at the beginning of a physical activity intervention.

In total, there seem to be indications that soccer physical activity interventions are a flow eliciting activity that has higher potential for initiating this state than running (for males) and Zumba (for females). There are several possible explanations for the advantages of soccer with regard to eliciting flow like good team

Table 21.2 Flow data for the two intervention groups over three measurements. Data are presented as means ± SD. * $p \leq .05$; ** $p \leq .01$; t1 = baseline, t2 = after 4 weeks, t3 = after 12 weeks

	Flow total (t1)		Flow total (t2)	Flow total (t3)
Sample				
Football (n=32)	3.90 ± 0.72	}*	4.03 ± 0.67	4.25 ± 0.81
Zumba (n=33)	3.50 ± 0.86		3.81 ± 0.98	4.24 ± 1.00

interactions, lower perceived worry and clear goals. The differences in flow experiences might be related to good team interactions (Jackson, 2007), which might be easier to establish in soccer than in an individual sport. With regard to male participants, the lower perceived worry while playing could be an advantage for achieving flow since higher experiences of worry can counteract the flow experience (Rheinberg et al., 2003). An additional explanation could be that the goals are clearer in soccer and that soccer offers more opportunities for receiving immediate feedback (e.g. was the pass successful, did I score a goal?). Immediate feedback is a specific characteristic of the flow state (Swann et al., 2012). Finally it is possible that soccer participants have more influence on the challenges they choose (e.g. which passes they play, how much they run), whereas in an activity like Zumba this is more strongly determined by the pace the instructor sets. According to Csikszentmihalyi and Csikszentmihalyi (1988) it is important that an individual perceives the challenge and his/her available skills as being in balance, so that the highly intrinsically motivated state of flow is experienced. The opportunities for finding this balance between skills and abilities might be greater in soccer.

This chapter described two studies investigating soccer as a physical activity intervention with regard to their possibility to elicit flow. The results with regard to flow experiences, gender differences as well as the relationship of flow to physiological improvement during and adherence to regular physical activity after the end of the intervention were reported. The results presented in this chapter indicate that flow is not related to physiological improvements during the intervention but is important for long term adherence to regular physical activity. Future research should focus on qualitative investigations of flow experiences in soccer. Qualitative studies could contribute to a better understanding of which factors exactly promote the higher flow experiences in soccer and could unfold the underlying factors for the gender differences that were found.

References

Bakker, A. B. (2005). Flow among music teachers and their students: The crossover of peak experiences. *Journal of Vocational Behavior, 66*, 26–44.

Bakker, A. B. (2008). The work-related flow inventory: Construction and initial validation of the WOLF. *Journal of Vocational Behavior, 72*, 400–414.

Bakker, A. B., Oerlemans, W., Demerouti, E., Slot, B. B., and Ali, D. K. (2011). Flow and performance: A study among talented Dutch soccer players. *Psychology of Sport and Exercise, 12*, 442–450.

Bangsbo, J. (1995). *The Yo-Yo Tests.* Copenhagen: HO + Strom, pp. 1–32.

Bangsbo, J., Mohr, M., Poulsen, A., Perez-Gomez, J., and Krustrup, P. (2006). Training and testing the elite athlete. *Journal of Exercise Science and Fitness, 4*, 1–10.

Borg G. A. (1982). Psychophysical bases of perceived exertion. *Medicine and Science in Sports and Exercise, 14*, 377–381.

Catley, D. and Duda, J. L. (1997). Psychological antecedents of the frequency and intensity of flow in golfers. *International Journal of Sport Psychology, 28*, 309–322.

Csikszentmihalyi, M. (1997). *Finding Flow: The Psychology of Engagement with Everyday Life.* New York: Harper Collins.

Csikszentmihalyi, M. and Csikszentmihalyi, I.S. (1988). *Optimal Experience: Psychological Studies of Flow in Consciousness.* Cambridge: Cambridge University Press.

Csikszentmihalyi, M. and Jackson, S.A. (2000). *Flow im Sport* [Flow in Sport]. München: BLV.

Csikszentmihalyi, M. and Rathunde, K. (1992). The measurement of flow in everyday life: Toward a theory of emergent motivation. In R. Dienstbier and J.E. Jacobs (eds.), *Nebraska Symposium on Motivation: Developmental Perspectives on Motivation* (vol. 40, pp. 57–97). Lincoln and London: University of Nebraska Press.

Demerouti, E. (2006). Job resources, work-related flow and performance. *Journal of Occupational Health Psychology, 11,* 266–280.

Elbe, A.-M., Barene, S., Strahler, K., Holtermann, A., and Krustrup, P. (2016). Experiencing flow in a workplace physical activity intervention for female health care workers: A longitudinal comparison between football and Zumba. *Women in Sport and Physical Activity Journal.*

Elbe, A.-M., Strahler, K., Krustrup, P., Wikman, J., and Stelter, R. (2010). Experiencing flow in different types of physical activity intervention programmes: Three randomised studies. *Scandinavian Journal of Medicine and Science in Sports, 20,* 111–117.

Engeser, S. and Rheinberg, F. (2008). Flow, performance, and moderators of challenge–skill balance. *Motivation and Emotion, 32,* 158–172.

Haworth, J. (1993). Skills–challenge relationships and psychological well-being in everyday life. *Society and Leisure, 16,* 115–128.

Jackson, S.A. (1996). Toward a conceptual understanding of the flow experience in elite athletes. *Research Quarterly for Exercise and Sport, 1,* 76–90.

Jackson, S.A. (2007). Factors influencing the occurrence of flow state in elite athletes. In D. Smith and M. Bar-Eli (eds.), *Essential Readings in Sport and Exercise Psychology* (pp. 144–154). Champaign, IL: Human Kinetics.

Jackson, S.A. and Csikszentmihalyi, M. (1999). *Flow in Sports: The Keys to Optimal Experiences and Performances.* Champaign, IL: Human Kinetics Publishers.

Jackson, S.A. and Marsh, H.W. (1996). Development and validation of a scale to measure optimal experience: The flow state scale. *Journal of Sport and Exercise Psychology, 18,* 17–35.

Jackson, S. and Kimiecik, J. (2008). Optimal experience in sport and exercise. In T. Horn (ed.), *Advances in Sport Psychology* (pp. 377–399). Champaign, IL: Human Kinetics.

Jackson, S., Thomas, H., Marsh, H., and Smethurst, C. (2001). Relationships between flow, self-concept, psychological skills, and performance. *Journal of Applied Sport Psychology, 13,* 129–153.

Kowal, J. and Fortier, M.S. (1999). Motivational determinants of flow: Contributions from self-determination theory. *Journal of Social Psychology, 3,* 355–368.

Krustrup, P., Nielsen, J.J., Krustrup, B., Christensen, J.F., Pedersen, H., Randers, M.B., Aagaard, P., Petersen, A.M., Nybo, L., and Bangsbo, J. (2009). Recreational soccer is an effective health promoting activity for untrained men. *British Journal of Sports Medicine, 43,* 825–831.

Moneta, G.B. and Csikszentmihalyi, M. (1996). The effect of perceived challenges and skills on the quality of subjective experience. *Journal of Personality, 2,* 275–310.

Murcia, J.A.M., Gimeno, E.C., and Coll, D.G.C. (2008). Relationships among goal orientations, motivational climate and flow in adolescent athletes: Differences by gender. *Spanish Journal of Psychology, 1,* 181–191.

Nybo, L., Sundstrup, E., Jakobsen, M.D., Mohr, M., Hornstrup, T., Simonsen, L., Bülow, J., Randers, M.B., Nielsen, J.J., Aagaard, P., and Krustrup, P. (2010). High-intensity training versus traditional exercise interventions for promoting health. *Medicine and Science in Sports and Exercise, 42*(10), 1951–1958.

Reinhardt, C., Lau, A., Hottenrott, K., and Stoll, O. (2006). Flow-Erleben unter kontrollierter Beanspruchungssteuerung – Ergebnisse einer Laufbandstudie [Flow experiences under controlled load – results of a treadmill study]. *Zeitschrift für Sportpsychologie, 4*, 140–146.

Reinhardt, C., Wiener, S., Heimbeck, A., Stoll, O., Lau, A., and Schliermann, R. (2008). Flow in der Sporttherapie der Depression – ein beanspruchungsorientierter Ansatz [Flow in the sport therapy of depression – an approach based on load]. *Bewegungstherapie und Gesundheitssport, 4*, 147–151.

Rheinberg, F., Vollmeyer, R., and Engeser, S. (2003). Die Erfassung des Flow-Erlebens. In J. Stiensmeier-Pelster and F. Rheinberg (eds.), *Diagnostik von Motivation und Selbstkonzept* [Diagnosing motivation and self-concept] (pp. 261–279). Göttingen: Hogrefe.

Russell, W. D. (2001). An examination of flow state occurrence in college athletes. *Journal of Sport Behavior, 1*, 83–107.

Schüler, J. and Brunner, S. (2009). The rewarding effect of flow experience on performance in a marathon race. *Psychology of Sport and Exerc*ise, *1*, 168–174.

Swann, C., Keegan, R.J., Piggott, D., and Crust, L. (2012). A systematic review of the experience, occurrence, and controllability of flow states in elite sport. *Psychology of Sport and Exercise, 13*, 807–819.

22 Coaching practice and player development

Donna O'Connor and Paul Larkin

Coaches perform a vital role in a player's acquisition of the skills necessary for performance (Ford et al., 2010). When considering player development, it is important to understand the coaching environment, as this is the primary teaching and learning medium for the development of player's technical and tactical skills (Cushion and Jones, 2001; Ford et al., 2010; Partington and Cushion, 2013; Woodman, 1993). Coaches are seen as teachers, who create meaningful teaching and learning activities while conveying important skills and concepts to their players. This can be achieved by creating and managing a positive learning environment, whereby specific performance-based objectives can be accomplished. Despite knowledge and understanding of the coaching environment to achieve these performance-based outcomes, coaches need to be aware of the developmental stages of their players and the impact this can have on player and team outcomes (Côté and Gilbert, 2009; Partington et al., 2014). For example, the coaching needs of a youth player will be different to senior professional level players. Therefore it has been recognized that differences in coaching is needed for players at different developmental stages, age and competition levels (Côté et al., 2010; Côté and Fraser-Thomas, 2007).

With respect to coaching, recent literature has identified two different coaching methods, a traditional coach-centered approach, and a modern athlete-centered approach (Cushion, 2010). In an athlete-centered training environment, the coach tries to use fewer instructions and allow athletes to problem solve and take responsibility for their own learning, by focusing on game-based activities. This method of coaching is informed by the Game Sense pedagogy (Pill, 2014) and often involves constraints-led practice (Passos, Araújo et al., 2008). It moves away from a practice session dominated by drills that don't involve decision-making (i.e. Training Form) and instead provides players with activities that replicate the demands of the game, and provides opportunities for developing decision-making and tactical skills (i.e. Playing Form).

Despite researchers indicating possible best practice methods (Harvey, Cushion, and Massa-Gonzalez, 2010; Kidman et al., 2005), coaches at all levels still generally emulate other coaches, resulting in the use of traditional or coach-centered approaches characterized by a direct and prescriptive approach (Partington and Cushion, 2013). This is supported by contemporary coach behavior research, which indicates the most frequently used coach behavior is instruction, with questioning, especially divergent questions (i.e. questions with the potential for multiple responses), used sparingly within a coaching session (Cushion and Jones, 2001; Ford et al., 2010; Partington and Cushion, 2013). Further, there is a general consensus in the literature that a larger proportion of youth practice time is invested to Training Form activities (65 percent Training Form, 35 percent Playing Form (Ford et al., 2010); 69 percent Training Form, 19 percent Playing Form (Low et al., 2013); 53 percent Training Form, 47 percent Playing Form (Partington and Cushion, 2013); 56 percent Training Form, 44 percent Playing Form (Partington et al., 2014)). In contrast however, recent findings at the elite senior level have indicated coaching sessions predominantly consist of 58 percent Playing Form and 42 percent Training Form (Hall et al., 2015). Despite the suggestion Playing Form may provide greater opportunities for player development, especially tactical awareness and decision-making ability, there is still a gap between research evidence and applied coaching (Ford et al., 2010).

Numerous sporting organizations, especially at the youth level, now promote an athlete-centered approach (e.g. Football Federation Australia's National Curriculum), however currently there is little evidence indicating whether coaches are implementing this philosophy and creating training environments that provide opportunities for players to enhance tactical and technical skills. Furthermore, there has been minimal comparison of the coaching behaviors between competitive levels (i.e. junior to senior). Therefore we aim to examine the coaching behaviors and practice activities of Australian coaches from various football codes (soccer, rugby league, rugby union, and Australian Rules Football) at the junior, youth, and senior (professional) levels.

Method

Participants

Australian male coaches currently coaching males in soccer, rugby union, rugby league, and Australian Rules football at differing levels of competition participated in the study. The three competitive levels were senior (first-grade, $n = 16$); youth (Under 16 – Under 18, $n = 24$); and junior (Under 10 – Under 12, $n = 118$) competitions.

Procedure

A total of 158 regular in-season practice sessions were observed by trained research assistants at the participants regular practice location. If permission was granted by the coach and the players or their parent/guardian, the practice session was video recorded and then coded, otherwise coding occurred in real time during the practice session. To assess the structure of the practice activities conducted during a session, an adapted version of Ford et al.'s (2010) soccer practice activity coding was used. The adapted instrument provided greater levels of information by categorizing the activity based on the organization, size of the groups, structure and type of activity. The size of groups was categorized according to the number of players involved and included (a) individual; (b) pairs; (c) 2–4 players; (d) five or more players; (e) the whole team. Table 22.1 provides the associated definition of each practice activity code. The adapted instrument measured the duration of various practice activities during the entire practice session.

For coding purposes, an adapted version of the Coach Analysis Intervention System (CAIS) (Cushion et al., 2012) was used to measure coach behavior. As this investigation involved live coding, the CAIS was reduced to three main behaviors; instruction (explanation or feedback); observation; and management and organization. To ensure consistent coding operational definitions were developed prior to coding. Instructions were defined as the information given to players before, during, or after and activity, and included all forms of feedback and explanations. Observation was defined as moments where the coach is not talking but rather observing players and analyzing their execution of the skill or activity, or observing the way in which the team is executing strategies in open play situations. Finally, management and organization was defined as the verbal statements related to the organizational details of a practice session that does not refer to strategy or fundamentals of the sport.

Table 22.1 The definitions of the practice activity codes used to describe the practice session environment

Activity	Operational definition
Whole group	When all the players were involved in the one activity at the same time
Divided group – same activities	Players were divided into small groups and were practicing the same activity
Divided group – different activities	Players were divided into small groups but were participating in different activities
Fitness	Fitness components of the game without a ball (e.g. warm-up, sprints, agility)
Isolated skill	Activities during coaching whereby the player is performing predetermined actions or movements. There is a set sequence to the activity with minimal options available to the player.
Drill	Player action involves at least two choices
Tactical plays	Practicing set plays, phase of play activities toward one goal
Small-sided games	Match play manipulating constraints (e.g. reduced players; rule variations)
Inactivity	Moments during the coaching session where players are not actively participating in any activities
Huddle	Coach stops the activity and gets the players to come together for a discussion near him/her
Freeze	Coach stops the activity to talk to the players and the players remain in their current position from when the activity stopped
Drink break	Coach stops the activity to allow the players to go and get a drink

Data analysis

Data were coded and quantified for each coach behavior and practice activity. To ensure consistency with previous coach behavior researchers, descriptive statistics (mean ± standard deviation) were used to describe the percentage of time allocated to the behaviors and activities conducted within practice sessions (Ford et al., 2010; Hall et al., 2015; Partington et al., 2014; Portrac et al., 2007). As the values for coach behavior and practice activity were significantly non-normal, non-parametric techniques were used. To assess differences between competitive levels for coach behaviors and practice activities, a one-way Kruskal Wallis test was conducted, with a significant alpha set at 0.05. Significant main effects were followed up with Bonferroni-corrected pairwise comparisons, with a significant corrected alpha set at 0.02 and effect sizes (r) denoted by a small ($r = 0.1 - 0.29$), medium ($r = 0.3 - 0.49$) or large effect ($r = 0.5 - 1$) (Cohen, 1992).

Results

Coach behaviors

The Kruskal Wallis test indicated a significant main effect for the coach behaviors of instruction, observation, and management and organization (see Table 22.2). Follow-up pairwise comparisons found significant differences between the senior and junior coaches for instruction ($p < 0.001$, $r = 0.43$), observation ($p < 0.001$, $r = 0.62$), and management and organization ($p < 0.001$, $r = 0.42$). There were also significant differences between the junior and youth coaches for instruction ($p = 0.001$, $r = 0.27$), observation ($p < 0.001$, $r = 0.63$), and management and organization ($p < 0.001$, $r = 0.42$). Finally, there were also significant differences between the senior and youth coaches for instruction ($p = 0.001$, $r = 0.52$).

Table 22.2 The mean and standard deviation of the average duration of the coach behaviors exhibited in a junior, youth and senior practice session

Competition level	Instructions		Observation		Management and organization	
	Mean	SD	Mean	SD	Mean	SD
Junior	41.28* †	16.08	27.16	15.14	16.54* †	6.42
Youth	30.12*	8.32	57.79‡	10.34	9.93	3.38
Senior	22.63	3.81	64.28‡	5.14	7.92	3.82
Chi-square	32.95		71.22		43.36	
p-value	<0.01		<0.01		<0.01	

* denotes significantly different from senior, p < 0.02
† denotes significantly different from youth, p < 0.02
‡ denotes significantly different from junior, p < 0.02

Practice activity

Table 22.3 presents the descriptive statistics, significant main effects and post-hoc analysis for the practice activity data. When considering the organization of practice, there were significant main effects for the time allocated to whole group activities ($H(2) = 16.97$, $p < 0.001$) and small groups conducting the same activity ($H(2) = 23.28$, $p < 0.001$). Post-hoc comparisons indicated youth coaches used significantly less whole group activities compared to the senior ($p < 0.001$, $r = 0.66$) and junior coaches ($p < 0.001$, $r = 0.42$). However, youth coaches invested significantly more time to small group activities where players were performing the same activity compared to senior ($p < 0.001$, $r = 0.83$) and junior coaches ($p < 0.001$, $r = 0.44$).

Table 22.3 The average percentage of practice time junior, youth and senior coaches allocated to practice activities when considered relative to the organization, structure, size of the groups and type of activity

	Junior		Youth		Senior		p-value
	Mean	SD	Mean	SD	Mean	SD	
Organization							
Whole group	61.10†	29.23	20.61	11.06	63.60†	24.87	<0.001
Small group – same activity	22.33	22.60	51.94* ‡	4.75	8.79	8.97	<0.001
Small group – different activity	16.51	25.22	27.45	11.44	27.26	28.43	0.028
Size of groups							
Individual	7.22*	8.73	7.75*	6.43	20.49	8.80	<0.001
Pairs	3.76	5.20	3.96	10.86	3.76	5.20	0.668
2–4 players	21.54	16.71	15.32	14.48	13.68	10.55	0.174
> 5 players	22.18	13.99	42.70‡	23.90	36.96	22.79	<0.001
Team	0.00	0.00	9.54	15.75	24.68	17.09	0.028
Structure							
Training form	45.69* †	23.16	18.85	14.02	28.89†	12.22	<0.001
Playing form	26.39	19.30	50.26‡	17.06	52.04‡	12.49	<0.001
Inactivity	26.55*	12.35	28.61*	6.54	19.07	3.00	0.003
Type of inactivity							
Huddle	10.83	6.50	9.49	3.35	9.43	3.14	<0.001
Freeze	14.94*	8.61	13.09*	5.62	1.89	1.97	<0.001
Drink break	4.65	2.62	6.03‡	2.10	7.74† ‡	1.58	<0.001
Type of activity							
Fitness	10.35†	11.77	2.38	3.95	16.52† ‡	5.77	<0.001
Isolated skill	48.90* †	31.08	13.73	16.58	19.18	15.83	<0.001
Drill > 2 options	13.77	2.89	30.30*	26.41	13.81	10.50	0.041
Tactical Play	0.00	0.00	42.31‡	30.55	41.63‡	15.25	<0.001
Small-sided games	27.80* †	22.61	11.63	14.57	8.86	10.82	<0.001

* denotes significantly different from senior, $p < 0.02$
† denotes significantly different from youth, $p < 0.02$
‡ denotes significantly different from junior, $p < 0.02$

When practice activity is considered relative to the size of the groups, Table 22.3 indicates significantly more time in senior practice sessions is allocated to individual activities compared to junior (p <0.001, r = 0.41) and youth (p <0.001, r = 0.68) practice sessions. Furthermore, youth coaches invested significantly more time in activities with greater than 5 players compared to junior coaches (p <0.001, r = 0.46). There were, however, no differences between competition levels for the period of time allocated to the other sized activities, however, it should be noted that junior training sessions did not include whole team activities.

There was also a significant main effect for the time allocated to fitness activities ($H(2)$ = 18.63, p <0.001), isolated skill activities ($H(2)$ = 34.23, p <0.001), drills with more than two options ($H(2)$ = 6.41, p = 0.041), tactical plays ($H(2)$ = 114.10, p <0.001), and small-sided games ($H(2)$ = 16.05, p <0.001) between competition levels. As indicated in Table 22.3, pairwise comparisons indicated significant differences on numerous activity types between the junior and senior sessions (fitness activities p = 0.02, r = 0.31; isolated skill activities p <0.001, r = 0.31; tactical plays p <0.001, r = 0.99; small-sided games p <0.001, r = 0.68) and junior and youth sessions (fitness activities p = 0.010, r = 0.26; isolated skill activities p <0.001, r = 0.42; tactical plays p <0.001, r = 0.88; small-sided games p = 0.20, r = 0.24).

Finally, as shown in Table 22.3 there were significant differences in the inactivity time allocated to freeze (see Table 22.1 for definition) and drink breaks between senior coaches and junior (freeze p <0.001, r = 0.70; drink break p <0.001, r = 0.59) and youth coaches (freeze p <0.001, r = 0.80; drink break p = 0.013, r = 0.39). There were, however, no differences between competition levels for the period of time players are inactive due to player huddles.

Discussion

The coaching environment is the primary teaching and learning medium for the development of players' technical and tactical skills (Cushion and Jones, 2001; Ford et al., 2010; Partington and Cushion, 2013; Woodman, 1993). Coaches have an important role as they need to create meaningful activities while conveying important skills and concepts to their players. Despite researchers identifying potentially better coaching methods to promote player development (Harvey et al., 2010; Kidman et al., 2005), coaches still generally emulate or mimic other coaches, resulting in practice sessions characterized by a direct and prescriptive approach (Partington and Cushion, 2013).

Findings from the systematic observation revealed junior coaches spend significantly more time instructing, organizing and managing their players compared to coaches of older players. In previous literature instruction has been reported to be the most frequently used coaching behavior regardless of the age or level of the athlete (Cushion and Jones, 2001; Ford et al., 2010; Partington and Cushion, 2013) and has been associated with athlete satisfaction and motivation (Becker, 2013). Effective instructions are clear, concise and simplified and do not lead to mixed messages being received by players (Becker, 2009). Instructional behavior also includes the use of demonstrations, explanations (e.g. relevance to game context), questioning and providing feedback with the aim to promote learning. The high level of instruction at the junior level may also be a reflection of the traditional coach centered approach where the coach spends the majority of his/ her time telling players what to do and correcting their actions explicitly. However coaches of older players rely less on instructions and spend more time observing players participating in various activities.

Observation is generally regarded as an effective coaching strategy as it allows coaches to reflect on the session and make adjustments when warranted and reduces the likelihood of 'over-coaching' (Cushion and Jones, 2001). The current results suggest youth and senior coaches utilized observation more than junior coaches. It has previously been reported that national and successful high school coaches tend to remain silent and observe players for greater amounts of time (Claxton, 1988; Horton and Deakin, 2007). While observation may be associated with successful coaches, it is still unclear how much coach observation is too much or too little. For example, some players may consider too much silence as the coach lacking knowledge or being disinterested, while a coach who constantly gives concurrent instruction may make players feel they are always making mistakes and wrong decisions (McGaha, 2000). Therefore, coaches considering implementing more observation within their session should be aware of their body language when observing players to reduce the likelihood of player misperception.

The current findings indicated coaches of older players were more effective in organizing and managing their players compared to coaches of young players. Research suggests age and skill level of the players may influence the amount of time a coach spends managing or organizing players, as less than 6 percent of senior elite level practice is managing and organizing compared to over 14 percent in high school practice sessions (Potrac et al., 2007; Stewart and Bengier, 2001). Possible reasons why junior coaches have difficulty with this aspect of coaching include: they may not have efficient transitions from one activity to the next; they may not set up their activities prior to practice commencing; they may have difficulty organizing the players into teams or groups; or they may have difficulty getting the players' attention. Therefore, coaches should consider becoming more efficient organizing and managing their session as this will help maximize learning opportunities for their players.

With respect to the structure of practice sessions, the majority of coaches preferred the players to participate in various activities as a whole group rather than using concurrent small group activities. An issue associated with junior coach's reliance on 'whole group' activities is it may reduce the opportunities players have to complete specific skills and make decisions as they often have to wait for their turn. This trend may suggest junior coaches lack confidence in their management and organizational skills and prefer to be working with all players collectively where they can keep an eye on them. Interestingly, senior coaches also allocated the majority of practice time to whole group activities although this was predominantly to perform team tactical plays and set moves. Youth coaches tended to organize players into small groups but still preferred to have the players complete the same task. This strategy has the potential to enhance skill learning and decision-making as concurrent small-sided games or activities gives players the opportunity to be more involved and have greater contact with the ball.

The final aspect of organization was the coaches' preference for the size of their group for each activity. Interestingly the two main differences were coaches of junior players were less likely to conduct activities with groups of more than five players whereas youth and senior coaches had over 50 percent of their session where players were in large groups or ran as a full team. Second, coaches of senior teams incorporated more individual practice perhaps reflecting player autonomy and empowerment as often they chose what to practice during this independent learning opportunity.

Coaches are responsible for planning and scheduling virtually all of a team's practice session. The current results suggest there is a shift by youth and senior coaches to predominantly playing form activities (Ford et al., 2010; Partington and Cushion, 2013; Partington et al., 2014). This learning environment promotes greater pressure and competition simulations and provided players with opportunities to develop their physiological, technical, tactical and perceptual cognitive skills. Unfortunately coaches of junior players still rely on training form activities. As junior players are in the sampling years (6–12 years), junior coaches should emphasize participation, enjoyment and play-like activities rather than deliberate practice (Côté and Fraser-Thomas, 2008). However, there still should be a balance between training form activities which may allow immediate success for novice players and game based or random practice which may result in greater errors and discourage these players from continued participation.

Coaches often complain they do not have enough practice time with their players. However it has previously been reported that players may be inactive for up to 48 percent of a practice session (Horton and Deakin, 2007). Findings form the current study suggest coaches at the high performance level use their allocated time more efficiently than youth and junior coaches with shorter periods of inactivity. However, coaches still need to be mindful that recovery periods are important if intensity and concentration levels are to remain high and often structure drink breaks during this time. Further analysis revealed junior and youth coaches chose to deliver more of their instructions and feedback to players frozen in position during a drill or activity rather than bringing them in together. Although this may have the benefit of saving time and immediacy of a teachable moment coaches need to ensure that all players can see and hear adequately.

Instruction and practice activities at the senior and youth level focus on the tactical aspects of the game. Coaches at this level utilized tactical play activities to practice set plays and simulate specific game scenarios with defensive players often adopting the traits of their upcoming opponents. This type of activity provides immediate feedback and opportunities for fine-tuning through repetition. This is likely to increase player confidence going into competitive matches when they feel they have prepared well for all potential situations. Although senior players are already technically proficient they still spent time practicing isolated skills such as accurate kicks and tackling.

As evidenced by the results junior level coaches predominantly use isolated skill drills to promote high levels of technical skill repetitions. However, youth coaches progress from this to instead use drills where players were required to make decisions (e.g. 3 attackers v 2 defenders). While these activities promote decision-making and are somewhat structured they allow numerous practice opportunities over a short time frame with players learning through self- reflection, trial and error and coach feedback. Also for junior players, coaches allocated approximately 25 percent of the session to small-sided games. Constraints-led practice (manipulating various constraints such as player numbers, field size and rules) and small-sided games incorporate random and variable practice where players have the opportunity to problem solve, make decisions and learn from mistakes rather than practicing skills in isolation (O'Connor, 2012). These games also provide opportunities for young players to develop an understanding of space, shape and time.

This preliminary analysis highlighted numerous differences in coach behavior and the microstructure of practice across the different competition levels. This study extends previous research by examining senior practice sessions as well as using more detailed descriptions for assessing the practice environment.

References

Becker, A. (2009). It's not what they do, it's how they do it: athlete experiences of great coaching. *International Journal of Sport Science and Coaching*, *4*(1), 93–119.

Becker, A. (2013). Quality coaching behaviours. In P. Potrac, W. Gilbert and J. Denison (eds.), *Routledge Handbook of Sports Coaching* (pp. 184–195). London: Routledge.

Claxton, A. (1988). Systematic observation of more and less successful high school tennis coaches. *Journal of Teaching in Physical Education*, *7*(4), 302–310.

Cohen, J. (1992). A power primer. *Psychological Bulletin*, *112*(1), 115–159.

Côté, J., Bruner, M., Erickson, K., Strachan, L., and Fraser-Thomas, J. (2010). Athlete development and coaching. In J. Lyle and C.J. Cushion (eds.), *Sports Coaching Professionalisation and Practice* (pp. 63–83). London: Elsevier.

Côté, J., and Fraser-Thomas, J. (2007). The health and developmental benefits of youth sport participation (pp. 266–294). In P. Crocker (eds.), *Sport Psychology: A Canadian Perspective*. Toronto: Pearson Education Canada.

Côté, J. and Gilbert, W. (2009). An integrative definition of coaching effectiveness and expertise. *International Journal of Sports Science and Coaching*, *4*(3), 307–323.

Cushion, C.J. (2010). Coach behaviour. In. J. Lyle and C.J. Cushion (eds.), *Sports Coaching Professionalization and Practice* (pp. 243–253). London: Elsevier.

Cushion, C., Harvey, S., Muir, B., and Nelson, L. (2012). Developing the Coach Analysis and Intervention System (CAIS): establishing validity and reliability of a computerised systematic observation instrument. *Journal of Sports Sciences*, *30*(2), 201–216.

Cushion, C.J. and Jones, R.L. (2001). A systematic observation of professional top-level youth soccer coaches. *Journal of Sport Behavior*, *24*(4), 354–376.

Ford, P.R., Yates, I., and Williams, A.M. (2010). An analysis of practice activities and instructional behaviours used by youth soccer coaches during practice: exploring the link between science and application. *Journal of Sports Sciences*, *28*(5), 483–495.

Hall, E.T., Gray, S., and Sproule, J. (2015). The microstructure of coaching practice: behaviours and activities of an elite rugby union head coach during preparation and competition. *Journal of Sports Sciences*, 1–10.

Harvey, S., Cushion, C.J., and Massa-Gonzalez, A.N. (2010). Learning a new method: teaching games for understanding in the coaches' eyes. *Physical Education and Sport Pedagogy*, *15*(4), 361–382.

Horton, S. and Deakin, J. (2007). Expert coaches in action. In D. Farrow, J. Baker, C. Mac-Mahon (eds.), *Developing Sport Expertise* (pp. 75–85). London: Routledge.

Kidman, L., Thorpe, R., and Hadfield, D. (2005). *Athlete-Centred Coaching: Developing Inspired and Inspiring People*. Christchurch, NZ: Innovative Print Communications.

Low, J., Williams, A.M., McRobert, A.P., and Ford, P.R. (2013). The microstructure of practice activities engaged in by elite and recreational youth cricket players. *Journal of Sports Sciences*, *31*(11), 1242–1250.

McGaha, P. (2000). A quantitative and qualitative exploration of coaching behaviours of successful high school baseball coaches. Unpublished doctoral thesis, Florida State University.

O'Connor, D. (2012). Challenges facing Youth Coaches. In J. O'Dea (ed.), *Current Issues and Controversies in School and Community Health, Sport and Physical Education* (pp. 283–294). New York: Nova Science.

Partington, M. and Cushion, C.J. (2013). An investigation of the practice activities and coaching behaviours of professional top-level youth soccer coaches. *Scandinavian Journal of Medicine and Science in Sports*, *23*(3), 374–382.

Partington, M., Cushion, C., and Harvey, S. (2014). An investigation of the effect of athletes' age on the coaching behaviours of professional top-level youth soccer coaches. *Journal of Sports Sciences*, *32*(5), 403–414.

Passos, P., Araújo, D., Davids, K., and Shuttleworth, R. (2008). Manipulating constraints to train decision making in rugby union. *International Journal of Sports Science and Coaching*, *3*(1), 125–140.

Pill, S. (2012). Teaching game sense in soccer. *Journal of Physical Education, Recreation and Dance*, *83*(3), 42–52.

Potrac, P., Jones, R., and Cushion, C. (2007). Understanding power and the coach's role in Professional English Soccer: A preliminary investigation of coach behaviour. *Soccer and Society*, *8*(1), 33–49.

Stewart, M. and Bengier, M. (2001). An analysis of volleyball coaches' coaching behaviour in a summer volleyball camp. *Physical Educator*, *58*(2), 86–99.

Woodman, L. (1993). Coaching: a science, an art, an emerging profession. *Sport Science Review*, *2*(2), 1–13.

23 Doping in soccer

A moral psychology perspective

Maria Kavussanu

The use of banned performance enhancing substances or methods to enhance performance, also known as doping, is a pervasive phenomenon in elite sport. The Council of Europe Committee for Out-of-School Education (1963) has defined doping as "the use by a healthy individual ... of any agent or substance not normally present in the body ... with the purpose of increasing artificially and in an *unfair manner* the performance of that individual during competition." A key aspect of this definition is the intention to increase performance in an unfair manner. Although other definitions of doping exist, this definition exemplifies that doping is a moral issue. Indeed, doping involves breaking the rules of the game and is therefore cheating. Thus, research on sport morality can inform our understanding of doping behavior in soccer.

Over the past 20 years, our understanding of moral behavior in sport has been considerably enhanced (see Kavussanu, 2012). Much of this research has been conducted in the context of soccer and has focused on understanding antisocial behavior, defined as behavior intended to harm or disadvantage another individual or group of individuals (Kavussanu, 2006; Sage et al., 2006). Antisocial behavior can have negative consequences for the recipient and includes verbal and physical aggression as well as cheating (Kavussanu, 2012). Examples of antisocial behavior in soccer are trying to injure an opponent, swearing at a teammate, and diving to fool the referee. Several variables have been consistently linked to antisocial behavior in soccer. Some of these variables are highly relevant to our understanding of doping and are discussed below. Research on three hypothesized distal predictors of doping is reviewed first, followed by work on three potential mediators. The chapter ends with a presentation of a conceptual model of doping in sport and the discussion of the findings of a large study examining this model in soccer players.

Distal predictors of doping

Based on research on morality in sport (see Kavussanu, 2012), three potential distal predictors of doping were identified: performance motivational climate, moral atmosphere, and moral identity. Motivational climate, a construct of achievement goal theory (Ames, 1992; Nicholls, 1989), refers to the situational goal structure, that is, the achievement goals emphasized and the criteria for success (in that context) that are conveyed to the participants by significant others, such as coaches, teachers, and parents (Ames, 1992). Those significant others determine important features of the achievement context, such as the evaluation procedures and the distribution of rewards, and, via their behavior, they communicate to participants what is valued in that context. Coaches create a performance motivational climate when they evaluate success using normative criteria such as winning, reward only the best athletes, and place emphasis on doing better than others. In this type of climate, players may be tempted to cheat or engage in other behaviors that could facilitate the goal of establishing superiority over others.

Several studies have shown that when soccer players perceive a performance motivational climate in their team, they are more likely to report higher frequency of antisocial behavior (e.g. Kavussanu and Spray, 2006; Miller et al., 2005). Performance motivational climate has been consistently associated with antisocial behaviors, such as diving to fool the referee, deliberate handball, and pretending to be injured (Kavussanu, 2006; Sage and Kavussanu, 2008; Sage et al., 2006), while in other research, this type of climate has been positively related to doping attitudes (e.g. Moran et al., 2008).

Moral atmosphere, the second distal predictor of doping, pertains to the collective group norms regarding moral action, that is, the type of behavior considered acceptable in a group by its group members. A construct that originated from the work of Kohlberg and colleagues (e.g. Power et al., 1989), moral atmosphere has been operationally defined as a set of collective norms regarding morally relevant action on the part of group members (Shields and Bredemeier, 1995). In a sports team, certain philosophies, which are partly the outcome of characteristics of the coach and team members, are developed over time regarding what is appropriate behavior. Teammates' perceptions of their peers' choices in situations that give rise to moral conflict are also part of the moral atmosphere (Shields and Bredemeier, 1995).

Previous research has examined moral atmosphere in relation to moral judgment, intention, and behavior (collectively referred to as moral functioning). This line of research has typically presented athletes with scenarios describing antisocial behaviors, such as faking an injury and intentionally injuring another player, and examined their perceptions of the number of teammates who would engage in these behaviors, as well as their perceptions of their coach as encouraging the behaviors in question. Soccer players, who perceived a moral atmosphere that condoned antisocial conduct in their team, also reported lower levels of moral functioning (Kavussanu and Spray, 2006; Miller et al., 2005). In another study, young female soccer players, who perceived that a large number of their teammates would behave aggressively in a hypothetical situation, also indicated greater likelihood to act aggressively (Stephens, 2000; Stephens and Bredemeier, 1996). These findings suggest that the athletes' immediate social environment may have a significant influence on their moral functioning.

Finally, moral identity refers to the cognitive schema a person holds about his or her moral character (Aquino et al., 2009) and can function as a self-regulatory mechanism that motivates moral action (Blasi, 1984). Individuals with a strong sense of moral identity consider being moral an important aspect of who they are (Aquino and Reed, 2002). Blasi (1984) proposed that a common set of moral traits are likely to be central to most people's moral self-definitions, and that being a moral person may occupy different levels of importance in each person's self-concept. Aquino and Reed (2002) identified nine traits (i.e. caring, compassionate, fair, friendly, generous, helpful, hardworking, honest, and kind) as being charac-teristic of a moral person and found variation in the degree to which these traits were central to one's self-concept. The extent to which the moral self-schema is experienced as being central to one's self-definition has been referred to as the internalization dimension of moral identity (Aquino and Reed, 2002) and has been the main focus of empirical research.

To date, only three studies have investigated moral identity in the sport context. Sage et al. (2006) presented adult male soccer players with the nine traits identi-fied as being characteristic of a moral person (Aquino and Reed, 2002) and asked them to respond to a measure of moral identity. They found that the more central moral identity was to the players' self-concept, the less likely the players were to report engaging in antisocial behavior while playing soccer. Similar findings were revealed in a second study with athletes from a variety of team sports including soccer (Kavussanu et al., 2013). Finally, in an experimental setting, moral identity led to reports of greater likelihood to aggress in a hypothetical situation, compared to a control group (Kavussanu et al., 2015).

In sum, research on morality in sport can assist our understanding of doping in soccer players. Performance motivational climate, moral atmosphere, and moral identity have been associated with antisocial behaviors, such as diving to fool the referee, and trying to injure another player, and all three variables could enhance our understanding of doping. Performance climate and moral atmosphere can reveal the extent of the group influence on doping, while moral identity can uncover the role of an individual difference moral variable on doping.

Mediating variables

As well as identifying distal predictors of doping, it is important to investigate mediators. A mediator is a variable that 'carries' or explains the effect of the pre-dictor on the outcome; by identifying mediators, we are able to better understand the relationship between a predictor and an outcome variable. Three variables could act as mediators of the effects of performance climate, moral atmosphere, and moral identity on doping. These are: ego orientation, moral disengagement, and anticipated guilt. In this section, these variables are described, and related research is discussed.

Ego orientation is one of two achievement goals assumed to operate in sport. Achievement goals reflect the criteria individuals use to define success and evalu-ate their competence, in achievement contexts (Nicholls, 1989). Athletes who are high in ego orientation tend to define their competence in relation to other peo-ple; they feel successful when they do better than others; and they endorse the belief that high ability, deception, and cheating lead to success in sport. Due to their focus on normative superiority, ego-oriented individuals may engage in rule-violating and cheating behaviors to facilitate their goal of establishing superiority over others (Nicholls, 1989). As Nicholls has put it, "When winning is everything, it is worth doing anything to win" (1989, p. 133).

These proposals have been supported by a number of studies. Specifically, university athletes recruited from soccer, hockey, rugby and netball teams, who were high in ego orientation, were also more likely to report low levels of moral functioning as reflected in their judgment, intention, and behavior (Kavussanu and Ntoumanis, 2003). Similarly, adolescent and adult soccer players high in ego orientation reported engaging in antisocial behavior while playing soccer (Boardley and Kavussanu, 2010; Kavussanu, 2006; Sage and Kavussanu, 2007a; Sage et al., 2006). In one experiment, Sage and Kavussanu (2007b) randomly assigned university students to a task, ego, or control group and recorded their behaviors (e.g. breaking the rules and deliberate cheating), via a hidden camera, during two table-soccer games. Participants in the ego-involving group displayed significantly more antisocial behaviors than did those in the control group. Finally, ego orientation has been associated with more favorable attitudes toward doping in elite athletes (Sas-Nowosielski and Swiatkowska, 2008; Moran et al., 2008). These findings suggest that ego orientation could be positively associated with doping.

Ego orientation is developed through socialization with significant others, who emphasize normative criteria for success, and could be influenced by performance motivational climate. In past research, this goal has been positively linked to performance motivational climate (e.g. Sage and Kavusanu, 2008). Thus, it is reasonable to expect that ego orientation would mediate the relationship between performance climate and doping, such that performance climate would lead to higher ego orientation, which in turn could facilitate doping.

The second mediator is moral disengagement, which is expected to mediate the effect of moral atmosphere on doping. Moral disengagement refers to eight cognitive mechanisms that individuals use to minimize anticipated negative affect (e.g. guilt, shame) when engaging in transgressive behavior (Bandura, 1999). These mechanisms act by: cognitively reconstructing harmful behaviors into benign ones; minimizing personal accountability for transgressive acts; misrepresenting the injurious effects that result from harmful conduct; or blaming the character or actions of the victim (Bandura, 1991). For example, players may blame their coach for their own behavior (displacement of responsibility); claim that they cheated to help their team (moral justification); claim that everyone in the team cheats or uses performance enhancing drugs (PEDs) (diffusion of responsibility), and therefore they should not be blamed for also doing this; or downplay the consequences of their actions for others (distortion of consequences).

Moral disengagement has received a lot of research attention in recent years, with abundant evidence attesting to its occurrence in sport (see Boardley and Kavussanu, 2011; Kavussanu, 2016). In the first study that provided quantitative evidence for the link between moral disengagement and antisocial behavior in sport, moral disengagement was positively associated with antisocial behavior among team sport athletes including soccer players (Boardley and Kavussanu, 2007). This finding has been replicated in many other studies (e.g. Boardley and Kavussanu, 2009, 2010; Kavussanu et al., 2013). Moral disengagement has also been positively associated with doping intention (e.g. Lucidi et al., 2004, 2008; Zelli et al., 2010), as well as acceptability and likelihood of cheating (d'Arripe-Longueville et al., 2010).

We hypothesized that moral disengagement would mediate the effect of moral atmosphere on doping. Specifically, if the coach encourages the use of PEDs and athletes perceive that their teammates are likely to use PEDs, they may be more likely to morally disengage, with subsequent effects on doping behavior.

Finally, anticipated guilt, which is a self-conscious moral emotion that plays an important role in regulating moral action (Tangney et al., 2007), could mediate the relationship between moral identity and doping. According to Bandura (1991), people avoid doing bad things because they want to avoid the negative feelings (e.g. guilt, shame) associated with transgressive behavior. Anticipated guilt has been negatively associated with team sport athletes' reported likelihood to behave aggressively, in a hypothetical sport situation (Kavussanu et al., 2015; Stanger et al., 2012). In another study, anticipated guilt for using human growth hormone (HGH) in a hypothetical situation was inversely associated with athletes' decision to use HGH (Strelan and Boeckmann, 2006). Thus, if athletes expect to feel bad after using PEDs, they are less likely to do it.

We hypothesized that anticipated guilt would mediate the effect of moral identity on doping. Specifically, athletes who feel that being a moral person is an important part of who they are should be more likely to feel guilt for using banned PEDs, which constitutes cheating; this in turn should deter athletes from doping.

A conceptual model of doping

It is evident from the literature reviewed above that several variables that have been associated with antisocial behavior in sport could influence doping. However, the measurement of doping behavior is rather challenging. Indeed, researchers have highlighted the difficulty of studying doping due to the sensitive issue of the topic (e.g. Moran et al., 2008). Essentially, athletes are asked to be honest about dishonest behavior! Although some studies have taken measures to facilitate honest responding (e.g. Lazuras et al., 2010), the problem of obtaining honest reports of doping behavior remains. To overcome this problem, we have developed and presented athletes with a hypothetical doping scenario and asked them to indicate the likelihood they would engage in the behavior if they were in the described hypothetical situation (Kavussanu et al., 2015). We refer to this variable as doping intention. In a project funded by the World Anti-Doping Agency (Kavussanu et al., 2015), we have proposed to test the model presented in Figure 23.1.

As can be seen in Figure 23.1, performance motivational climate, moral atmosphere (i.e. a team environment that condones doping) and moral identity were hypothesized to be positive predictors of ego orientation, moral disengagement, and anticipated guilt, respectively. In turn, ego orientation and moral

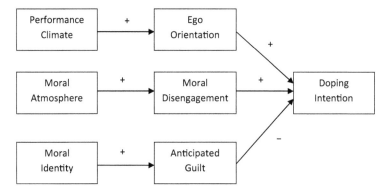

Figure 23.1 The hypothesized effects of performance climate, moral atmosphere and moral identity on doping intention are mediated by ego orientation, moral disengagement and anticipated guilt

disengagement were expected to positively predict doping intention, whereas anticipated guilt is expected to be a negative predictor of doping intention. Thus, the effects of performance climate, moral atmosphere and moral identity on doping intention were expected to occur via ego orientation, moral disengagement, and anticipated guilt, respectively.

For this project, we recruited a large sample of male and female soccer players from three European countries: UK, Denmark, and Greece. We asked participants to respond to the following scenario describing a hypothetical situation, likely to occur in soccer:

> It is the day before *the most important game* of the season. The winner of this game will win the league. The team against which you will compete is of similar ability level to your team, and they are just one point ahead of your team in the league. Lately, your performance has been below your best. You don't feel you have the necessary fitness for this important game, and you are concerned about how you will perform. You mention this to one of your teammates, who tells you that he/she has been using a new substance, which has enhanced his/her fitness and, as a result, his/her performance. The substance is banned for use in sport, but the chance that you will be caught is *extremely small*.
>
> (Kavussanu et al., 2015)

Following this scenario, we asked soccer players to imagine that they are in the hypothetical situation described in the scenario, and indicate how likely it is that they would use the banned substance (doping intention). We also asked them to imagine that they did use the banned substance to improve their performance and indicate how guilty they would feel, if they were in this hypothetical situation. As this pertained to a hypothetical situation, we refer to this variable as anticipated guilt. We measured moral atmosphere by asking participants to indicate how many of their teammates would use the banned substance and the extent to which their coach would encourage them to use the banned substance (in this hypothetical situation). Finally, we measured moral disengagement, ego orientation, performance climate, and moral identity using established or adapted measures of these variables.

Our findings were consistent with the hypothesized model, with the exception of the link between ego orientation and doping intention (Kavussanu et al., 2015). Specifically, when our soccer players perceived in their team a moral atmosphere that condoned doping, they reported higher moral disengagement, which in turn was a positive predictor of doping intention. As hypothesized, moral identity was a positive predictor of anticipated guilt, which in turn negatively predicted doping intention. Performance climate had a small positive effect on ego orientation, but contrary to our hypothesis, ego orientation did not predict doping intention.

These findings suggest that much of the research on morality in sport is highly relevant to doping. This is not surprising, as the use of banned substances to enhance performance involves breaking the rules of the game, thus it is clearly a transgressive behavior with moral connotations. This is further underlined by the fact that all 'moral' variables were strong predictors of doping intention.

The fact that ego orientation did not predict doping intention suggests that doping is also distinct from other moral behaviors examined in previous research. For example, behaviors such as diving, shirt pulling, or dangerous tackles might be considered part of the game, and as such might be legitimized among soccer players. In contrast, doping is clearly labelled as illegal behavior that breaks the rules of the game. This might explain why motivational variables such as motivational climate and ego orientation did not strongly predict doping intention, a finding that is in line with previous research (see Ntoumanis et al., 2014).

Conclusion

In conclusion, research on morality in sport can inform our understanding of doping behavior in soccer. The moral atmosphere of the team, reflected in players' perceptions of their coach and teammates' behavior, together with their moral identity could have a profound influence on one's intention to use banned substances and subsequent doping behavior. A moral atmosphere that condones doping could facilitate justifications of this behavior, which in turn can make it easier for the player to dope. In contrast, a strong moral identity could lead one to experience guilt, an emotion that can dissuade players from using banned PEDs. These forces act in opposite ways, and suggest that in order to deter players from doping we need to strengthen their moral identity and intervene at the level of the team.

Acknowledgment

The author would like to acknowledge the financial support of the World Anti-Doping Agency for some of the research discussed in this chapter.

References

Ames, C. (1992). Achievement goals, motivational climate, and motivational processes. In G. C. Roberts (ed.), *Motivation in Sport and Exercise* (pp. 161–176). Champaign, IL: Human Kinetics.

Aquino, K. and Reed, A. (2002). The self-importance of moral identity. *Journal of Personality and Social Psychology*, *83*, 1423–1440.

Aquino, K., Freeman, D., Reed, A., Lim, V. K. G., and Felps, W. (2009). Testing a social cognitive model of moral behavior: The interactive influence of situations and moral identity centrality. *Journal of Personality and Social Psychology*, *97*, 123–141.

Bandura, A. (1991). Social cognitive theory of moral thought and action. In W. M. Kurtines and J. L. Gewirtz (eds.), *Handbook of Moral Behavior and Development: Theory, Research, and Applications* (vol. 1, pp. 71–129). Hillsdale, NJ: Lawrence Erlbaum.

Bandura, A. (1999). Moral disengagement in the perpetration of inhumanities. *Personality and Social Psychology Review*, *3*, 193–209.

Blasi, A. (1984). Moral identity: Its role in moral functioning. In W. Kurtines and J. Gewirtz (eds.), *Morality, Moral Behaviour and Moral Development* (pp. 128–139). New York: Wiley.

Boardley, I. D. and Kavussanu, M. (2007). The moral disengagement in sport scale. *Journal of Sport and Exercise Psychology*, *29*, 608–628.

Boardley, I. D. and Kavussanu, M. (2009). The influence of social variables and moral disengagement on prosocial and antisocial behaviours in field hockey and netball. *Journal of Sports Sciences*, *27*(8), 843–854.

Boardley, I. D. and Kavussanu, M. (2010). Effects of goal orientation and perceived value of toughness on antisocial behavior: The mediating role of moral disengagement. *Journal of Sport and Exercise Psychology*, *33*, 176–192.

Boardley, I. D. and Kavussanu, M. (2011). Moral disengagement in sport. *International Review of Sport and Exercise Psychology*, *4(2)*, 93–108.

d'Arripe-Longueville, F., Corrion, K., Scoffier, S., Roussel, P., and Chalabaev, A. (2010). Socio-cognitive self-regulatory mechanisms governing judgments of the acceptability and likelihood of sport cheating. *Journal of Sport and Exercise Psychology*, *32*, 595–618.

Elbe, A.M., Kavussanu, M., and Hatzigeorgiadis, A. (2015). Psycho-social factors and doping attitudes in football players: A cross-cultural investigation. Paper presented at the 14th European Congress of Psychology, Milano, July 7–10.

Kavussanu, M. (2006). Motivational predictors of prosocial and antisocial behaviour in football. *Journal of Sports Sciences*, *24*, 575–588.

Kavussanu, M. (2012). Moral behavior in sport. In S. Murphy (ed.), *The Oxford Handbook of Sport and Performance Psychology* (pp. 364–383). Oxford: Oxford University Press.

Kavussanu, M. (2016). Moral disengagement and doping. In V. Barkoukis, L. Lazuras, and H. Tsorbatzoudis (eds.), *The Psychology of Doping in Sport* (pp. 151–164). London and New York: Routledge.

Kavussanu, M., Elbe, A.M., and Hatzigeorgiadis, A. (2015). *A Cross-cultural Approach to a Cross-cultural Issue: Psychosocial Factors and Doping in Young Athletes*. Final report submitted to the World Anti-Doping Agency.

Kavussanu M., Hatzigeorgiadis, A., and Elbe, A.M. (2015). *A Conceptual Model of Doping Intentions in Sport.* Paper presented at the 14th European Congress of Sport Psychology, Bern, Switzerland, July 12–15.

Kavussanu, M. and Ntoumanis, N. (2003). Participation in sport and moral functioning: Does ego orientation mediate their relationship? *Journal of Sport and Exercise Psychology*, *25*, 1–18.

Kavussanu, M. and Spray, C.M. (2006). Contextual influences on moral functioning of male football players. *Sport Psychologist, 20*, 1–23.

Kavussanu, M., Stanger, N., and Boardley, I.D. (2013). The prosocial and antisocial behavior in sport scale: Further evidence for construct validity and reliability. *Journal of Sports Sciences, 31*, 1208–1221.

Kavussanu, M., Stanger, N., and Ring, C. (2015). The effects of moral identity on moral emotion and antisocial behavior in sport. *Sport, Exercise and Performance Psychology, 4*(4), 268–279.

Lazuras, L., Barkoukis, V., Rodafinos, A., and Tsorbatzoudis, H. (2010). Predictors of doping intentions in elite-level athletes: A social cognition approach. *Journal of Sport and Exercise Psychology, 32*, 694–710.

Lucidi, F., Grano, C., Leone, L., Lombardo, C., and Pesce, C. (2004). Determinants of the intention to use doping substances: An empirical contribution in a sample of Italian adolescents. *International Journal of Sport Psychology, 35*, 133–148.

Lucidi, F., Zelli, A., Mallia, L., Grano, C., Russo, P.M., and Violani, C. (2008). The social–cognitive mechanisms regulating adolescents' use of doping substances. *Journal of Sports Sciences, 26*, 447–456.

Miller, B.W., Roberts, G.C., and Ommundsen, Y. (2005). Effect of perceived motivational climate on moral functioning, team moral atmosphere perceptions, and the legitimacy of intentionally injurious acts among competitive youth soccer players. *Psychology of Sport and Exercise, 6*, 461–477.

Moran, A., Guerin, S., and Kirby, K. (2008). *The development and validation of a doping attitudes and behavior scale.* Report submitted to the World Anti-Doping Agency.

Nicholls, J.G. (1989). *The Competitive Ethos and Democratic Education.* Cambridge, MA: Harvard University Press.

Ntoumanis, N., Ng, J.Y.Y., Barkoukis, V., Backhouse, S. (2014). Personal and psychosocial predictors of doping use in physical activity settings: A meta-analysis. *Sports Medicine, 44*, 1603–1624.

Power, C., Higgins, A., and Kohlberg, L.A. (1989). *Lawrence Kohlberg's Approach to Moral Education.* New York: Columbia University Press.

Sage, L. and Kavussanu, M. (2007a). Multiple goal orientations as predictors of moral behavior in youth soccer. *Sport Psychologist, 21*, 417–437.

Sage, L. and Kavussanu, M. (2007b). The effects of goal involvement on moral behavior in an experimentally manipulated competitive setting. *Journal of Sport and Exercise Psychology, 29*, 190–207.

Sage, L. and Kavussanu, M. (2008). Goal orientations, motivational climate, and prosocial and antisocial behaviour in youth football: Exploring their temporal stability and reciprocal relationships. *Journal of Sports Sciences, 26*, 717–732.

Sage, L., Kavussanu, M., and Duda, J.L. (2006). Goal orientations and moral identity as predictors of prosocial and antisocial functioning in male association football players. *Journal of Sports Sciences, 24*, 455–466.

Sas-Nowosielski, L. and Swiatkowska, K. (2008). Goal orientations and attitudes toward doping. *International Journal of Sports Medicine, 29*, 607–612.

Shields, D.L. and Bredemeier, B.J.L. (1995). *Character Development and Physical Activity.* Champaign IL: Human Kinetics.

Stanger, N., Kavussanu, M., and Ring, C. (2012). Put yourself in their boots: Effects of empathy on emotion and aggression. *Journal of Sport and Exercise Psychology, 34*, 208–222.

Stephens, D.E. (2000). Predictors of likelihood to aggress in youth soccer: An examination of coed and all-girls teams. *Journal of Sport Behavior, 23*, 311–325.

Stephens, D. E. and Bredemeier, B. J. L. (1996). Moral atmosphere and judgments about aggression in girls' soccer: Relationships among moral and motivational variables. *Journal of Sport and Exercise Psychology*, *18*, 158–173.

Strelan, P. and Boeckmann, R. J. (2006). Why drug testing in elite sport does not work: Perceptual deterrence theory and the role of personal moral beliefs. *Journal of Applied Social Psychology*, *36*, 2909–2934.

Tangney, J. P., Stuewig, J., and Mashek, D. J. (2007). Moral emotions and moral behavior. *Annual Review of Psychology*, *58*, 345–372.

Zelli, A., Mallia, L., and Lucidi, F. (2010). The contribution of interpersonal appraisals to a social–cognitive analysis of adolescents' doping use. *Psychology of Sport and Exercise*, *11*, 304–311.

Index

Note: italic page numbers indicate tables and figures.

232 *Index*

For Product Safety Concerns and Information please contact our EU
representative GPSR@taylorandfrancis.com
Taylor & Francis Verlag GmbH, Kaufingerstraße 24, 80331 München, Germany